Spine and Joint Articulation for Manual Therapists

Giles Gyer

BSc (Hons) Osteopathy, Diploma Medical Acupuncture, Diploma Sports Massage

Jimmy Michael

BSc (Hons) Osteopathy, BSc (Hons) Sports & Exercise Science, Diploma Medical Acupuncture, Diploma Sports Massage

Ben Calvert-Painter

BSc (Hons) Osteopathy, PGCAP

Spine and Joint Articulation for Manual Therapists

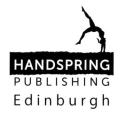

HANDSPRING
PUBLISHING
Edinburgh

HANDSPRING PUBLISHING LIMITED
The Old Manse, Fountainhall,
Pencaitland, East Lothian
EH34 5EY, United Kingdom
Tel: +44 1875 341 859
Website: www.handspringpublishing.com

First published 2016 in the United Kingdom by Handspring Publishing
Reprinted 2019, 2020

ISBN 978-1-909141-31-5

British Library Cataloguing in Publication Data
A catalogue record for this book is available from the British Library.

Important notice
It is the responsibility of the clinician/practitioner, employing a range of sources of information, their personal experience, and their understanding of the particular needs of the patient/client, to determine the best approach to treatment.
Neither the publishers nor the authors will be liable for any loss or damage of any nature occasioned to or suffered by any person or property in regard to product liability, negligence or otherwise, or through acting or refraining from acting as a result of adherence to the material contained in this book.

Publisher Mary Law
Design Direction, Illustrations and Cover Design Bruce Hogarth, kinesis-creative.com
Typesetter DSMSoft
Printed in India by Replika Press Pvt. Ltd.

The
Publisher's
policy is to use
paper manufactured
from sustainable forests

Contents

Acknowledgments

We would like to thank the following individuals who helped with the creation of this book. Without their input it wold not have been possible.

The individuals who modelled for the photographs:

Abby Flint

Roy MacDonald

Franziska Trbola

Daniela Witten

The photographer: Bradley Chippington of Bradley Chippington Photography

www.bradleychippington.co.uk

The professional practitioners and colleagues who advised on the structuring and content of the technique chapters:

Fatimah Ayoade, MOst, Bsc and Msc in Biomedical sciences

Stuart Bishop, MOst

Raj Chatwal, MOst

Sian Cook, MOst

Gurkartar Deoora, MOst

Sarah Gray, MOst

Richard Lewis, MOst

Siham Louzri, MOst DO ND

Arjun Mehra, MOst

Lynn Peters, MOst

Nandip Sehra, MOst

Bobby Qureshi, MOst

It is important to start by defining clearly what we mean by articulation. The word articulation (ar•tic•u•la•tion, *noun* \är-ti-kyə-lā-shən\) originates from the Latin meaning 'jointed' or 'divided into joints'. Several definitions may be used (Webster 2015):

1. a. a joint or juncture between bones or cartilages in the skeleton of a vertebrate
   b. a movable joint between rigid parts of an animal

2. a. the action or manner of jointing or interrelating
   b. the state of being jointed or interrelated

Articulation is a cornerstone of most manual therapies, including physiotherapy, osteopathy, chiropractic, sports therapy and many others. We have written this book in an attempt to enhance the understanding of what articulation is and what it can achieve when used appropriately and correctly. We also wanted to provide a clinical handbook which would discuss in depth the use of articulation techniques in relation to each musculoskeletal area. Our aim has been to provide an informed, evidence-based guide to articulation that will help any manual therapist, from student to qualified practitioner, to develop a thoughtful approach to their practice. The information we have presented here, which is supported by references to the latest research, will give the reader the knowledge of when to use these techniques and the correct force or amplitude to use when applying them. This will ensure that they have the information they need to be able to treat their patients safely, confidently and effectively.

The book is divided into two parts and is illustrated with over 300 photographs and line drawings.

Section 1 introduces movement and the basic anatomy of joints; the effects of articulation; patient handling and practitioner posture; identifying red flags and contraindications to treatment.

Section 2 comprises chapters each looking at a specific joint. All chapters in Section 2 have a similar structure and sequence of headings, and they describe the etiology, anatomy, common injuries, special tests, red flags and specific joint assessments and articulations relating to the joint being discussed. Each technique is clearly described and illustrated, with annotations for ease of understanding. The standard structure of each chapter makes the book easy to follow and to dip into.

Manual therapy practitioners have shown for many years that articulation techniques can help to relieve pain and increase the range of movement in joints (Maitland 1986, Kaltenborn & Evjenth 1989, Powers et al 2008). Manual therapy and articulation have been shown to be effective in the treatment of five symptom groups (Maitland et al 2005):

- pain
- stiffness
- pain associated with stiffness
- momentary jabs of pain
- disorders directly related to a specific diagnosis.

Therapeutic articulation of joints has also been observed to lead to improvements in rehabilitation (Lederman 1997), including:

- improved range of movement
- better quality of recovery
- decreased pain medication levels
- increased speed of recovery to patient's normal levels of activity.

One of the systems used to grade therapeutic articulation of the joint, which we refer to in the book, was developed by Maitland (1986). It is as follows:

- **Grade 1** – slow, small amplitude movements performed at the initial range of movement
- **Grade 2** – slow, larger amplitude movements executed through the range of movement, but not at the full end range of movement
- **Grade 3** – slow, large amplitude movements executed at the end range of movement
- **Grade 4** – slow, small amplitude movements executed at the end range of movement and into the resistance
- **Grade 5** – fast, small amplitude movements, high velocity movement (or High Velocity Low Amplitude (HVLA) thrust), which is executed into the pathological limits of movement.

Preface

Spine and Joint Articulation for Manual Therapists is aimed at the use of grades 1–4. Grades 1–2 are aimed mainly at achieving tissue healing, relieving pain, maintaining mobility and helping in the general health and mechanics of the joint. Grades 3–4 are aimed more at increasing the range of movement of the joint (Saunders & Saunders 2004).

In writing this book our aim has been to discuss these manual techniques in depth, with reference to the latest research, and to provide the basis for a better understanding of the role of articulation in clinical practice. We hope it will give you the guidance, confidence and understanding to develop as a confident and safe practitioner and to use these techniques effectively within the clinical environment.

Enjoy!

Giles Gyer, Jimmy Michael, Ben Calvert-Painter

London, May 2016

REFERENCES

Kaltenborn FM, Evjenth O (1989). Manual Mobilization of the Extremity Joints: Basic Examination and Treatment Techniques, 4th ed. Oslo, Norway: Olaf Norlis Bokhandel Universitatsgaten.

Lederman E (1997). Fundamentals of Manual Therapy: Physiology, Neurology and Psychology. London: Churchill Livingstone.

Maitland GD (1986). Vertebral Manipulation, 5th ed. London: Butterworth.

Maitland GD, Hengeveld E, Banks K et al (2005). Vertebral Manipulation, 7th ed. London: Butterworth-Heinemann.

Powers CM, Beneck GJ, Hulig K et al (2008). Effects of a single session of posterior to anterior spinal mobilisation and press-up exercise on pain and response with lumbar spine extension in people with nonspecific low back pain. Journal of the American Physical Therapy Association 88:485-493.

Saunders HD, Saunders R (2004). Evaluation, Treatment, and Prevention of Musculoskeletal Disorders. Chaska, MN: Saunders Group.

Webster M (2015). Articulation. Available at: http://www.merriam-webster.com/dictionary/articulation [Accessed 9 May 2016].

Abduction
Movement of an outlying joint away from the midline

Adduction
Movement of an outlying joint towards the midline

Active motion
Patient's voluntary movement

Amplitude
Distance of articulation

Appendicular skeleton
The part of the skeleton consisting of the bones or cartilage that support the appendages

Applicator
A part of the operator's body which is placed on the contact point of the patient

Arthrokinematics
The specific simultaneous movement of joint surfaces (classed as roll, glide and spin). Sometimes also called arthrokinematic movement or joint play

Articulation
Place where two or more bones unite
The active or passive progress of moving a joint through its allowed physiological range of motion. Sometimes called joint mobilization

Axial skeleton
The part of the skeleton that consists of the bones of the head and trunk

Biaxial
Having or relating to two axes, a biaxial joint has the articular surface where one bone is oval (ellipsoid) and fits into an identically shaped socket on the other bone. All movements except rotation can occur in this shape of joint.

Caudal/Caudad
Towards the tail/inferiorly

Cervical (C)
Neck

Circumduction
The active or passive movement of a limb in a circular fashion (e.g. the circular motion of the ball-and-socket joint)

Coccyx
Tip or end of the tailbone

Contact point
The part of the patient's body where the operator places the applicator

Coronal/Frontal
Plane dividing the body into anterior and posterior parts by passing through it longitudinally from one side to the other

Cranial/Cephalad/ Cephalic
Towards the head/superiorly

Cross fiber/Kneading
Soft-tissue technique: Intermittent force that is applied transversely to the long axis of muscle

Deep pressure/Inhibition
Soft-tissue technique: A local sustained force that is applied to a specific joint

Deviation
Movement of the joint either laterally or medially from the anatomical midline

Distraction
Force acting along a perpendicular to longitudinal axis to draw the structures apart

Dorsum
Back of the hand or the top surface of the foot

Effleurage
Soft-tissue technique: A stroking movement performed in order to encourage the return of fluid from distal to proximal

Eversion
Foot-related movement in a lateral direction

Extension
Backward motion in a sagittal plane about a transverse axis
Straightening of a spinal curve (exception: cervical and lumbar spines) or internal angle

Flexion
Bending movement that decreases a spinal curve (exception: thoracic spine) and internal angle

Basic techniques

Gapping
Medial and lateral – opening one side of a joint

Hypoalgesia
Decreased sensitivity to pain

Hypothenar eminence
The medial side of the hand palmar surface

Inferior (inf)
Bottom

Inversion
Foot-related movement in a medial direction

Lateral (lat)
Further away from the midline

Lateral flexion
Movement in a coronal (frontal) plane about an anterior–posterior axis. Also called side bending

Longitudinal stretch
Soft-tissue technique: Stretch force that is applied along the long axis of muscle

Lower extremity
Thigh, leg and foot

Lumbar (L)
Lower back

Medial (med)
Closer to the midline

Meniscoid
Intercapsular synovial fold formed either in the embryo or as a result of trauma to the joint

Mobilization
See Articulation

Multiaxial
All movement is possible in this type of joint, it is commonly known as a ball and socket joint (e.g hip and shoulder joints)

Nociceptor
Sensory receptor (neuron) that sends signals that cause the perception of pain in response to potentially damaging stimuli

Operator
Practitioner, therapist

Osteokinematics
The basic movements of a joint (e.g. flexion, extension, abduction, adduction). Sometimes also called osteokinematic movement or physiologic movement

Palmar
Palm surface of the hand

Passive motion
Movement made by the operator while the patient is relaxed or passive

Patient
Individual receiving treatment

Plantar
Sole surface of the foot

Plicae
Embryological synovial folds that occur mainly in the knee joint

Posterior (post)
Back

Pronation
Applied to the hand: An act of turning the palmar surface/medial rotation
Applied to the foot: A combination of abduction or eversion in the tarsal or metatarsal joints

Reinforce
Applying extra pressure in order to focus specifically on or protect another part of the body by placing the applicator

Rotation
Movement about an axis – internal, external or medial, lateral

Sacroiliac joints
Joints between the sacrum and the ilia

Sacrum
Tail bone between the two halves of the pelvis

Sagittal
Plane dividing the body into left and right portions by passing through it longitudinally from the front to the back

Shearing
Action or force inclining to lead to two adjoining parts of an articulation to slide in the direction of their plane of contact relative to each other

Shifting
Anteroposterior (A/P) and lateral (Lat). Sliding movement

Side bending
See Lateral flexion

Soft tissue
Tissue other than bone or joint

Springing
Application of repetitive and subtle force to a targeted point

Superior (sup)
Top

Supination
Applied to the hand: Turning the palm forward or upward by lateral external rotation of the forearm
Applied to the foot: Applying adduction and inversion movement to the medial margin of the foot

Synovial
Relating to or denoting a type of joint which is surrounded by thick flexible membrane forming a sack into which is secreted a viscous fluid that lubricates the joint.

Synovial fold
A fold or a ridge or projection of a synovial membrane of a joint extending towards or between the two articular surfaces.

Thenar eminence
The lateral side of the hand palmar surface at the base of the thumb

Thoracic (T)/Dorsal (D)
Mid and upper back

Traction
Force acting along a longitudinal axis in order to draw the structures apart

Translation
Motion along an axis

Transverse
Plane dividing the body to upper and lower portions by passing perpendicular to sagittal and frontal planes horizontally through the body

Upper extremity
Arm, forearm and hand

Basic techniques

Osteopathic techniques

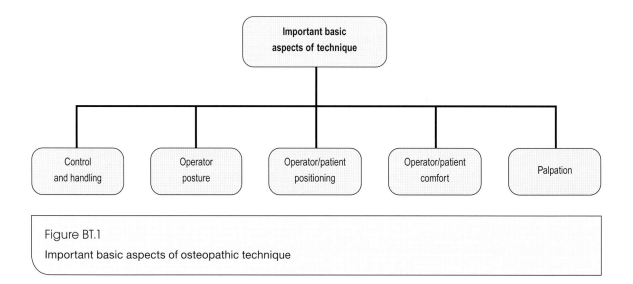

Figure BT.1

Important basic aspects of osteopathic technique

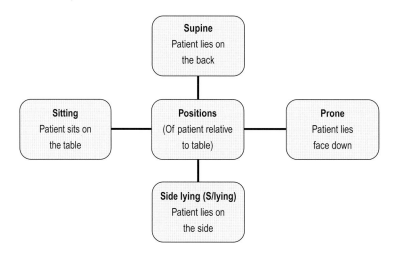

Figure BT.2

Positioning the patient

Joint or tissue	Techniques
Elbow joint	Passive supine extension, flexion, pronation and supination, and gapping
	Soft tissue extensor and flexor muscles
Wrist joints	Passive palmarflexion and dorsiflexion, and ulnar and radial deviation (the operator must be able to locate these bones)
	Anterior and posterior shift at the radiocarpal, intercarpcal and carpometacarpal rows. Lateral shift to the radiocarpal and carpometacarpal rows
Sacroiliac joints	Passive side-lying shearing and gapping to the uppermost joint. Anterior and posterior articulation to the uppermost joint that supports the uppermost extremity
	Passive likely to short-lever anterior and posterior rotation of the ilium on the sacrum and vice versa
Cervical spine	Passive supine extension and flexion, and side bending and rotation
	Soft tissue CES – X fiber
Soft tissues	Lateral and linear stretching, deep pressure, traction and/or separation of muscle origin and insertion – while monitoring the motion changes and tissue response by palpation
	Cross fiber/kneading: Intermittent force that is applied transversely to the long axis of muscle
	Longitudinal stretch: Stretch force that is applied along the long axis of muscle
	Deep pressure/Inhibition: A local sustained force that is applied to a specific joint
	Effleurage: A stroking movement performed in order to encourage the return of fluid from distal to proximal

Table BT.1

Joint and soft-tissue techniques

1

Articulation – theory and evidence

Articulation techniques in the treatment of pain and movement

1

In this chapter we will discuss the biomechanics and individual components of movement. We will present a general overview but will concentrate in particular on synovial joints, which are the joints that manual therapists engage with most.

Movement and stress

Human joints have to withstand considerable forces day to day from compression, shearing and tension. To do this they have evolved layers of tissues and mechanisms to protect against and dissipate the forces that daily activities generate.

Movement and stress always result in mechanical deformation of tissues and structures in the body because tissues undergo an elastic deformation when they are stretched. This deformation allows the tissue to rebound to its original shape and length if it is stretched within normal limits. However, if the tissue is stressed beyond its physical limitations of the elastic phase, it will fail to return to its original structure and will be lengthened. We call this the plastic phase of deformation (Threlkeld 1992).

Stressing the tissue beyond its maximum capacity will result in a tear of that tissue. It is, however, important to note that joint tissues typically work in the elastic phase of tissue deformation as this is vital for normal tissue homeostasis. Not undergoing a healthy deformation within the elastic phase because of lack of activity or immobilization will inhibit joints from regenerating optimally. The end result is tissue thickening, insufficient water in the tissue matrix, loss of tissue elasticity, collagen cross-bridging and shortening of tissue (Threlkeld 1992). There will be a loss of range of motion of joints and the patient will experience joint stiffness and difficulty in moving.

Joint articulation techniques which involve movements that exceed the natural motion barrier stress the tissues excessively and force them into the plastic phase of deformation and so should be avoided.

Movement and tissue repair

Healthy movement through the joint tissues can aid tissue repair and recovery. Khan and Scott (2009) discuss the theory of mechanotransduction and its stages of mechanocoupling, cell–cell communication and effector cell response. Mechanotransduction is described as 'the process whereby cells convert physiological mechanical stimuli into biochemical responses' (Khan & Scott 2009) or 'the mechanical and structural cues that encourage cell behaviour' (Ingber 2006). An example is the effect on bone mineral density in astronauts living in zero-gravity conditions and the reintroduction of gravity and loading to the skeletal system upon their return to Earth. This area is of interest because it can help our understanding of how the mechanical forces involved in distorting and stressing tissues can influence healing and promote tissue recovery by affecting their chemical structure. It also helps us to understand how poor mechanical forces can have the opposite effect, converting mechanical energy into biochemical energy. Manual therapy can aid mechanotherapy by enabling the patient to return to physical activity as quickly as possible and promoting healthy cellular homeostasis (Huang et al 2013).

Joint articulation is commonly used as a technique in manual therapy that has been shown to be effective at reducing musculoskeletal pain (Shum et al 2012). Articulations are often used with the objective to increase the range of motion of the joint through stretching of fibrous tissue and by affecting the stretch reflex excitability (Cook 2007). One theory is that repetitive movement and stretching may cause the tissue to elongate (Refshauge & Gass 2004).

This elongation relates to the ability of tissues to change shape over time as a constant load is applied (Threlkeld 1992). It is thought that this effect on the tissues can increase the range of motion at the joint (McCollam & Cindy 1993, Arnoczky et al 2002, Powers et al 2008, Shum et al 2012). In addition, rhythmical movement causes a pumping action within the joint which influences the intra-articular pressure (Rice & McNair 2009), improving quality and quantity of motion. Saunders and Saunders (2004) demonstrated that articulation of the joint can also increase the vascular circulation to and from the joint during and after treatment. Bortnem and Zavertnik (2009) hypothesized that this may assist in the removal of metabolic waste products and help to balance pH levels within the joint, thus aiding the health, stability and integrity of the joint.

Given the nature of the loading, the pressure inside synovial joints and the need to achieve a low-friction environment, it is important to develop the optimum mechanical conditions after an injury to aid a joint's recovery (Buckwalter 1998). The application of early controlled movement through a joint can aid recovery and also prevent degenerative changes to the articular surfaces (Buckwalter 1995, Buckwalter et al 1996). Buckwalter (1995) also postulated that early mobilization of the joint stimulated the recovery of the proteoglycan matrix, a theory supported by the work of Williams and colleagues (1994). Although getting patients to return to activity has been demonstrated to help articular cartilage recovery (Salter 1993, Mankin & Buckwalter 1997), loading the cartilage too soon can cause delayed recovery in the cartilage (Williams & Brandt 1984, Sun 2010). It is also suggested that the early introduction of movement helps in fluid drainage, preventing the build-up of fluid and distension forces upon the tissues and joint (Lederman 1997). In addition, prolonged distension of a joint caused by effusion could potentially decrease the blood supply to the synovial membrane, leading to damage of the chondrocytes and thus the articular cartilage (Geborek et al 1989, Lafeber et al 1992, Rice & McNair 2009). Beattie et al (2009) found that articulation of L5/S1 caused an increase in water diffusion at the associated intervertebral disc. It was postulated that an increase in diffusion to the intervertebral disc would cause an increase in

intradiscal cell activity and elevated oxygen levels, thus increasing the formation of collagen and proteoglycans within the disc. Although these effects were noted to happen several hours after articulation of the joint, they would still aid in the health and structural stability of the disc.

Joint articulation has been shown to influence the sympathetic nervous activity of the body, thus affecting blood flow, blood pressure, heart rate or respiratory rate (Jowsey & Perry 2010, Zusman 2011, Moutzouri et al 2012, Kingston et al 2014). These sympathetic responses may be associated with changes in blood component levels caused by articulation reducing inflammatory proteins (Teodorczyk-Injeyan et al 2006).

Thus early articulation and management of a joint and injury are essential in the recovery and long-term management of the patient (Hockenbury & Sammarco 2001, Wolfe et al 2001). A study by Green et al (2001) found that passive articulation to the ankle joint after an acute ankle sprain greatly improved the recovery of pain-free movement compared to a control group, providing evidence for the importance of passive joint articulation at the acute stage. This was also supported by Collins et al (2004) who found that articulation of the ankle joint caused an increase in joint range of movement, although this study found no significant hypoalgesic effect from the articulation. However, Yeo & Wright (2011) did find a decrease in pain threshold as well as an increase in range of movement with passive articulation.

Structure of synovial joints

Synovial joints are formed from two opposing bones that are connected by a joint capsule which surrounds the joint cavity. The joint capsule is made up of two distinct layers: the first is an outer fibrous coating around the joint; the second is an inner layer of synovial membrane. This second layer is important in the secretion of synovial fluid into the joint (synovial) cavity. The surfaces of the opposing bones are each covered by a layer of articular cartilage, which aids shock absorbency and fluidity of movement in the joint. This synovial cavity, which is found only in synovial joints, permits movement within the joint.

Cartilage

There are three main types of cartilage: hyaline, white fibrocartilage and yellow fibrocartilage.

- **Hyaline cartilage** forms the fetal skeleton and can also be found in the articular cartilage of synovial joints. In articular cartilage it helps to provide some of the elasticity needed to withstand articular stresses.

- **White fibrocartilage** has great tensile strength. It is found in the intervertebral discs, the menisci of the knee and the articular discs of the temporomandibular and wrist joints, and it also helps form the labrum of the glenohumeral and hip joints.

- **Yellow fibrocartilage** is elastic in nature and, unlike hyaline cartilage, does not ossify or calcify. It is found mainly in the external ear and some cartilages of the larynx and epiglottis.

Articular cartilage is the load-bearing material of synovial joints. It is important in the distribution of contact forces and the reduction of friction and wear. It can be compressed by 5–20% of its overall thickness (Eckstein et al 2000, Kersting et al 2005). Articular cartilage is an avascular structure, i.e. lacking blood vessels, lymph channels and nerves. Nutritional supply to the cartilage is predominately from the synovial fluid, so movement through the joint, both passively and actively, is important not only for the optimal health of the articular cartilage but also in its recovery from damage (da Gracca Macoris & Bertone 2001, Viitanen et al 2003, Bertone 2008) and for the smooth lubrication of the articular surfaces. This lubrication and the surface architecture create a smooth and low-friction surface which is five times smoother than ice (O'Meara 1993).

Articular cartilage can be difficult to analyze from a technical bio-movement model due to its composition of a permeable solid medium distended with fluid (Mow & Lai 1980). The major components of the cartilage matrix are collagen (type II), proteoglycans (60–87%) and other minor proteins and lipids (Armstrong & Mow 1982, Poole et al 2001). Histologically, the cartilage is formed of three layers with different directional fibers which deliver a structure that is resistant to load bearing (Mow et al 1989). These are classified into the superficial zone (10–20% of the cartilage depth), the transitional zone (40–60%) and the deep zone (30%). This layering allows the movement of fluid within the cartilage matrix, making the cartilage a rapid viscoelastic responsive tissue that is able to deform in response to stress without trauma (Mow et al 1980). The hydration of the cartilage causes it to swell moderately and provides extra shock absorbency (Lai et al 1991, Khalsa & Eisenberg 1997, Bursac et al 2000). The change in orientation of the fibers between the layers allows the cartilage to respond to tensile and compressive forces without structural damage, but the layering of the proteoglycans within these tissues is still dictated by the direction of forces through them, even down to the chondrocytes (Guilak 1995, Quinn et al 2001). Therefore it is essential for the nutritional health and potential healing of the cartilage for there to be movement through the joint, whether it is active or passive.

Synovial membrane and fluid

On the inner side of the capsule of the joint is an important membrane called the synovial membrane, which secretes synovial fluid into the joint cavity. An articular joint's resistance to wear and tear is due in part to the lubrication of the joint with this synovial fluid. One of the purposes of the fluid is to create a layer between the articular cartilages to prevent direct contact. This is particularly effective when the joint is under stress: when the cartilage is compressed and deforms, it expresses fluid to create this layer (Mansour & Mow 1976). Due to its macromolecular contents with polyanionic hyaluronic acid and the fact that it is a dialysate of blood plasma, synovial fluid can be difficult to characterize quantitatively (Mow & Lai 1980, Forster & Fisher 1996).

There have been several theories regarding lubrication of the joints such as fluid film lubrication (Macconaill 1932, Dowson et al 1969) and boundary lubrication (Charnley 1960, Hills 1989, Jay et al 2001, Schmidt et al 2007). In their study, Caligaris and colleagues (2009) suggested that the effectiveness of the synovial fluid is from boundary lubrication rather than from fluid film lubrication and lubrication via fluid cartilage pressurization (Forster & Fisher 1996, Krishnan et al 2004).

The three main theories as to how synovial fluid lubricates joints are:

- interstitial (weeping) lubrication
- fluid film lubrication
- boundary lubrication.

Interstitial (weeping) lubrication

In early studies, McCutchen (1959) pressed a large, flat glass against cartilage and noted what he proposed was interstitial (weeping) lubrication, which caused a decrease in friction and thus allowed ease of movement. This was later supported by his studies on the hypothetical effects of a 'weeping bearing' joint in animals (McCutchen 1962). In 2004, Krishnan and colleagues hypothesized that articular cartilage lubrication is dependent on the pressurization of the joint and the 'cartilage interstitial water' (Krishnan et al 2004), thus this loading of the joint shifts to a low-friction articular matrix (Forster & Fisher 1996, Ateshian et al 1998, Krishnan et al 2004, Caligaris et al 2009). McCutchen (1962) and Forster & Fisher (1996) termed this 'self-pressurized hydrostatic lubrication' and 'biphasic lubrication', respectively.

Fluid film lubrication

Fluid film lubrication takes place when opposing articular surfaces are entirely separated by a lubricant film (Hamrock et al 2004). In this theory the layer of synovial fluid over the cartilage is pressurized and disperses mechanical forces across the articular surfaces of the joint. An example of this is motor oil lubricating pistons within a car engine, resulting in low friction while under high stresses. However, this theory has not been proven within synovial joints, possibly due to the porous nature of articular cartilage (Ateshian 2009), and there is currently more evidence to support the boundary lubrication theory (Jahn et al 2016).

Boundary lubrication

Boundary lubrication occurs where there is surface-to-surface contact and it is dependent on the lubricating qualities of the surrounding fluid (Schmidt et al 2007). In a study by Caligaris et al (2009) the authors postulated that, although boundary lubrication would seem more effective than weeping lubrication, both are needed to effectively lubricate the synovial joint. This is confirmed by several studies (Jay et al 1992, Hills & Monds 1998a, Forsey et al 2006, Zappone et al 2007) that show that the boundary lubricants in synovial fluid are more effective than saline lubrication at lubricating articular cartilage. This is evidence for the importance of articulating joints through injury and recovery to ensure effective lubrication of the joint, as stated above and supported by da Gracca Macoris & Bertone (2001), Viitanen et al (2003) and Bertone (2008).

On the other hand, it has been suggested that disuse and degeneration are interconnected (Rapperport et al 1985, Salter 1989, Responte et al 2012). This is due to reduced nutritional input caused by a lack of lubrication during immobility, so movement and articulation of a joint are important for joints, especially if a patient has limited mobility. The potential reduction in interstitial lubrication could explain the increase in friction of a joint that is undergoing osteoarthritic changes (Basalo et al 2004, 2005). In addition, where osteoarthritis affects the production of components of synovial fluid, it can also affect the production of boundary lubricants (Hills & Monds 1998b, Elsaid et al 2007, 2008, Teeple et al 2008, Caligaris et al 2009). This effect again supports the idea that traction and articulation of the joint in a controlled therapeutic manner aid the lubrication of the joint, by what is sometimes called the trans-synovial pump (Fernandez et al 2010). This trans-synovial pump action is made up of three mechanisms that are enhanced with movement:

1. Fluctuation of the intra-articular pressure increases the lubrication of the joint

2. Upsurge in blood flow to the joint

3. Facilitation of drainage of the area via the lymphatic system.

The combined effect of these mechanisms aids in the optimization of synovial elements and their passage in and out of the joint. Therefore, when we undertake articulation of synovial joints as part of manual therapy, we can assume we are encouraging this trans-synovial pump, and potentially the healing within the joint and its surrounding tissues, by aiding the fluid circulation to and from the joint.

Tendons and ligaments

Ligaments (the word 'ligament' comes from the Latin word *'ligare'* which means to bind) and tendons, as well as the joint capsule, surround and encase the joints of the skeletal system. The purpose of the ligaments and joint capsule is to connect and stabilize the bones of the joint and also help in the guiding of movement through the joint (Frank & Shrive 1999). They give the joint stability, and rigidity when needed, and they restrict the range of movement of the joint. Most ligaments are found around the outside of joints and are referred to as extra-articular. Less commonly they are found within the joint and are referred to as intra-articular (e.g. the cruciate ligaments of the knee).

Connective tissues such as tendons and ligaments are formed of approximately parallel collagen fibers which run in the direction of the tensile stress with some elastic fibers mixed in with them. What is interesting is that the ligamentum flavum between the vertebrae has higher elastin content than other ligaments (Nachemson & Evans 1968, Williams et al 1989). Although the fibers are laid parallel, they lie in a wave-like crumpled configuration, without loss of structural integrity. As a joint is put through its range of movement, the connective tissue straightens

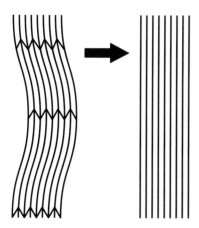

Figure 1.1
The configuration of collagen fibers in a tendon changes from wave-like (left) to straight (right) during joint movement

(see Figure 1.1). Some manual therapists consider this to be 'taking up the slack' in the tissues (Maitland 1986, Kaltenborn 1989).

Following trauma to ligaments and tendons, it is important to encourage movement through them, either passively or actively, along the lines of mechanical stress, in order to aid their recovery (Sawhney & Howard 2002). Physical strain can affect the kinetic chain of protein strands and protein ligands in cells. Applying stress through connective and muscular tissue prolongs the strength and resistance of the tissues (Veigel et al 2003). This structural positioning to mechanical stressors can be found in the majority of tissues in the human body (Schmidt & Wrisberg 2008). Tendons are an excellent example of this structural arrangement of tissue, but it is not only the tendon that responds in this manner: blood vessels, nerve tracts and muscle bundles are all shaped and arranged to withstand and support stress through the tissues and joints, even down to the cellular arrangement of the basement membranes of the cells (Ralphs et al 2002, Huijing & Jaspers 2005).

Evidence would suggest that placing stress on connective tissue is important for its nutritional and vascular health (Noel et al 2000, Schild & Trueb 2002, Heinemeier et al 2007). In addition, movement of the joint has been shown to aid in its lubrication. This, in turn, increases the metabolic actions caused during inflammation and recovery (Hargens & Akeson 1986, Hawley 2010). Some studies have shown that early articulation of a joint after injury can help to develop higher tensile strength of the ligaments, as long as the movement is not too great (Takai et al 1991, Thomopoulos et al 2009).

Joint articulation is often employed to alleviate pain and increase range of motion of the joint by stretching fibrous tissue (Refshauge & Gass 2004). This causes the tissue to change its shape over time as persistent load is applied to it. Prompt articulation of a joint has similarly been shown to reduce the formation of fibrous tissue and adhesions between the tendon and its sheath that could interfere with the normal gliding of the tissues (Thomopoulos et al 2009).

To cause a physical change and lengthen connective tissue, joints need to be articulated at the end range of movement (Threlkeld 1992). When they are placed under stress, tendons and ligaments remodel to the pressures placed through them within their anatomical limits (Herzog & Gal 1999). They strengthen and become stiffer when placed under strain and weaken with less strain (Wang et al 2012). As the body ages, so do the ligaments and tendons, by forming more cross-links in the collagen fibers (Couppe et al 2009). As the tissues age, the collagen content of the fibers decreases, thus decreasing the flexibility of the tissues, decreasing the strength and increasing the diameter of the fibers (Dressler et al 2002, Karamanidis & Arampatzis 2006, Couppe et al 2009). Tendon-related injuries therefore increase as you get older (Dressler et al 2002). When you are articulating a joint, you must reflect on what you are trying to achieve with the individual patient.

Synovial folds (meniscoids)

Intercapsular synovial folds (meniscoids) can be formed either in the embryo or as a result of trauma to the joint. Meniscoids of the spinal facet joints were originally thought to be present mainly in the facet joints of the cervical and lumbar spine, but subsequent studies have shown that they can be found in most intervertebral joints (Kos et al 2001, Webb et al 2009). Farrell et al (2015) discovered that 86% of the cervical facet joints they examined had meniscoids inside them. Meniscoids vary in size and shape (Kos et al 2001), and are not specific to size, gender or joint type (Farrell et al 2015). Meniscoids of the facet joints are of embryological origin, but in other synovial joints they can also be a result of trauma to the joint. The ankle joint is a site where meniscoids regularly occur after trauma to the joint (Lahm et al 1998, Baums et al 2006, Glazebrook et al 2009), and this will be discussed in more detail in Chapter 14, The ankle and foot.

Meniscoids can be divided into three types (Schulte et al 2010):

- **Type 1** (90%; mean length 3.1 mm) are classified as being thin, solid folds extending between the articular surfaces, developing with a connective tissue base extending from the joint capsule with numerous vessels.

- **Type 2** (6%) are situated in the recess of the joint and do not extend between the articular surfaces of the joint. They are formed of loose connective tissue.

- **Type 3** (4%) are thickenings of the synovial joint capsule.

Early thinking about meniscoid injuries (extrapment or entrapment) was that, although the resulting problem of the meniscoid was not necessarily painful, pain was caused by the pull of this dysfunction on the joint capsule (Kos & Wolf 1972). This proposal has since been discredited by Bogduk and Jull (1985) who stated that the distortion caused by a meniscoid injury is not strong enough to cause an issue with the joint capsule. Instead, it is thought that a loose body can be formed from material torn from the apex of the meniscoid or subcapsular hemorrhage due to a basal tear of the meniscoid, resulting in pain and an acute facet lock (Bogduk & Engel 1984, Mercer & Bogduk 1993).

In cases of meniscoid problems, the aim for the manual therapist is to open the joint surfaces to allow the meniscoid to return to its normal position and to restore the range of movement to the joint (Lewit 2010), as illustrated in Figure 1.2. In the scenario of the subcapsular hemorrhage, articulation of the joint is important in the improvement of the trans-synovial pump, which helps the creation and drainage of synovial fluid (Fernandez et al 2010).

Plicae

Plicae are embryological synovial folds that occur mainly in the knee joint although they can also be found in other synovial joints, such as the elbow joint (Kim et al 2006, Steinert et al 2010). They are a common structural occurrence but rarely symptomatic (Dupont 1997, Kenta & Khandujab 2010). As they are most often associated with the knee joint, the anatomy and clinical relevance of plicae are discussed in more detail in Chapter 13, The knee.

Menisci and articular discs

The congruency of some joints is increased by the presence of fibrocartilage intra-articular structures that help make best use of the opposing joint surfaces. Examples include the temporomandibular and knee joints. By improving the congruency of the joint, mobility in a joint that would otherwise be unstable and mechanically at

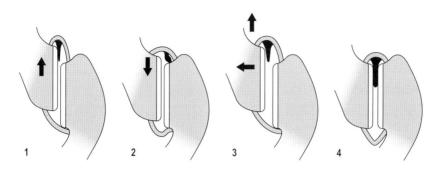

Figure 1.2

Meniscoid extrapment. **1** As the joint surfaces separate, the meniscoid moves with the joint capsule. **2** As the joint surfaces return, the meniscoid contacts the side of the joint so that, instead of returning to its original starting position, it becomes compressed between the bone of the joint and the capsule. **3** Reopening of the joint with an articulation technique decompresses the meniscoid and opens up the articular space, allowing it to reposition into its normal neutral position (**4**). (Adapted from Bogduk 1997)

a disadvantage is improved. In addition, these fibrocartilage structures increase the cushioning that absorbs and distributes forces in the joint, especially in the example of the menisci in the knee joint.

Occasionally, damage to the joint causes tags and tears to the intra-articular structures that can become trapped or folded between the articular surfaces of the joints, causing pain or restriction of the joint. Articulation of these joints can be extremely beneficial in these situations, opening out the joint and allowing the intra-articular structure to sit in a neutral position, for example unfolding the temporomandibular disc. Obviously, if the damage to the joint is extreme, surgical intervention may be needed; you will need to use your clinical judgment on whether to treat or refer.

Neurological effects of articulation

Active and passive movements of the joints stimulate mechanoreceptors in joint tissues, ligaments and the joint capsule (Dutton 2002). When joint tissue is stressed within the normal tissue extensibility limits, pain nerve receptors called nociceptors are activated and cause a pain response.

Joint articulation techniques can be employed in order to highlight mechanical effects that will result in improved extensibility of targeted joint tissues, enhanced mobility and better joint alignment. Thus, pain and muscle spasm can be reduced, and joint range

of motion and flexibility can be enhanced. Note that an individual cannot move a joint properly, either actively or passively, without stimulating the nervous system.

Several studies have shown that articulation can greatly decrease the pain response and increase the pain-free range of movement of joints. Moss and colleagues (2007) found that articulation of an osteoarthritic knee had immediate hypoalgesic effects, both locally and distally. Sluka et al (2006) found that rhythmical articulation of knee joints in rats decreased the pain thresholds in the area of chronically inflamed joints and muscle. They also found that this joint articulation caused a bilateral reduction in hyperalgesia, suggesting that a central neural mediator affected the analgesia of the areas. Courtney and colleagues (2010) suggested that joint mobilization/articulation caused a significant decrease in flexor withdrawal responses in osteoarthritic knees when compared to control groups, again illustrating that articulation can lower the pain threshold in joints. Pain threshold lowering effects post-treatment have also been reported after articulation of the cervical spine (Vicenzino 1995, Sterling et al 2001, Coppieters et al 2003) and lumbar spine (Krouwel et al 2010, Willett et al 2010, Pentelka et al 2012).

Pain gate theory

Patrick Wall and Roland Melzack were the first to develop the pain gate theory, which supposes that not all pain signals freely reach the brain. Melzack and

Wall (1965) proposed the idea of a series of 'gates' that the pain signal has to travel through if it is to move up the spinal cord, and that pain is therefore perceived only if all these gates are 'open'.

The thinking behind this is as follows:

- Afferent (sensory) transmissions travel to the spinal cord and are 'gated' at the dorsal horn. If the stimulus is strong enough, it will progress to the next neuron.

- Gating is controlled by large-diameter neurofibers that close the gates and are opened by small neurofibers.

- The gating organization is controlled via the descending pathways from the central nervous system.

- When the stimulus is strong enough to traverse the gated neural threshold, the ascending fibers activate and the brain perceives the pain. The opposite can happen in hypersensitivity, when the gated system is left open and the neural threshold is lowered. This is one of the ideas relating to central sensitization (Dickenson 2002).

The theory is that, when we massage or articulate an area, we are activating large myelinated fibers that cause a dampening effect on the neurological C-fiber pain fibers, resulting in a change in the pain threshold of the nervous system and a 'closing' of the gating system.

Another theoretical part of the pain gate theory is the descending pathway inhibition via the periaqueductal grey (PAG). This suggests that stimulation of the periaqueductal grey matter of the midbrain causes a response in the descending pathways to the dorsal horn of the spinal cord that stimulates inhibiting interconnecting neurons situated in the substantia gelatinosa (Figure 1.3). This in turn restricts the release of substance P from the first-order neurons, resulting in an inhibition of second-order neurons and thus an interruption in signals to the spinothalamic tract and thalamus (Bee & Dickenson 2007, Staud et al 2007, Apkarian et al 2009). This pathway can be influenced with manual therapy (Schmid et al 2008), causing a neurophysiological response. Kandel et al (2000) found that stimulation of the periaqueductal grey matter has a profound effect in causing selective analgesia.

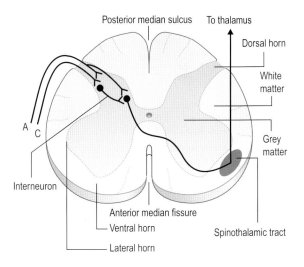

Figure 1.3
Cross section of the spinal cord, illustrating the position of the substantia gelatinosa within the II laminae and the location of the inhibitory neurons

Lundberg (2000) discusses how mental stress causes increases in the excretion of adrenaline and noradrenaline. This results in an increase in blood glucose levels, which then cause an increase in inflammation because of the pro-inflammatory effects of glucose (Dandona et al 2013). Together with increased sympathetic arousal, this causes heightened sensitivity in the tissues and in damaged nerves (Chabal et al 1992, Raja & Treede 2012), thus contributing to the central sensitive state. Studies by Watkins and Maier (1999, 2000), Black (1995) and Sternberg and Gold (1997) review the effects of the immune system and pain. As our understanding of pain and central sensitization expands, we realize that the central sensitized state is caused via a multi-system response to pain, and our treatments must take this into consideration.

Amplitude of articulation

The amplitude (or distance) of articulation is as important as the technique itself. It should be great enough to generate movement but not so great that it causes pain. As the symptoms subside, the amplitude should be gradually increased, with the patient providing feedback. So far, there is no definitive evidence for the optimum duration, frequency or amplitude for articulation techniques. Research investigating subject responses to three cycles of 60-second articulations has shown immediate responses in both local and widespread analgesia (Goodsell et al 2000, Krouwel et al 2010, Willett et al 2010). Pentelka et al (2012) also observed that articulation of the lumbar spine decreased patients' pain thresholds but found that at least four sets of articulation were needed over either 30 seconds or 60 seconds to achieve a change in threshold. However, the rate, duration, amplitude and frequency of the articulation should be tailored to the individual patient, joint and therapist (Maitland et al 2005). For this reason, it is impossible to give absolute values for the amount of force or range of movement needed when examining or articulating a joint.

Articulation of the synovial joints can have a profound effect on range of movement and pain threshold, but it is also important to consider how articulation can affect the cellular structure of a tissue. Whether it is muscle, tendon, ligament, synovial membrane or bone, articulation, hands-on manual therapy and rehabilitation all affect the scaffold effect of the cells. Intervention after injury is therefore advised at an early stage, but it also important in the treatment of chronic patients, especially those who have had restricted mobility as a result of physical difficulties, pain or avoidance of movement.

REFERENCES

Apkarian AV, Baliki MN, Geha PY (2009). Towards a theory of chronic pain. Progress in Neurobiology 87(2):81-97.

Arnoczky SP, Tian T, Lavagnino M et al (2002). Activation of stress-activated protein kinases (SAPK) in tendon cells following cyclic strain: the effects of strain frequency, strain magnitude, and cytosolic calcium. Journal of Orthopaedic Research 20(5):947-52.

Armstrong CG, Mow VC (1982). Variations in the intrinsic mechanical properties of human articular cartilage with age, degeneration, and water content. Journal of Bone and Joint Surgery 64A:88-94.

Ateshian GA (2009). The role of interstitial fluid pressurization in articular cartilage lubrication. Journal of Biomechanics 42(9):1163-1176.

Ateshian GA, Wang H, Lai WM (1998). The role of interstitial fluid pressurization and surface porosities on the boundary friction of articular cartilage. Journal of Tribology 120:241-248.

Basalo IM, Mauck RL, Kelly TA et al (2004). Cartilage interstitial fluid load support in unconfined compression following enzymatic digestion. Journal of Biomechanical Engineering 126(6):779-786.

Basalo IM, Raj D, Krishnan R et al (2005). Effects of enzymatic degradation on the frictional response of articular cartilage in stress relaxation. Journal of Biomechanics 38(6):1343-1349.

Baums MH, Kahl E, Schultz W et al (2006). Clinical outcome of the arthroscopic management of sports-related 'anterior ankle pain': a prospective study. Knee Surgery, Sports Traumatology, Arthroscopy 14(5):482-486.

Beattie PF, Donley JW, Arnot CF et al (2009). The change in the diffusion of water in normal and degenerative lumbar intervertebral discs following joint mobilization compared to prone lying. Journal of Orthopaedic and Sports Physical Therapy 39(1):4-11.

Bee LA, Dickenson AH (2007). Rostral ventromedial medulla control of spinal sensory processing in normal and pathophysiological states. Neuroscience 147(3):786-793.

Bertone AL (2008). Joint physiology: responses to exercise and training. In: KW Hinchcliff, RJ Geor, AJ Kaneps eds. Equine Exercise Physiology. Elsevier Limited; 132-142.

Black PH (1995). Psychoneuroimmunology: brain and immunity. Science and Medicine 2:16-27.

Bogduk N (1997). Clinical Anatomy of the Lumbar Spine and Sacrum, 3rd ed. Edinburgh: Churchill Livingstone.

Bogduk N, Engel R (1984). The menisci of the lumbar zygapophyseal joints: a review of their anatomy and clinical significance. Spine 9(5):454-460.

Bogduk N, Jull G (1985). The theoretical pathology of acute locked back: a basis for manipulative therapy. Manual Medicine 1:78-82.

Bortnem G, Zavertnik J (2009). Neuromuscular Effects of Joint Mobilizations and Manipulations. Oregon: Pacific University Oregon.

Buckwalter JA (1995). Activity vs rest in the treatment of bone, soft tissue and joint injuries. Iowa Orthopaedic Journal 15:29-42.

Buckwalter JA (1998). Articular cartilage: injuries and potential for healing. Journal of Orthopaedic and Sports Physical Therapy 28(4):192-202.

Buckwalter JA, Einhorn TA, Bolander ME et al (1996). Healing of musculo-skeletal tissue. In: CA Rockwood, D Green eds. Fractures. Philadelphia: JB Lippincott; 261-304.

Bursac P, McGrath CV, Eisenberg SR et al (2000). A microstructural model of elastostatic properties of articular cartilage in confined compression. Journal of Biomechanical Engineering 122:347-353.

Caligaris M, Canal CE, Ahmad CS et al (2009). Investigation of the frictional response of osteoarthritic human tibiofemoral joints and the potential beneficial tribological effect of healthy synovial fluid. Osteoarthritis and Cartilage 17(10):1327-1332.

Chabal C, Jacobson L, Russell LC et al (1992). Pain response to perineuromal injection of normal saline, epinephrine and lidocaine into humans. Pain 49:9-12.

Charnley J (1960). The lubrication of animal joints in relation to surgical reconstruction by arthroplasty. Annals of the Rheumatic Diseases 19:10-19.

Collins N, Teys P, Vicenzino B (2004). The initial effects of a Mulligan's mobilization with movement technique on dorsiflexion and pain in subacute ankle sprains. Manual Therapy 9(2):77-82.

Cook C (2007). Orthopedic Manual Therapy: An Evidence-based Approach. Upper Saddle River, NJ: Pearson/Prentice Hall.

Coppieters MW, Stappaerts KH, Wouters LL et al (2003). The immediate effects of a cervical lateral glide treatment technique in patients with neurogenic cervicobrachial pain. Journal of Orthopaedic and Sports Physical Therapy 33(7):369-378.

Couppe C, Hansen P, Kongsgaard M et al (2009). Mechanical properties and collagen cross-linking of the patellar tendon in old and young men. Journal of Applied Physiology 107(3):880-886.

Courtney CA, Witte PO, Chmell SJ et al (2010). Heightened flexor withdrawal response in individuals with knee osteoarthritis is modulated by joint compression and joint mobilization. The Journal of Pain 11(2):179-185.

da Gracca Macoris D, Bertone A (2001). Intra-articular pressure profiles of the cadaveric equine fetlock joint in motion. Equine Veterinary Journal 33(2):184-190.

Dandona P, Ghanim H, Green K et al (2013). Insulin infusion suppresses while glucose infusion induces Toll-like receptors and high-mobility group-B1 protein expression in mononuclear cells of type 1 diabetes patients. American Journal of Physiology: Endocrinology and Metabolism 304(8):E810-E818 doi: 10.1152/ajpendo.00566.2012.

Dickenson AH (2002). Editorial I: Gate Control Theory of pain stands the test of time. British Journal of Anaesthesia 88(6):755-757.

Dowson D, Wright V, Longfield MD (1969). Human joint lubrication. Biomedical Engineering 4:160-165.

Dressler MR, Butler DL, Wenstrup R et al (2002). A potential mechanism for age-related declines in patellar tendon biomechanics. Journal of Orthopaedic Research 20(6):1315-1322.

Dupont JY (1997). Synovial plicae of the knee: controversies and review. Clinics in Sports Medicine 16(1):87-122.

Dutton M (2002). Manual Therapy of the Spine: an integrated approach. New York: McGraw-Hill.

Eckstein F, Lemberger B, Stammberger T et al (2000). Patellar cartilage deformation in vivo after static versus dynamic loading. Journal of Biomechanics 33:819-825.

Elsaid KA, Jay GD, Chichester CO (2007). Reduced expression and proteolytic susceptibility of lubricin/superficial zone protein may explain early elevation in the coefficient of friction in the joints of rats with antigen-induced arthritis. Arthritis and Rheumatism 56(1):108-116.

Elsaid KA, Fleming BC, Oksendahl HL et al (2008). Decreased lubricin concentrations and markers of joint inflammation in the synovial fluid of patients with anterior cruciate ligament injury. Arthritis and Rheumatism 58(6):1707-1715.

Farrell SF, Osmotherly PG, Cornwall J et al (2015). The anatomy and morphometry of cervical zygapophyseal joint meniscoids. Surgical and Radiologic Anatomy 37(7):799-807.

Fernandez C, Arendt-Nielsen L, Gerwin R (2010). Tension-type and Cervicogenic Headache: Pathophysiology, Diagnosis, and Management. Burlington, MA: Jones & Bartlett Learning.

Forsey RW, Fisher J, Thompson J et al (2006). The effect of hyaluronic acid and phospholipid-based lubricants on friction within a human cartilage damage model. Biomaterials 27(26):4581-4590.

Forster H, Fisher J (1996). The influence of loading time and lubricant on the friction of articular cartilage. Proceedings of the Institution of Mechanical Engineers, Part H 210(2):109-119.

Frank CB, Shrive NG (1999). Ligament. In: BM Nigg, W Herzog eds. Biomechanics of the Musculoskeletal System, 2nd ed. New York: John Wiley & Sons; 107-126.

Geborek P, Moritz U, Wollheim FA (1989). Joint capsular stiffness in knee arthritis. Relationship to intra-articular volume, hydrostatic pressures, and extensor muscle function. Journal of Rheumatology 16(10):1351-1358.

Glazebrook MA, Ganapathy V, Bridge MA et al (2009). Evidence-based indications for ankle arthroscopy. Arthroscopy 25(12):1478-1490.

Goodsell M, Lee M, Latimer J (2000). Short-term effects of lumbar posteroanterior mobilisation in individuals with low back pain. Journal of Manipulative and Physiological Therapeutics 23(5):332-342.

Green T, Refshauge K, Crosbie J et al (2001). A randomised controlled trial of a passive accessory joint mobilisation on acute ankle inversion sprains. Physical Therapy 81(4):984-994.

Guilak F (1995). Compression-induced changes in the shape and volume of the chondrocyte nucleus. Journal of Biomechanics 28:1529-1541.

Hamrock BJ, Schmid SR, Jacobson BO (2004). Fundamentals of Fluid Film Lubrication. Boca Raton, FL: CRC Press.

Hargens AR, Akeson WH (1986). Stress effects on tissue nutrition and viability. In: AR Hargens ed. Tissue Nutrition and Viability. New York: Springer-Verlag.

Hawley B (2010). Joint motion and motion therapy. Dynamic Chiropractic, August 26, vol. 28, issue 18.

Heinemeier KM, Olesen JL, Haddad F et al (2007). Expression of collagen and related growth factors in rat tendon and skeletal muscle in response to specific contraction types. Journal of Physiology Aug 1, 582(Pt 3):1303-1316.

Herzog W, Gal J (1999). Tendon. In: BM Nigg, W Herzog eds. Biomechanics of the Musculoskeletal System, 2nd ed. New York: John Wiley & Sons; 127-147.

Hills BA (1989). Oligolamellar lubrication of joints by surface active phospholipid. Journal of Rheumatology 16:82-91.

Hills BA, Monds MK (1998a). Deficiency of lubricating surfactant lining the articular surfaces of replaced hips and knees. British Journal of Rheumatology 37(2):143-147.

Hills BA, Monds MK (1998b). Enzymatic identification of the load-bearing boundary lubricant in the joint. British Journal of Rheumatology 37(2):137-142.

Hockenbury RT, Sammarco GJ (2001). Evaluation and treatment of ankle sprains. The Physician and Sports Medicine 29(2):57-64.

Huang C, Holfeld J, Schaden W et al (2013). Mechanotherapy: revisiting physical therapy and recruiting mechanobiology for a new era in medicine. Trends in Molecular Medicine 19(9):555-564.

Huijing PA, Jaspers RT (2005). Adaptation of muscle size and myofascial force transmission: a review and some new experimental results. Scandinavian Journal of Medicine and Science in Sports 15:349-380.

Ingber DE (2006). Cellular mechanotransduction: putting all the pieces together again. FASEB Journal 20(7):811-827.

Jahn S, Seror J, Klein J (2016). Lubrication of articular cartilage. Annual Review of Biomedical Engineering 18(1).

Jay GD, Lane BP, Sokoloff L (1992). Characterization of a bovine synovial fluid lubricating factor. III. The interaction with hyaluronic acid. Connective Tissue Research 28(4):245-255.

Jay GD, Tantravahi U, Britt DE et al (2001). Homology of lubricin and superficial zone protein (SZP): products of megakaryocyte stimulating factor (MSF) gene expression by human synovial fibroblasts and articular chondrocytes localized to chromosome 1q25. Journal of Orthopaedic Research 19:677-687.

Jowsey P, Perry J (2010). Sympathetic nervous system effects in the hands following a grade III postero-anterior rotatory mobilisation technique applied to T4: a randomised, placebo-controlled trial. Manual Therapy 15(3):248-253.

Kaltenborn FM (1989). Manual Mobilization of the Extremity Joints: Basic Examination and Treatment Techniques, 4th ed. Oslo, Norway: Olaf Norlis Bokhandel Universitatsgaten.

Kandel E, Schwartz J, Jessell T (2000). Principles of Neural Science, 4th ed. New York: McGraw-Hill.

Karamanidis K, Arampatzis A (2006). Mechanical and morphological properties of human quadriceps femoris and triceps surae muscle–tendon unit in relation to aging and running. Journal of Biomechanics 39(3):406-417.

Kenta M, Khandujab V (2010). Synovial plicae around the knee. The Knee 17(2):97-102.

Kersting UG, Stubendorff JJ, Schmidt MC et al (2005). Changes in knee cartilage volume and serum COMP concentration after running exercise. Osteoarthritis Cartilage 13:925-934.

Khalsa PS, Eisenberg SR (1997). Compressive behaviour of articular cartilage is not completely explained by proteoglycan osmotic pressure. Journal of Biomechanics 30:589-594.

Khan KM, Scott A (2009). Mechanotherapy: how physical therapists' prescription of exercise promotes tissue repair. British Journal of Sports Medicine 43(4):247-252.

Kim DH, Gambardella RA, ElAttrache NS et al (2006). Arthroscopic treatment of posterolateral elbow impingement from lateral synovial plicae in throwing athletes and golfers. The American Journal of Sports Medicine 34(3):438-444.

Kingston L, Claydon L, Tumilty S (2014). The effects of spinal mobilizations on the sympathetic nervous system: a systematic review. Manual Therapy, 19(4):281-287.

Kos J, Hert J, Sevcik P (2001). Meniscoids of the intervertebral joints. Acta Chirurgiae Orthopaedicae et Traumatologiae Cechoslovaca 69(3):149-157.

Kos J, Wolf J (1972). Les menisques intervertebraux et leur role possible dans les blocages vertebraux. Annales de Medicine Physique 15:203-218.

Krishnan R, Kopacz M, Ateshian GA (2004). Experimental verification of the role of interstitial fluid pressurization in cartilage lubrication. Journal of Orthopaedic Research 22:565-570.

Krouwel O, Hebron C, Willett E (2010). An investigation into the potential hypoalgesic effects of different amplitudes of PA mobilisations on the lumbar spine as measured by pressure pain thresholds (PPT). Manual Therapy 15:7-12.

Lafeber FPJG, Veldhuijzen JP, Vanroy JLAM et al (1992). Intermittent hydrostatic compressive force stimulates exclusively the proteoglycan synthesis of osteoarthritic human cartilage. Rheumatology 31(7):437-442.

Lahm A, Erggelet C, Reichelt A (1998). Ankle joint arthroscopy for meniscoid lesions in athletes. Arthroscopy 14(6):572-575.

Lai WM, Hou JS, Mow VC (1991). A triphasic theory for the swelling and deformation behaviors of articular cartilage. Journal of Biomechanical Engineering 113:245-258.

Lederman E (1997). Fundamentals of Manual Therapy: Physiology, Neurology and Psychology. London: Churchill Livingstone.

Lewit K (2010). Manipulative Therapy: Musculoskeletal Medicine. Philadelphia: Elsevier Health Sciences.

Lundberg U (2000). Catecholamines. In: G Fink ed. Encyclopedia of Stress. San Diego: Academic Press.

McCollam RL, Cindy BJ (1993). Effects of posterio-anterior mobilisation on lumbar extension and flexion. Journal of Manual and Manipulative Therapy vol. 1, no. 4.

Macconaill MA (1932). The function of intra-articular fibrocartilages, with special reference to the knee and inferior radio-ulnar joints. Journal of Anatomy 66:210-227.

McCutchen CW (1959). Sponge-hydrostatic and weeping bearings. Nature 184:1284-1285.

McCutchen CW (1962). The frictional properties of animal joints. Wear 5(1):1-17.

Maitland GD (1986). Vertebral Manipulation, 5th ed. London: Butterworth.

Maitland GD, Hengeveld E, Banks K et al (2005). Vertebral Manipulation, 7th ed. London: Butterworth–Heinemann.

Mankin HJ, Buckwalter JA (1997). Articular cartilage. II. Degeneration and osteoathrosis, repair, regeneration and transplantation. Journal of Bone and Joint Surgery 79A(4):612-632.

Mansour JM, Mow VC (1976). The permeability of articular cartilage under compressive strain and at high pressures. Journal of Bone and Joint Surgery 58A:509-516.

Melzack R, Wall PD (1965). Pain mechanisms: a new theory. Science (New York) 150(3699):971-979 PMID: 5320816.

Mercer S, Bogduk N (1993). Intra-articular inclusions of the cervical synovial joints. Rheumatology 32(8):705-710.

Moss P, Sluka K, Wright A (2007). The initial effects of knee joint mobilisations on osteoarthritic hyperalgesia. Manual Therapy 12:109-118.

Moutzour, M, Perry J, Billis E (2012). Investigation of the effects of a centrally applied lumbar sustained natural apophyseal glide mobilization on lower limb sympathetic nervous system activity in asymptomatic subjects. Journal of Manipulative and Physiological Therapeutics 35(4):286-294.

Mow VC, Kuei SC, Lai WM et al (1980). Biphasic creep and stress relaxation of articular cartilage in compression: theory and experiments. Journal of Biomechanical Engineering 102:73-84.

Mow V, Lai M (1980). Recent developments in synovial joint biomechanics. SIAM Review vol. 22, no. 3 (Society for Industrial and Applied Mathematics).

Mow VC, Proctor CS, Kelly MA (1989). Biomechanics of articular cartilage. In: M Nordin, VH Frankel eds. Basic Biomechanics of the Musculoskeletal System, 2nd ed. Philadelphia, PA: Lea & Febiger; 31-58.

Nachemson AL, Evans JH (1968). Some mechanical properties of the third human lumbar interlaminar ligament (ligamentum flavum). Journal of Biomechanics 1:211-220.

Noel G, Verbruggen LA, Barbaix E et al (2000). Adding compression to mobilization in a rehabilitation program after knee surgery. A preliminary clinical observational study. Manual Therapy 5(2):102-107.

O'Meara PM (1993). The basic science of meniscus repair. Orthopaedic Review 22(6):681-686.

Pentelka L, Hebron C, Shapleski R et al (2012). The effect of increasing sets (within one treatment session) and different set durations (between treatment sessions) of lumbar spine posteroanterior mobilisations on pressure pain thresholds. Manual Therapy 17(6):526-530.

Poole AR, Kojima T, Yasuda T et al (2001). Composition and structure of articular cartilage: a template for tissue repair. Clinical Orthopaedics 391(suppl):S26-33.

Powers CM, Beneck GJ, Hulig K et al (2008). Effects of a single session of posterior to anterior spinal mobilisation and press-up exercise on pain and response with lumbar spine extension in people with nonspecific low back pain. Journal of the American Physical Therapy Association 88:485-493.

Quinn TM, Dierickx P, Grodzinsky AJ (2001). Glycosaminoglycan network geometry may contribute to anisotropic hydraulic permeability in cartilage under compression. Journal of Biomechanics 34:1483-1490.

Raja SN, Treede RD (2012). Testing the link between sympathetic efferent and sensory afferent fibers in neuropathic pain. The Journal of the American Society of Anesthesiologists 117(1):173-177.

Ralphs JR, Waggett AD, Benjamin M (2002). Actin stress fibers and cell–cell adhesion molecules in tendons: organisation *in vivo* and response to mechanical loading of tendon cells *in vitro*. Matrix Biology 21:67-74.

Rapperport DJ, Carter DR, Schurman DJ (1985). Contact finite element stress analysis of the hip joint. Journal of Orthopaedic Research 3(4):435-446.

Refshauge K, Gass E (2004). Musculoskeletal Physiotherapy: Clinical Science and Evidence-based Practice, 2nd ed. Oxford: Butterworth–Heinemann.

Responte DJ, Lee JK, Hu JC et al (2012). Biomechanics-driven chondrogenesis: from embryo to adult. FASEB Journal 26(9):3614-3624.

Rice D, McNair P (2009). Quadriceps arthrogenic muscle inhibition: neural mechanisms and treatment perspectives. Seminars in Arthritis and Rheumatism 40(3):250-266.

Salter RB (1989). The biologic concept of continuous passive motion of synovial joints. The first 18 years of basic research and its clinical application. Clinical Orthopaedics and Related Research 242:12-25.

Salter RB (1993). Continuous passive motion (CPM): a biological concept for the healing and regeneration of articular cartilage, ligaments and tendons. In: Original Research to Clinical Applications. Baltimore: Williams & Wilkins; 419.

Saunders HD, Saunders R (2004). Evaluation, Treatment, and Prevention of Musculoskeletal Disorders. Chaska, MN: Saunders Group.

Sawhney RK, Howard J (2002). Slow local movements of collagen fibers by fibroblasts drive the rapid global self-organization of collagen gels. Journal of Cell Biology 157(6):1083-1092. doi: 10.1083/jcb.200203069.

Schild C, Trueb B (2002). Mechanical stress is required for high-level expression of connective tissue growth factor. Experimental Cell Research 274(1):83-91.

Schmid A, Brunner F, Wright A et al (2008). Paradigm shift in manual therapy? Evidence for a central nervous system component in the response to passive cervical joint mobilization. Manual Therapy 13(5):387-396.

Schmidt TA, Gastelum NS, Nguyen QT et al (2007). Boundary lubrication of articular cartilage: role of synovial fluid constituents. *Arthritis and Rheumatism* 56:882-891.

Schmidt RA, Wrisberg CA (2008). Motor Learning and Performance: A Situation-based Learning Approach. Human Kinetics.

Schulte TL, Filler TJ, Struwe P et al (2010). Intra-articular meniscoid folds in thoracic zygapophysial joints. Spine 35(6):E191-E197.

Shum GL, Tsung BY, Lee RL (2012). Immediate effect of posteroanterior mobilisation on reducing back pain and the stiffness of the lumbar spine. Archive of Physical Medicine and Rehabilitation doi:10,1016/j.amr.2012.11.020.

Sluka KA, Skyba DA, Radhakrishnan R et al (2006). Joint mobilization reduces hyperalgesia associated with chronic muscle and joint inflammation in rats. The Journal of Pain 7(8):602-607.

Staud R, Craggs JG, Robinson ME et al (2007). Brain activity related to temporal summation of C-fiber evoked pain. Pain 129:130-142.

Steinert AF, Goebel S, Rucker A et al (2010). Snapping elbow caused by hypertrophic synovial plica in the radiohumeral joint: a report of three cases and review of literature. Archives of Orthopaedic and Trauma Surgery 130(3):347-351.

Sterling M, Jull G, Wright A (2001). Cervical mobilisation: concurrent effects on pain, sympathetic nervous system activity and motor activity. Manual Therapy 6:72-81.

Sternberg EM, Gold PW (1997). The mind–body interaction in disease. Scientific American 7, Special Issue, Mysteries of the Mind:8-17.

Sun HB (2010). Mechanical loading, cartilage degradation, and arthritis. Annals of the New York Academy of Sciences 1211(1):37-50.

Takai S, Woo SL, Horibe S et al (1991). The effect of frequency and duration of controlled passive mobilization on tendon healing. Journal of Orthopaedic Research 9(5):705-713.

Teeple E, Elsaid KA, Fleming BC et al (2008). Coefficients of friction, lubricin, and cartilage damage in the anterior cruciate ligament-deficient guinea pig knee. Journal of Orthopaedic Research 26(2):231-237.

Teodorczyk-Injeyan J, Injeyan H, Ruegg R (2006). Spinal manipulative therapy reduces inflammatory cytokines but not substance P production in normal subjects. Journal of Manipulative and Physiological Therapeutics 29:14-21.

Thomopoulos S, Das R, Silva M et al (2009). Enhanced flexor tendon healing through controlled delivery of PDGF-BB. *Journal of Orthopaedic Research* September, 27(9):1209-1215. doi:10.1002/jor.20875.

Threlkeld A (1992). The effects of manual therapy on connective tissue. Physical Therapy 72(12):893-902.

Veigel C, Molloy JE, Schmitz S et al (2003). Load-dependent kinetics of force production by smooth muscle myosin measured with optical tweezers. Nature Cell Biology 5:980-986.

Vicenzino B (1995). An investigation of the effects of spinal manual therapy on forequarter pressure and thermal pain thresholds and sympathetic nervous system activity in asymptomatic patients: a preliminary study. In: M Shacklock ed. Moving in on Pain. Melbourne, Australia: Butterworth–Heinemann; 185-193.

Viitanen MJ, Wilson AM, McGuigan HP et al (2003). Effect of foot balance on the intra articular pressure in the distal interphalangeal joint in vitro. Equine Veterinary Journal 35(2):184-189.

Wang JH, Guo Q, Li B (2012). Tendon biomechanics and mechanobiology – a mini review of basic concepts and recent advancements. Journal of Hand Therapy 25(2):133-141.

Watkins LR, Maier SF (1999). Cytokines and Pain. Basel: Birkhauser.

Watkins LR, Maier SF (2000). The pain of being sick: implications of immune-to-brain communication for understanding pain. Annual Review of Psychology 51:29-57.

Webb AL, Darekar AA, Sampson M et al (2009). Synovial folds of the lateral atlantoaxial joints: *in vivo* quantitative assessment using magnetic resonance imaging in healthy volunteers. Spine 34(19):E697-E702.

Willett E, Hebron C, Krouwel O (2010). The initial effects of different rates of lumbar mobilisations on pressure pain thresholds in asymptomatic subjects. Manual Therapy 15(2):173-178.

Williams JM, Brandt KD (1984). Immobilization ameliorates chemically induces articular cartilage damage. Arthritis and Rheumatism 27:208-216.

Williams JM, Moran M, Thonar EJ et al (1994). Continuous passive motion stimulates repair of rabbit knee articular cartilage after matrix proteoglycan loss. Clinical Orthopaedics 304:252-262.

Williams PL, Warwick R, Dyson M et al (1989). Gray's Anatomy, 37th ed. New York: Churchill Livingstone; 69-70.

Wolfe MW, Uhl TL, Mattacola CG et al (2001). Management of ankle sprains. American Family Physician 63(1):93-104.

Yeo HK, Wright A (2011). Hypoalgesic effect of a passive accessory mobilisation technique in patients with lateral ankle pain. Manual Therapy 16(4):373-377.

Zappone B, Greene GW, Oroudjev E et al (2007). Molecular aspects of boundary lubrication by human lubricin: effect of disulfide bonds and enzymatic digestion. Langmuir 24(4):1495-1508.

Zusman M (2011). Mechanism of mobilization. Physical Therapy Reviews 16(4):233-236.

Introduction to movement and joints 2

In this chapter we will present an overview of the different types of joint, their classification and joint movement(s).

Describing movement

To help describe movement, we use the terminology of 'planes'. There are three planes of movement in the human body (the frontal and sagittal planes are shown in Figure 2.1a):

- **Frontal plane** – divides the body into anterior and posterior portions. An example of this movement would be lifting your arms and legs out to the side while doing a star jump: your arms and legs would be moving in the *frontal plane*.

- **Transverse plane** – divides the body through a line parallel to the floor in the horizontal position. Twisting and rotational movements such as turning your head to look over your shoulder occur in the *transverse plane*.

- **Sagittal plane** – divides the body into left and right portions with a line that goes from anterior to posterior. For example, when you are walking, your feet are moving in a *sagittal plane*.

Directions of movement are described using the terms superior/inferior, anterior/ventral and posterior/dorsal (Figure 2.1b).

What are joints?

The main purposes of the musculoskeletal system are movement and support. It is joints that enable movement. Joint mobility varies greatly and depends on a multitude of factors, such as the type of joint, ligament and muscular tension, and the apposition of connective tissue inside the joint. The structure of the joint dictates the angle and direction of the movement that takes place, but the joint must be sufficiently

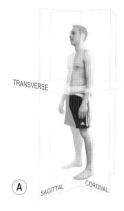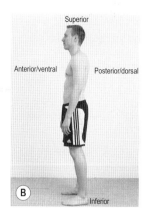

Figure 2.1
Planes and directions of movement

stable to maintain its integrity. For every joint there is an integral balance between stability and mobility: the more mobile a joint is, the less stable it is, and vice versa.

Joints are not only responsible for allowing movement; they also aid shock absorbency. Some of this shock absorbency is effected by the dynamics of the fluid and cartilage inside the joints (see Chapter 1). It is particularly important in the spine and lower extremities to help in the dissipation of forces that could potentially damage other parts of the body, for example when we run, jump or exercise. The mechanism is similar to shock absorbers in vehicles, which reduce damage or wear caused to the vehicle by the forces of the road.

When examining joints, the two components we are looking for are the 'quantity' and the 'quality' of the movement. The quantity refers to the range of movement of the joint. Through examination, our aim is to assess the amount of movement the joint can achieve within a particular plane until the movement stops. The limitation of the movement can be caused by pain or muscular contraction, or by the approximation of bone, connective tissue or soft tissue.

When a bony approximation is present, it is felt as a sudden ending of movement through the joint. Bony approximation can be due to natural anatomical approximation of the joint surfaces or to bony hypertrophy, either intra- or extracapsular. A connective tissue cause of the end of range of movement will give a firm end feel but it will also give an element of spring when tensioned. This spring end of range element is caused by the joint capsule or ligaments around the joint. Restriction of a joint movement due to soft tissue approximation gives a much softer end feel, with no definite end to the range of movement. This uncertainty about the exact end of range of movement may be an issue when examining larger patients.

Arthrokinematics

Arthrokinematics or arthrokinematic movement (sometimes also called joint play) refer to the specific simultaneous movements of joint surfaces. These are classed as roll, glide and spin.

- **Roll** is when one surface of a bone 'rolls' across another, similar to a wheel rolling along the ground.

- **Glide** happens when one articular surface moves parallel to another while keeping the space equal between the two surfaces.

- **Spin** occurs when one bone/joint surface 'spins' on another around a central axis.

The shape of the articular surfaces of the joints helps to dictate how these movements can occur (see 'Types of joint' later in the chapter). Individual joints are described in more detail in separate chapters, but a very brief summary of the mechanics of the knee here will serve to illustrate how different movements can occur in one joint.

The knee is classified as a modified hinge joint because the joint allows all the movements of roll, spin and glide. As the knee bends, forces of roll and glide occur as the condyles of the femur articulate with the tibial plateau. These movements are guided by the shape of the meniscus of the knee and the pull of the ligamentous tissues. Spin also occurs as the knee approaches full extension, when the tibia externally rotates (or spins) along its long axis to achieve a close-packed position in knee-joint extension. This is important as the forces involved in achieving this position cause an energy-saving biomechanical tension on the supportive structures of the knee when the person is standing. (We will discuss this in more detail in Chapter 13, The knee.)

Types of joint

Joints can be divided into three types:

- fibrous

- cartilaginous

- synovial.

Fibrous joints

Fibrous joints are strong joints that allow either small ranges of movement or, in some cases, no movement to occur. They can be subdivided into three groups:

- suture – e.g. of the cranial bones in the adult skull (Figure 2.2)

- gomphosis – e.g. the root of a tooth attaching to the bone

- syndesmosis – e.g. tibia and fibula (Figure 2.3).

Suture and gomphosis type joints generally have no movement. Syndesmosis joints (such as between the tibia and the fibula) have a small amount of movement. (We will discuss this further in Chapter 13, The knee.)

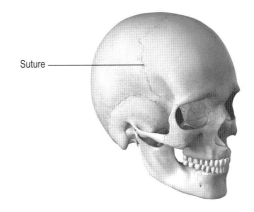

Suture

Figure 2.2
Sutures of the cranium. The arrow indicates the suture between the frontal and temporal bones

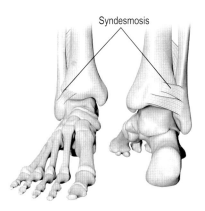

Figure 2.3
The syndesmosis joint of the distal tibia and fibula

Cartilaginous joints

Cartilaginous joints are generally flexible, strong, shock-absorbing joints that have no direct blood supply and no space between the cartilaginous and the skeletal tissues. They are of two types:

- synchondrosis – e.g. first rib and the sternum (Figure 2.4)

- symphysis – e.g. pubic symphysis, vertebral disc and vertebra (Figure 2.5).

Synovial joints

Synovial joints are the most common type of joint in the human body and, when they are healthy, they are

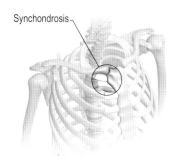

Figure 2.4
The synchondrosis joint between the first rib and the sternum

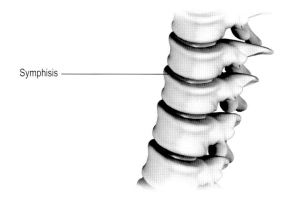

Figure 2.5
Symphysis joints in the vertebral column

generally mobile. The articular part of the skeletal tissue is covered with smooth articular/synovial cartilage. The joint is then supported by ligamentous tissue and a synovial joint capsule. These structures are important in allowing smooth fluid movement of the healthy joint while maintaining the stability and integrity of the joint.

Synovial joints can be subdivided into six different types of joint, according to their shape and structure, which dictate the movement that happens at the joint:

- planar
- hinge
- pivot
- condyloid
- saddle
- ball-and-socket.

Synovial joints are the main joints of the human body and they are the joints which manual therapists will treat most frequently. We will therefore discuss them now in more detail.

Planar joints

Planar joints have articular surfaces which are slightly curved and allow gliding movements to occur. For this reason they are occasionally referred to as 'gliding joints'. The range of movement within a planar joint is limited. Examples of planar joints are the carpal and tarsal joints in the hands and feet (Figure 2.6).

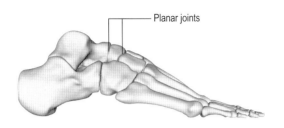

Figure 2.6
Planar joints in the foot

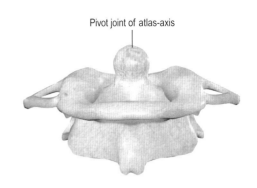

Figure 2.8
The atlanto-axial (pivot) joint

Hinge joints

Hinge joints allow only one primary movement to occur. One bone in the joint is slightly convex in shape and articulates with the concave surface of the opposing bone. This means that, when moving the joint, one bone appears stationary while the other is moving, similar to the hinge of a door. The humeroulnar (elbow) joint is a classic example of this (Figure 2.7).

Pivot joints

These joints consist of one bone fitting into another ring-shaped bone. This structure allows a rotational function to occur. An example of a pivot joint is the atlanto-axial joint (between the first and second vertebrae of the neck) (Figure 2.8).

Condyloid joints

Condyloid joints are also referred to as ellipsoidal joints. They have an oval-shaped end to one of the articular surfaces which articulates with a similar oval-shaped hollow on the other articular surface. These types of joint allow primary movement to occur along primary axes. Examples include the interphalangeal joints of the fingers (Figure 2.9) and toes.

Saddle joints

Saddle joints move in a similar way to condyloid joints but the saddle shape of the articular surfaces (hence the name) allows a greater range of mobility in the joint. An example of this is the thumb joint, which, because of the shape of the articular surfaces, has a greater range of movement than the interphalangeal joints (Figure 2.10).

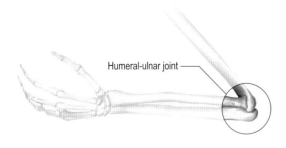

Figure 2.7
The humeroulnar hinge joint of the elbow

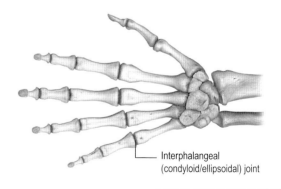

Figure 2.9
Interphalangeal joints in the fingers

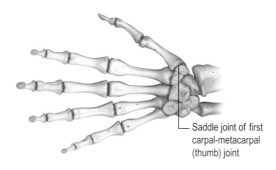

Figure 2.10
The saddle joint in the thumb

Ball-and-socket joints

Ball-and-socket joints are the most mobile of the synovial joints and allow movement in all directions. They have the greatest range of movement of all joints. They are formed by a rounded sphere-shaped articular surface on one bone which articulates into a cup-like socket in the opposing articular surface. Examples of this type of joint are the hip and glenohumeral joint (Figure 2.10).

Osteokinematics

Osteokinematics or osteokinematic movement (sometimes also called physiologic movement) refers to the basic movements of a joint. Examples are flexion, extension, abduction and adduction. Being able to understand and describe how the body moves, ranges

of movement and actions is critical in the evaluation of the patient and in the communication between patients, teachers and other professionals.

When discussing planes of movement and actions, our starting point is the neutral anatomical position (see Figure 2.12).

The terms we use to describe movement can also be used to describe a position – for example, 'holding the joint in a flexed position' or 'starting from a medially rotated position'. These terms are used as a measurement when making a comparison with the neutral anatomical position.

Nearly all movements are paired. This is because most movements have an opposite, moving the joint in the opposite direction but in the same plane of movement. We will discuss them in the following order:

- Flexion and extension
- Horizontal flexion and extension
- Lateral flexion
- Adduction and abduction

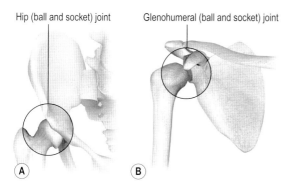

Figure 2.11
Ball-and-socket joints: **A** hip joint;
B glenohumeral joint

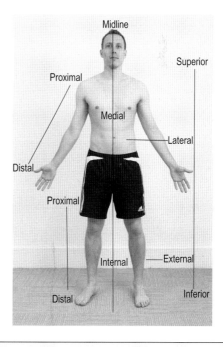

Figure 2.12
The neutral anatomical position

- Medial and lateral rotation
- Elevation and depression
- Protraction and retraction
- Pronation and supination
- Eversion and inversion
- Medial and lateral deviation
- Opposition and apposition
- Dorsiflexion and plantarflexion
- Circumduction
- Traction and distraction

Flexion and extension (Figure 2.13)

Flexion and extension are movements that happen in the sagittal plane.

Flexion is generally classed as a bending movement, for example when the knee bends, bringing the heel towards the buttock. In this example, the angle of the joint decreases as the heel moves towards the buttock.

Extension is the return of the joint back into the anatomical resting position from the flexed position. Staying with the example of the knee, the angle of the joint increases in extension as the leg is straightened. Hyperextension is when this movement passes the neutral anatomical position.

Horizontal flexion and extension (Figure 2.14)

These movements occur in the horizontal plane.

Horizontal flexion is the movement where the angle of the joint decreases in the horizontal plane.

Horizontal extension refers to movement where the angle of the joint increases in the horizontal plane.

Lateral flexion (Figure 2.15)

Lateral flexion is a term of movement that is used by some therapists that refers to the spine moving laterally away from the midline. It is also known as side bending.

Adduction and abduction (Figure 2.16)

Abduction and adduction are two terms used to describe movements that occur in the frontal plane either towards or away from the midline of the body.

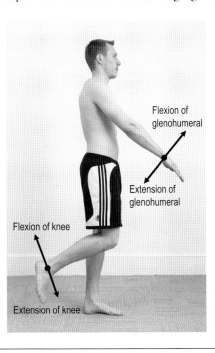

Figure 2.13
Flexion/extension of the knee and of the glenohumeral joint

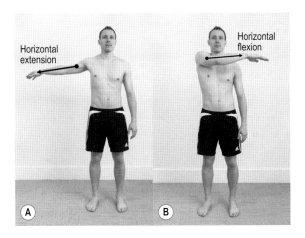

Figure 2.14
Horizontal extension and flexion of the shoulder

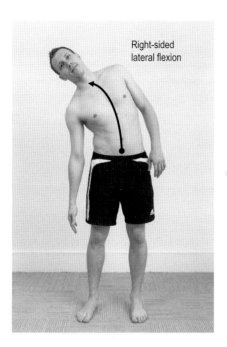

Figure 2.15
Lateral flexion (side bending), in this example right-sided

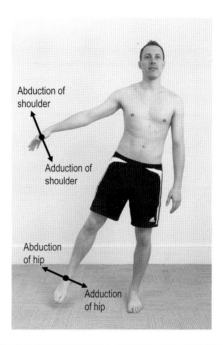

Figure 2.16
Adduction/abduction of the shoulder and of the hip

Adduction is the movement of the joint towards the midline.

Abduction is the movement of the joint away from the midline.

Medial and lateral rotation (Figure 2.17)

Medial rotation and lateral rotation are terms used to describe the movements of the limbs along their long axis.

Medial (internal) rotation occurs as the joint is moving towards the midline.

Lateral (external) rotation is the movement when the joint moves away from the midline.

Elevation and depression (Figure 2.18)

Elevation and depression normally refer to the movement of the scapula (shoulder blade).

Elevation is the movement of the scapula in a superior or upward direction (e.g. when you shrug your shoulders).

Depression is the opposite movement to elevation and refers to the scapula moving in an inferior or downward direction.

Protraction and retraction (Figure 2.19)

These are additional movements that occur in the shoulder complex, with the major part of the movement happening in the scapulothoracic pseudo joint.

Protraction is the movement of the shoulder forward (anteriorly) in the frontal plane.

Retraction is the backward (posterior) movement of the scapula, as it moves towards the midline of the body.

Pronation and supination
(Figures 2.20 and 2.21)

Pronation and supination are movements that occur in the elbow and the subtalar joints in the foot. In the elbow, pronation and supination relate to the position of the forearm when the elbow is in the semi-flexed position.

Pronation refers to the movement or position of the forearm when the elbow is flexed at 90° and the palm

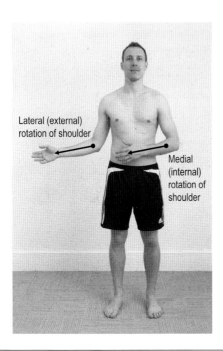

Figure 2.17
Medial and lateral rotation of the shoulder

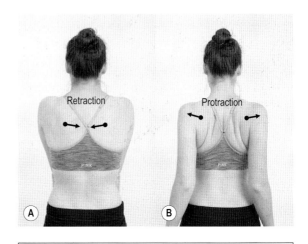

Figure 2.19
Retraction and protraction of the scapula

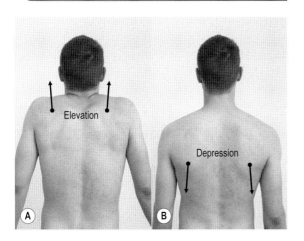

Figure 2.18
Elevation and depression of the scapula

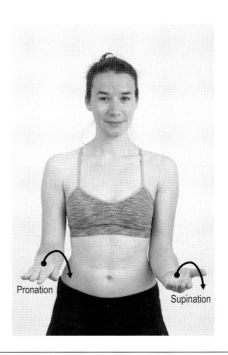

Figure 2.20
Pronation and supination of the elbow

of the hand is facing towards the floor. In the subtalar joint, it refers to the movement of the foot turning outwards (laterally).

Supination is the movement or position of the forearm when the elbow is flexed at 90° and the palm is

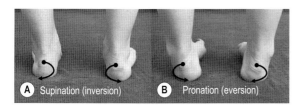

Figure 2.21
Supination (inversion) and pronation (eversion) of the subtalar joint in the foot

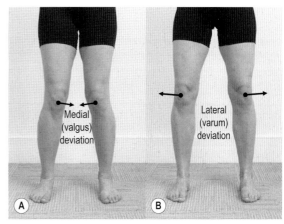

Figure 2.23
Medial (valgus) and lateral (varum) deviation of the knee

facing towards the sky. In the subtalar joint, it is when the foot is turned inwards (medially).

Medial and lateral deviation
(Figures 2.22 and 2.23)

Deviation refers to the movement of the joint either laterally or medially from the anatomical midline.

In relation to the wrist, we speak about medial or lateral deviation of the wrist or hand. These can also be classified as ulnar and radial deviation respectively (Figure 2.22).

Medial and lateral deviation can also relate to the knee, although deviations of the knee are more usually described using the terms valgus (medial

deviation or knock-kneed, Figure 2.23a) and varum (lateral deviation or bow-legged, Figure 2.23b).

Opposition and apposition (Figure 2.24)

These movements are unique to humans and some primates and occur at the thumb (pollex) at the carpometacarpal joint.

Opposition allows the thumb to cross the palm and bring the thumb and little finger together.

Apposition (also known as reposition) is a movement that returns the thumb back in the neutral

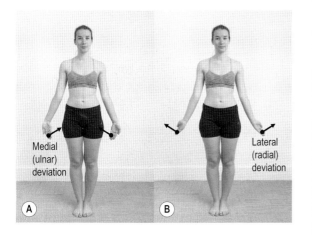

Figure 2.22
Medial (ulnar) and lateral (radial) deviation of the wrist/hand

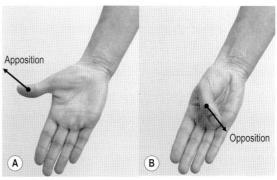

Figure 2.24
Apposition and opposition of the thumb

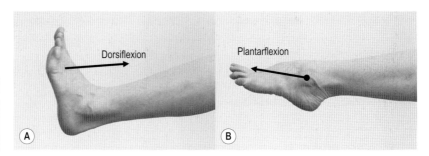

Figure 2.25
Dorsiflexion and plantarflexion of the foot

anatomical position from an oppositional position, allowing the thumb to move back across the palm.

Dorsiflexion and plantarflexion (Figure 2.25)

Dorsiflexion and plantarflexion are movements that take place at the ankle (talocrural) joint. The descriptions of the movement refer to the parts of the foot: the dorsum (superior surface) and the plantar surface (the sole).

Dorsiflexion is the movement when the foot rises towards the head. Some therapists class this movement as flexion of the ankle.

Plantarflexion refers to the foot moving towards the floor, thus 'planting' the foot to the floor. This can also be classed as extension of the ankle.

Circumduction (Figure 2.26)

Circumduction is a movement that occurs in ball-and-socket joints. It is actually a combination of movements that causes pivoting through the joint in a circular direction: moving from flexion, adduction and internal rotation towards extension, abduction and external rotation.

Traction and distraction (Figure 2.27)

Traction and **distraction** are therapeutic movements that are generated through the joint from an external force on the joint rather than by direct muscle control. They are classed as the separation of the joint surfaces, without anatomical damage to the surrounding soft tissue.

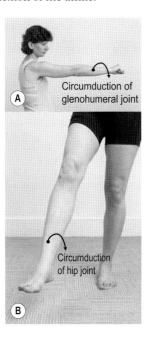

Figure 2.26
Circumduction of the glenohumeral joint and of the hip joint

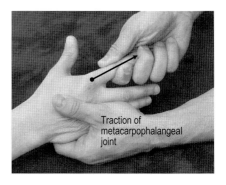

Figure 2.27
Traction of the metacarpophalangeal joint of the index finger

Contraindications and considerations for articulation techniques

> In this chapter we will look at contraindications and considerations that the practitioner should weigh up before undertaking articulation techniques.

It is a professional practitioner's duty to identify the treatment that will be most advantageous to the patient, and it should be borne in mind that not all cases can be helped by treatment with manual therapy. Indications offer reasons to choose a particular treatment in order to benefit the patient; contraindications are reasons why certain treatments may be risky or inappropriate.

All medical treatment methods have at least one contraindication associated with their use. Most skilled professionals develop the ability to detect warning signs that help them take necessary precautions when addressing a certain condition. Experienced manual therapists will immediately be aware that there is a problem when they put their hands on the patient, so allowing them to deal with the issue with caution. Experience is just as important as being educated about the problem being treated.

There are warning signs that may give you cause to stop for a moment and to rethink your decision to employ a particular technique. Is this the best possible treatment for this patient or should you consider a different modality? It is much better to be cautious and decide not to act when you could have done so than to act without caution and be wrong about your judgment – the latter leads to more harm than good (Hartman 1997).

Absolute and relative contraindications

By definition, a contraindication is a situation in which a procedure, drug, therapy or surgery should not be used because it may cause the patient harm. In medicine, contraindications are classified into two subsets: absolute contraindications and relative contraindications.

Certain conditions do not allow a particular treatment to be used because there is no reasonable justification for taking that route. For example, people with severe food allergies should not be given foods that they are allergic to as this may lead to an anaphylactic attack. This is a contraindication that is referred to as **absolute**.

Not all contraindications are absolute, however. Some contraindications are **relative**. This means that a patient may have a high risk of adverse effects or complications but these risks are outweighed or reduced by other treatment approaches (Figure 3.1). For example, X-rays are strictly inadvisable during pregnancy as they can negatively affect the developing fetus inside the mother's womb. However, on occasions, X-ray may be necessary because the woman or fetus may be in danger – for instance, in the case of tuberculosis. In that situation X-rays are advised

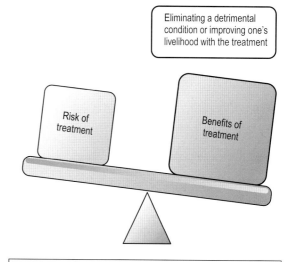

Figure 3.1
Diagrammatic representation of a relative contraindication: the benefits of a treatment outweigh the risk(s)

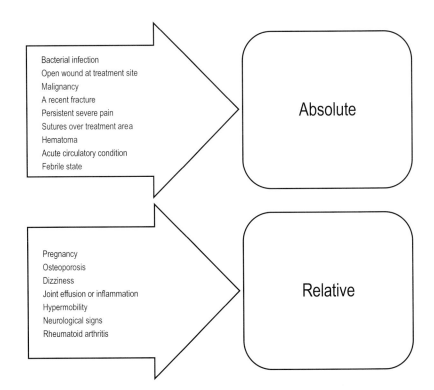

Bacterial infection
Open wound at treatment site
Malignancy
A recent fracture
Persistent severe pain
Sutures over treatment area
Hematoma
Acute circulatory condition
Febrile state

Absolute

Pregnancy
Osteoporosis
Dizziness
Joint effusion or inflammation
Hypermobility
Neurological signs
Rheumatoid arthritis

Relative

Figure 3.2
Contraindications to
manual therapy

(Starke 1997). These are *cautions* that the practitioner needs to keep in mind when determining the best possible treatment for any individual patient.

Indications are reasons to choose a certain treatment in order to benefit the patient; they are the opposite of contraindications. A professional practitioner must find the treatment that will be most advantageous to the patient and which will cause minimal side effects, if any.

Not all cases can be helped by treatment with manual therapy (Figure 3.2 and Table 3.1). The procedures

Treatment method	Indication	Contraindication
Joint articulation	Restriction of joint movement	Signs of vertebral artery disease
	Malalignment of joints	Increased pain with manual therapy
	Mechanical joint pain which worsens with movement	Signs and symptoms of spinal cord lesions
		Fracture or dislocation
	Muscle tightness and imbalance	Instability of joint or ligament
	Nerve root compression, disc lesions, spondylosis	Pain from non-mechanical causes
		Active bone disease/malignancy
Manual traction	Joint stiffness or compressive stress	Same as above
	Nerve root compression or disk herniation that responds positively to manual traction	

Table 3.1
Indications and contraindications to joint articulation and other modalities

that are chosen will be expected to cause no damage. However, if the seriousness of the patient's current condition outweighs the risk of any possible long-term damage or side effect, the patient will be informed about risks and side effects relevant to the area that will be treated and/or their condition prior to the start of any treatment (Hartman 1997).

Joint articulation

Joint articulation is referred to as a manual therapy intervention – a passive movement of an articular surface or skeletal joint performed by a skilled manual therapist. Joint articulation focuses on providing a therapeutic effect to the patient. The techniques involved are used by a wide variety of manual therapists to improve joint alignment, increase flexibility and improve mobility. Their use is also aimed at reducing pain and discomfort and muscle spasms. This, in turn, helps to increase joint range of motion (ROM) (Mulligan 2010).

When joint articulation is applied to the spine, it is called spinal or vertebral articulation. The human spine has 24 articulating or movable vertebrae. When all 24 vertebrae articulate in a free manner, they are able to move load up and down the spine. There are a number of specific contraindications to undertaking spinal and joint articulations (see Table 3.2). It is important to be aware of these.

The flag system for musculoskeletal disorders

The origin of pain may sometimes be more psychological than physical. For example, a person may come to the therapist describing his pain as 'excruciating' but still be able to walk properly and to perform certain physical activities at a level which seems to be inconsistent for a person with that level of pain. In order to determine the physical intensity of pain in such a situation, the therapist can make use of the 'flag system', which employs 'flags' as markers of risk factors in musculoskeletal disorders.

There are five flags currently in clinical use: red, yellow, blue, black and orange. The colors allow the therapist to determine the risk of disability in the patient and to work out appropriate interventions to help prevent the risk. The flags also help the therapist evaluate how potential barriers to rehabilitation treatment may be addressed (Table 3.3).

Contraindications	Precautions
Hypermobility	Care must be taken in order to avoid applying too much strain on the vertebra in the spine if it is hypermobile compared to other joints in the spine
Neurological effects	Spinal cord symptoms
	Disturbance in bladder and bowel functions
	Arm pain from two nerve roots
Radiological changes	Osteoporosis and rheumatoid arthritis – contraindications to high-force articulations
	Patients with vertigo require special supervision
	A pathology that leads to substantial bone weakening such as infections, tumors, fractures and long-term corticosteroid medications
Vascular	Bleeding into joints, such as in the case of severe hemophilia and aortic aneurysm
Musculoskeletal deformity	Spondylolysis and spondylolisthesis
Pregnancy	Diabetic mother
	Cardiac disorders – heart disease
	Chronic hypertension
	Previous problem in pregnancy – previous miscarriage
	History of systemic conditions

Table 3.2
Contraindications to and considerations in spinal or vertebral joint articulations

Flag color	Use
Red	Signs of a serious pathology that requires immediate surgical opinion
Yellow	Psychological factors such as depression and the individual's beliefs of their condition
Blue	Individual's perception of work
Black	Work conditions that may inhibit rehabilitation, such as an occupation which requires heavy lifting
Orange	Abnormal psychological processes or drug abuse. Referral to a specialist may be required

Table 3.3
Use of the flag system for assessing low back pain

Fear-Avoidance Beliefs Questionnaire

The Fear-Avoidance Beliefs Questionnaire (FABQ) was developed by Waddell and colleagues in order to investigate fear-avoidance beliefs among patients suffering from low back pain (Waddell et al 1993). Its use helps therapists to predict patients with high pain-avoidance behavior. These patients may have to be supervised more closely than those who are able to confront their pain and state of discomfort.

The questionnaire is made up of two subscales which are presented in two separate sections: the physical activity subscale (FABQPA) and the work subscale (FABQW). Each subscale is scored by summing the responses given by the individuals, as follows:

- To score the physical activity subscale, sum items 2, 3, 4 and 5.

- To score the work subscale, sum items 6, 7, 9, 10, 11, 12 and 15.

An example of an FABQ is shown in Figure 3.3.

Patient history taking

The importance of history taking

Three factors play a role in establishing a working diagnosis: the history you obtain from your patient; the signs you notice when you perform a physical assessment; and the results of laboratory investigation. In the past, some experts believed that clinical diagnoses for most patients should be based on history taking alone. Some books for medical students concentrate on determining physical signs rather than on thorough history taking. And today the increasing trend towards dependence on laboratory investigations can be demonstrated simply by looking at how much the workload of medical service departments has increased in recent years. We are at risk of losing the art of clinical history taking, but it is a skill we need to keep and its importance cannot be over-emphasized.

In clinical practice the ability to take a good detailed and accurate patient history is perhaps the most important skill for us to possess. It is one that evolves with time – it requires experience, concentration and understanding to achieve results. Through the history taking and consultation, your ultimate aim is to ensure that every treatment is safe. As the practitioner, you are looking for any contraindications to manual therapy treatment, i.e. anything that may make your treatment unsafe. You are also looking for anything in the case history which may indicate that you may have to modify your treatment. Inaccurate or incomplete history taking may negatively affect the clinical diagnosis, and the lack of accurate data can negate the criteria for the treatment the therapist proposes.

Good history taking is also essential for building a good patient–practitioner relationship. It will help you to get to know your patient and their concerns, thus helping to win their trust and enabling them to understand their problems at a deeper level. A successful consultation can increase the confidence of the patient and allow them to feel more at ease as they get the opportunity to release their frustrations and concerns and simply to vent their feelings about their problem (Bub 2004).

Some people like to think of the occasion when the medical history is taken as being a meeting of experts, where the patient is the expert at experiencing their

Name: _____ Date: _____

The following lists a few things other patients have talked about regarding pain. Circle any number on the scale of 0 to 6 telling us how much physical activities such as walking, lifting, bending or driving would affect your low back pain.

Physical activity		Completely disagree		Unsure			Completely agree	
1.	Pain is caused by physical activity	0	1	2	3	4	5	6
2.	Pain worsens with physical activity	0	1	2	3	4	5	6
3.	Physical activity may harm my back	0	1	2	3	4	5	6
4.	I should avoid physical activities that (might) worsen my pain	0	1	2	3	4	5	6
5.	I cannot perform physical activities that worsen my pain	0	1	2	3	4	5	6

In the same manner, tell us how your work may or does affect your low back pain.

Work		Completely disagree		Unsure			Completely agree	
6.	My pain is caused by work or an accident at work	0	1	2	3	4	5	6
7.	My work aggravated my pain	0	1	2	3	4	5	6
8.	I have a claim for compensation for my pain	0	1	2	3	4	5	6
9.	My work is too heavy for me	0	1	2	3	4	5	6
10.	My work makes or would make my pain worse	0	1	2	3	4	5	6
11.	My work might harm my back	0	1	2	3	4	5	6
12.	I should not do my work with my present pain	0	1	2	3	4	5	6
13.	I cannot do my normal work with my present pain	0	1	2	3	4	5	6
14.	I cannot do my normal work until my pain resolves	0	1	2	3	4	5	6
15.	I do not think I will be back to work within 3 months	0	1	2	3	4	5	6
16.	I do not think I will ever be able to go back to that work	0	1	2	3	4	5	6

Figure 3.3

Example of Fear-Avoidance Beliefs Questionnaire

Adapted from Waddell et al 1993

illness and explaining it in their own way, and the healthcare provider is the expert in diagnosis and managing the illness.

History taking has three main aims:

1. To identify the vital organ systems that are responsible for the symptoms of the illness

2. To clarify the nature of the musculodysfunction in the patient's body

3. To characterize the patient's illness in a social context, including their own interpretation of their symptoms and illness, their beliefs about their condition and the limitations in their daily life caused by the illness (Bickley 1999).

Gathering information

Explore every aspect of the problem presented by the patient who enters your clinic. Figure 3.4 summarizes the information that you should aim to obtain through taking their history.

Active listening

It is important to allow the patient to tell you the story they have been storing up for you prior to their visit. You need to employ the skills of active listening, developed through education and by learning from your own experiences, both good and bad.

In active listening, you must be seen to be attentive and interested in what the patient has to say. Allow the patient time to present their own pre-prepared narrative of their ailment to you, rather than immediately asking them a series of questions. This will help you to understand their personal perspective of their experi-

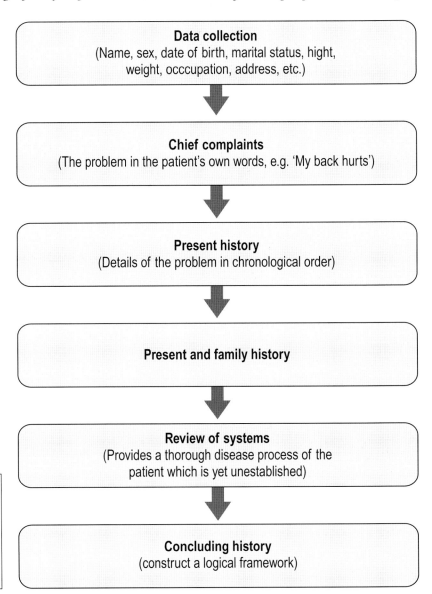

Figure 3.4
Summary of the information that should be obtained through history taking from the patient

ence with the problem which you will be attempting to treat. That said, try to keep the patient on track and do not allow them to ramble on about things that are not relevant. Allow them time to speak but do not be afraid to interrupt if they are going off the point.

Asking questions

Then move on to ask delineating and discriminating questions regarding the symptoms the patient is experiencing. The answers to these will help you to establish the true nature of the symptoms and should provide sufficient details to inform the process of diagnosis. Attention to timing is crucial. Make sure that you record each of the symptoms in the order presented by the patient. This will enable you to build the chronological sequence of symptoms and hopefully help to clarify the 'cause' of the problem. A clear timeline record is one sign of an experienced practitioner.

Some patients will not come prepared with a story about their illness. In these cases you need to ask questions from the start and seek clarification to establish a full patient history. If this sparks a story from the patient, make sure you listen to it carefully as it may contain important information.

You must use your skills as a practitioner to elicit as much relevant information as you can. If direct communication is difficult, consider using aids such as sign language interpreters, translators, drawings and picture boards to allow the patient to describe or show where their pain is located. Adapt your approach as necessary to get the information you need.

Observation

You will not acquire information during a history-taking session solely from what you hear. It is also important to observe – from the moment the patient enters the room. Make sure you pick up all possible clues from the patient, such as changes in facial expression, verbal fluency and body language. This can be particularly useful if there is a psychological basis for the patient's physical symptoms (the patient will be unaware of this aspect, of course). You may, for example, notice that the patient becomes uncomfortable or hesitant when talking about a certain aspect of their problem.

The accuracy of the results you obtain from this vital information-gathering will contribute towards devising an appropriate and safe treatment plan for your patient.

REFERENCES

Bickley LS (1999). Bates' Guide to Physical Exam and History Taking, 7th ed. Philadelphia: Lippincott; 1-42.

Bub B (2004). The patient's lament: hidden key to effective communication: how to recognise and transform. Medical Humanities 30:63-69.

Hartman L (1997). Handbook of Osteopathic Technique, 3rd ed. Oxford: Chapman & Hall.

Mulligan BR (2010). Manual Therapy: Nags, Snags, MWMs, 6th ed. Orthopedic Physical Therapy & Rehabilitation.

Starke JR (1997). Tuberculosis. An old disease but a new threat to the mother, foetus and neonate. Clinics in Perinatology 24(1): 107-127.

Waddell G, Newton M, Henderson I et al (1993). A Fear-Avoidance Beliefs Questionnaire (FABQ) and the role of fear-avoidance beliefs in chronic low back pain and disability. Pain 52:157-168.

Therapist posture and stance 4

In order to treat patients successfully, the manual therapist requires high levels of knowledge and skill. Of vital importance in this skill mix is knowing how to use and protect your own body while you work. In this chapter we will offer guidance on the treatment postures and stances best adopted by the practitioner.

Working as a manual therapy practitioner is challenging, and it requires the development and practice of a range of complex skills prior to application in the clinical context. Apart from developing the ability to apply a technique skilfully and appropriately, you also need to learn and practice how to move your own body with an understanding of the laws of physics. This will enable you to work more efficiently on your client with less effort, using stronger forces with less fatigue while exposing your body to less force (Domholdt 2000). Irrespective of how a technique is used with a client, it is of critical importance that you understand and apply the fundamentals of good body mechanics. Your efficiency in using your body during the delivery of the therapy is crucial, not only for the quality of care you provide to the client but also for your own well-being and long-term fitness to practice. Once you understand how to use your body parts as a single entity, you will be able to perform techniques with maximum efficiency (Muscolino 2008).

In the world of manual therapy, however, the study of body mechanics has not yet received much attention. Because of this, many established practitioners, as well as new graduates, often work harder, instead of working smarter; as a result, a good number of them are at risk of incurring career-ending injuries (Muscolino 2006). This chapter will discuss one of the principal concerns of healthy body mechanics: the positioning of your body, particularly your posture and stance, while delivering a therapeutic procedure.

Treatment posture

In manual therapy, good treatment posture means that the practitioner's body is positioned in a way that allows the whole body to move efficiently and to work effortlessly, without requiring the muscles to generate extra effort. Poor posture causes muscle imbalances and inefficient movement throughout the body. This can lead to the overworking of muscles and unnecessary fatigue when generating greater force (Di Fabio 1992).

Assuming the correct posture during the therapy session enables the practitioner to shift their body weight efficiently from side to side, or forwards and backwards. It also allows for more coordinated action between the practitioner's body and hands. Taken together, it can be said that a good posture is one in which you feel well-grounded while having the liberty to turn or move (Cassar 2005).

Adjusting or correcting posture is not as easy a task as it sounds; it takes extensive practice and constant reminding. To adopt a correct posture prior to employing a technique, you need to use a combination of components including your body weight, body position and transfer of force (Cassar 2005). In finding your correct posture, you should focus primarily on the following factors:

- your own physical structure

- your body weight and gravity

- your head position

- the height and width of the treatment table relative to the client's body part being treated

- your contact with the ground or table

- your preferred therapeutic technique.

Physical structure

Your posture must suit your own physical structure. Everyone is different and you cannot simply duplicate another practitioner's posture; if you try to do so, you may fail to apply the technique correctly. As a practitioner, you have to appreciate your own individual morphology when you apply a technique. Observe other practitioners' styles and then adapt them to suit you. Finding a style suitable for your own physical structure and build will allow you to have more control over the technique you are practicing in terms of the transfer of force. It will also make the force applied to the patient more consistent and precise, giving greater sensation to the patient while giving you, the practitioner, accurate feedback from the joints and soft tissue in which you are trying to effect a change (Osteopathic Technique 2016).

Body weight and gravity

The practitioner's body weight plays a significant role in generating force to work on a patient. Usually, this force can be produced in one of two ways: internally and externally (Muscolino 2006). The internal force is created within the body by musculature, but this can be fatiguing as it requires more effort on the part of the practitioner. The external force, on the other hand, is generated with the help of gravity and so requires less effort and causes less fatigue. Therefore, if your goal is to generate greater force with the minimum possible effort, you should learn and practice how to use gravity together with your body weight as much as possible (Clay & Pounds 2003).

Since gravity only works vertically downward, in order to take advantage of it, your body weight should be higher than the patient. This requires setting the table low, so that the client is positioned below the practitioner (Peterson & Bergmann 2002). Because the whole weight of the body is located in the core (i.e. the trunk), your trunk should be positioned above the patient, as much as possible, when you lean to generate forceful thrust/pressure (Muscolino 2006).

Head position

The position of the practitioner's head has no effect on the delivery of thrust while performing a technique. For this reason, you can keep your head in whatever position is the least stressful for you (Muscolino 2014).

However, it has been suggested that holding the head over the trunk is the healthiest posture during a therapy, as this position balances the core weight of the head over the trunk and does not require the neck muscles to support the head (Frye 2004) (Figure 4.1a). Unfortunately, many practitioners have a habit of flexing down the neck and head at the spinal joints in order to observe their client (Figure 4.1b). This leads to an imbalance of the head position and thereby requires isometric contraction of the extensor muscles of the neck to prevent the head from falling anteriorly into flexion (Nordin & Frankel 2001). Eventually, this results in pain and spasm in the posterior neck.

Table height

Correct table height is probably the single most important factor in determining the efficiency of a practitioner's force delivery. How low or how high a table should be depends on a number of factors:

- **The height of the practitioner** helps in calculating the appropriate table height. There is some debate about this but the correct height of the treatment table is usually considered to be the half the practitioner's own height. However, practitioners with longer legs may need to make the table slightly higher. Conversely, practitioners with a longer torso may need to adjust the table slightly down (American Massage Therapy Association 2014).

- **The size of the client** is another important factor, because choosing a correct table height based on the client's size helps to reduce strain on the practitioner's body (Muscolino 2006).

- **The client's positioning on the table** (i.e. prone, supine or side lying) also plays a major part in determining the table height. For example, the hips of a client in a side-lying position would be higher than their head and neck. In order to work on the hips in this position, the table would need to be lowered (Frye 2004).

- **The therapeutic technique being used** on the patient will necessitate adjustment of the table height. If the practitioner needs to create stronger force with less effort, the table needs to be low. However, a higher table height is more desirable when light thrust/force is being applied (Fritz 2004).

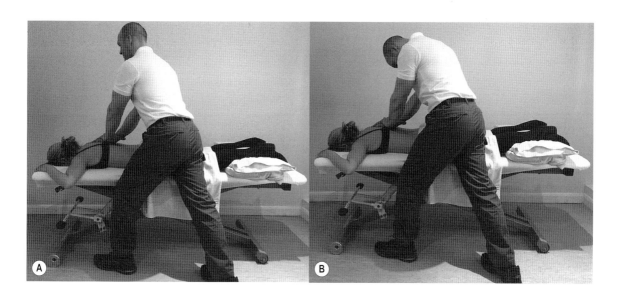

Figure 4.1
A Good head position, with the head held over the trunk; **B** bad head position, with the neck flexed

Table width

For a good treatment posture, the width of the table must be considered in addition to its height. If the table is wide, it will require the practitioner to bend and twist more to reach the client. This will increase the stress on the practitioner's shoulders and lower back. Moreover, it will be difficult for the practitioner to position their body weight over the patient. A narrow table is therefore often desirable, providing better access to the midline of the client and allowing better utilization of the practitioner's body weight (Goggins 2007, Muscolino 2008), as well as being lighter and less bulky to lift and reposition.

Correct stance

In physical therapy, stance is the manner and/or position in which the practitioner arranges their hands and feet prior to delivery of the technique. Although stance and posture are to some extent mutually dependent, they are not interchangeable terms (see Figure 4.2). Stance describes your position relative to the table and the patient. You may have a good posture in relation to balance but your positioning may be unsuitable for appropriate execution of the technique (Osteopathic Technique 2016). You need to maintain a correct stance so that you are able to transfer the force of the technique you are applying in the most appropriate way.

To achieve a proper stance, you should start from the ground. You must always make sure that your feet are correctly positioned for the technique being employed to efficiently transfer your body weight through your hands to the patient. This will allow you to use your body in the most effective way, and to apply

Posture	Therapist's weight in relation to gravity Head position Contact with the ground/table Weight and force distribution
Stance	Positioning to carry out a technique Where the feet point Operator balance

Figure 4.2
Posture versus stance

your hands to perform the technique effortlessly. In addition, with a correct stance, you will be able to work more efficiently and with less fatigue resulting from treating your client (American Massage Therapy Association 2014).

Types of stance

The practitioner's stance can be broadly divided into two categories: longitudinal stance and transverse stance. The longitudinal stance is taken by positioning the feet parallel to the table length. This stance works when you are aiming to deliver force longitudinally across the client's body because it orients your body weight in the same direction; this stance is fruitless when you work transversely up the client's body because your body weight is not orienting in the same direction. Conversely, the transverse stance is taken by lining up the feet at right angles to the table length. This stance is effective when you deliver force transversely along the client's body because it orients your body weight in the same direction; the stance is ineffective when you work longitudinally along the client's body because your body weight is not orienting in the same direction (Muscolino 2006).

Orientation of the practitioner's feet

There has been some debate regarding the optimal positioning of the feet while delivering the technique. An asymmetric stance is often preferable, where one foot is forward and the other back (Figure 4.3), but there are three possible orientations of the feet relative to each other (Muscolino 2008):

- **feet aligned position** – both feet aligned next to each other and parallel (Figure 4.4a)

- **feet staggered, position I** – both feet facing in nearly the same direction (i.e. approximately parallel) (Figure 4.4b)

- **feet staggered, position II** – the orientation of the rear foot is approximately perpendicular to the front foot (Figure 4.4c).

Although these positions are recommended, the feet do not have to remain fixed throughout a treatment procedure (i.e. from the beginning to the end of a force delivery). There is no rule that states that you cannot move them! You will inevitably want to make some fine tuning of your positioning while performing a technique (Fritz 2004).

Elbow and hand positioning

Elbows

The positioning of the elbows is crucial to the efficient delivery of many of the techniques performed by the manual practitioner. If you pull your elbows as close to the sides of your body as possible, you will be able to perform most of the procedures with better accuracy and greater ease.

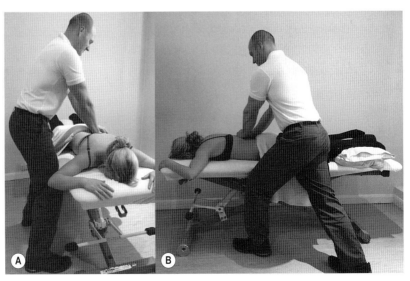

Figure 4.3
A Symmetric stance;
B asymmetric stance

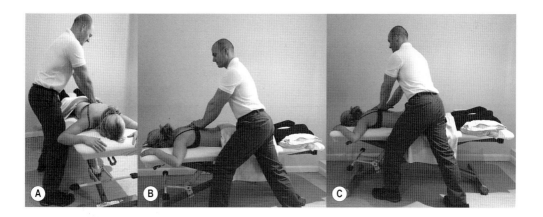

Figure 4.4
Recommended positions for the feet: **A** feet aligned; **B** feet staggered, position I; **C** feet staggered, position II

Hands

The therapist's hands are the body part most often used to contact the client. For example, when a thrust is being delivered, practitioners usually use their hands to transfer that thrust into the client. This repeated use of the hands to contact the client makes them prone to a number of injuries, and you should take all necessary precautions to protect your hands. Overstrain of the hands can be avoided by minimizing the level at which the wrist is flexed or extended when your hands are placed on the client (see Figure 4.5). To avoid injuries to the fingers or thumb, you can use the palm of your hand for deeper thrust. If a technique requires your thumb to apply pressure, the best approach is to apply it with as little abduction as possible.

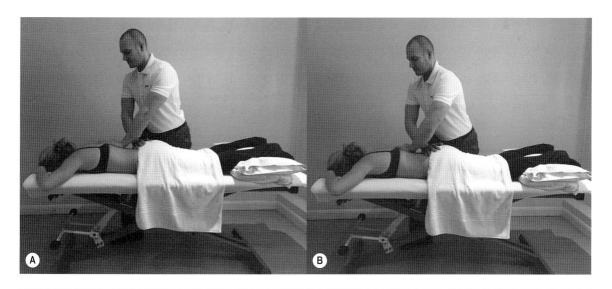

Figure 4.5
Hand and elbow positioning: **A** correct; **B** incorrect

Importance of breathing

The breathing cycle of the practitioner while they perform a technique is as important a consideration as the force being applied to the client. Some practitioners tend to hold their breath, creating strain against their thorax and abdomen to firm up the procedure. This can elevate blood pressure and therefore it is best to avoid holding your breath during a technique.

Conclusion

In order for you to establish good posture and stance during a procedure, it is important to be efficient with your balance and with the transfer of your body weight and grip. These components can be adjusted by making some simple changes in the technique you are employing. Over time, making this effort to have correct posture and stance will not only maximize your efficiency to deliver various techniques but also benefit you by minimizing the long-term occupational stress on your body. Good working posture and stance need to be practiced on a regular basis to achieve success. You should spend as much time on this aspect of giving treatment as you do on practicing the actual techniques, as this is the basis of your longevity as a practicing manual therapist.

REFERENCES

American Massage Therapy Association (2014). Work smarter, not harder. Available from: https://www.amtamassage.org/articles/3/MTJ/detail/2901 [Accessed 19 April 2016].

Cassar M-P (2005). The importance of good posture in bodywork part I. Available from: http://www.positivehealth.com/article/bodywork/the-importance-of-good-posture-in-bodywork-part-i [Accessed 19 April 2016].

Clay J, Pounds D (2003). Basic Clinical Massage Therapy – Integrating Anatomy and Treatment. Philadelphia: Lippincott Williams & Wilkins.

Di Fabio RP (1992). Efficacy of manual therapy. Physical Therapy 72(12):853-864.

Domholdt E (2000). Physical Therapy Research: Principles and Applications. Philadelphia: WB Saunders.

Fritz S (2004). Fundamentals of Therapeutic Massage, 3rd ed. Philadelphia: Elsevier Science.

Frye B (2004). Body Mechanics for Manual Therapists: A Functional Approach to Self-care, 2nd ed. Stanwood.

Goggins R (2007). Ergonomics for MTs and bodyworkers. Massage Bodywork. Available from: http://www.massagetherapy.com/articles/index.php/article_id/1275 [Accessed 19 April 2016].

Muscolino JE (2006). Work smarter, not harder. Body mechanics for massage therapists. Massage Therapy Journal, winter 2006.

Muscolino JE (2008). The Muscle and Bone Palpation Manual with Trigger Points, Referral Patterns and Stretching. New York: Elsevier Health Sciences.

Muscolino JE (2014). Kinesiology: The Skeletal System and Muscle Function. New York: Elsevier Health Sciences.

Nordin M, Frankel VH eds (2001). Basic Biomechanics of the Musculoskeletal System. Philadelphia: Lippincott Williams & Wilkins.

Osteopathic Technique (2016). Operator posture and stance. Available from: http://www.doctorabel.us/osteopathic-technique/operator-posture-and-stance.html [Accessed: 18 April 2016].

Peterson D, Bergmann T (2002). Chiropractic Technique – Principles and Procedures. Philadelphia: Elsevier Science.

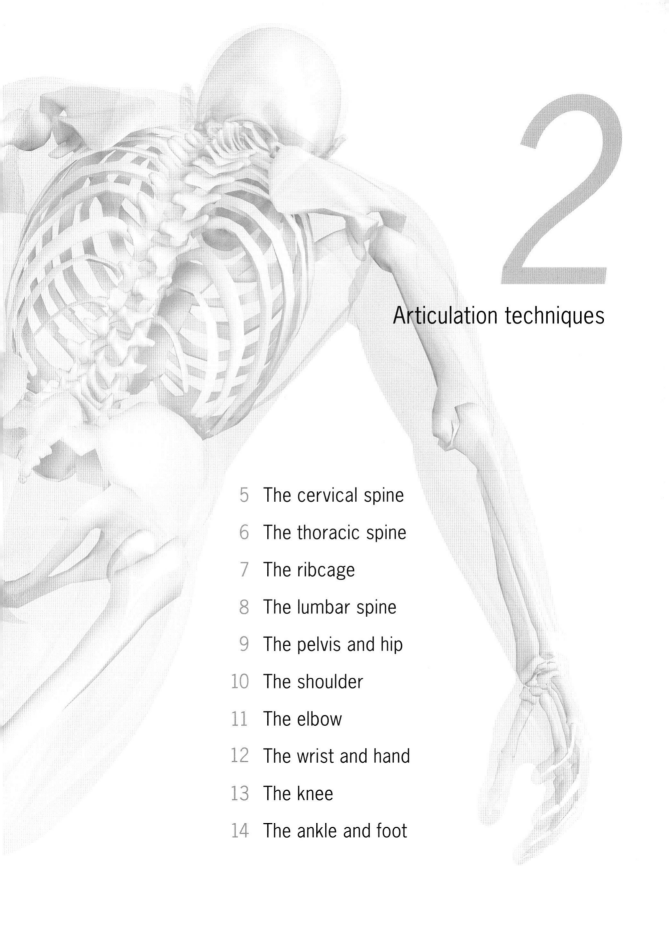

2

Articulation techniques

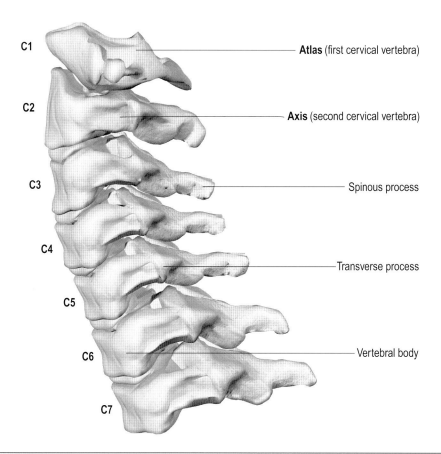

C1

C2

C3

C4

C5

C6

C7

Atlas (first cervical vertebra)

Axis (second cervical vertebra)

Spinous process

Transverse process

Vertebral body

Figure 5.1
The cervical spine

Introduction

Neck pain is one of the most common reasons people visit manual therapists, with 54% of Americans visiting complementary therapists for either neck or back pain compared to 37% seeking conventional care (Wolsko et al 2003). Another study by Bassols et al (2002) found that 29.4% would seek complementary help, compared to 22.8% who self-medicated.

Vernon et al (2007) found moderate to high evidence that manual therapy to chronic neck pain not due to whiplash-associated disorders (WAD) and without arm pain or headaches had clinically reported improvements in the patients' symptoms. However, the research did not report the same for massage as a stand-alone treatment modality.

In their study 'Effectiveness of manual therapies: the UK evidence report' Bronfort et al (2010) found that there are several studies supporting the beneficial effects of manual therapy including articulation of the cervical spine in the treatment of mechanical neck disorders (MND), WAD and chronic neck pain. There is also evidence to suggest that cervical spine articulation and exercise can be beneficial in relieving pain and increasing the range of motion in MND and WAD (Allison et al 2002, Hoving et al 2002, 2006, Jull et al 2002, Korthals-de Bos et al 2003). Persson and Lilja (2001) found that manual therapy was more beneficial in relieving patients' symptoms than surgery or immobilizing the neck in a collar. Gross and colleagues (2007) found strong evidence for the sustained reduction of pain, improvement in mobility and a positive mental attitude change in response to exercise with manual therapy. The clinical practice guidelines for neck pain from the Orthopaedic Section of the American Physical Therapy Association (Childs et al 2008) 'concluded that the most beneficial manipulative interventions for patients with mechanical neck pain with or without headaches should be combined with exercise to reduce pain and increase patient satisfaction'.

Studies by Hall et al (2010) and Zito et al (2006) have shown that articulation to the atlas–axis (C1–C2) can have a beneficial effect on headaches, neck pain and range of movement. This is of particular importance because 39–45% of cervical rotation occurs at C1–C2 with only 4–8% rotation occuring at each other cervical segment (Hall & Robinson 2004, Ogince et al 2007). Dunning et al (2012) found in their study that treating into the upper thoracic spine as well as the cervical spine achieved better outcomes in pain levels and range of movement than treating into the cervical spine alone.

One of the main concerns that therapists and patients have with treating the cervical spine is the risk of vertebrobasilar stroke. In a study by Cassidy et al (2008) no evidence was found that there is an excessive risk of vertebrobasilar stroke with manual therapy of the cervical spine. In addition, Carlesso et al (2010) found no strong evidence of any link between manual therapy of the cervical spine and the occurrence of serious adverse events. Haldeman et al (1999) found the groups that had the highest risk of adverse reaction were patients with hypertension or migraines, those using oral contraceptives, and smokers, but they found that these risk factors were roughly the same or lower than in the general population. Although the risks of adverse reactions for manipulation or high-velocity thrusts to the cervical spine are viewed to be low by most studies, some studies advise that articulation is the preferred method of treatment with lower potential risk factors than manipulation or high-velocity thrusts (Di Fabio 1999, Hurwitz et al 2005).

Anatomy

The cervical spine consists of the first seven vertebrae (C1–C7) of the spinal column, beginning just below the skull and ending just above the thoracic vertebrae. It includes the atlanto-occipital joint (A–O or C0–C1 joint), the atlanto-axial joint (A–A or C1–C2 joint) and the lower cervical joints (C3–C7). It is the shortest section of the spinal column, but it is the most mobile segment of the entire spine and supports a high degree of movement. It plays several important functions in the body, such as providing support to the skull, allowing full range of motion of the head, and protecting the spinal cord, vertebral artery and nerve roots. In addition, the craniocervical junction (i.e. the junction between the skull and the upper cervical spine (C0–C2)) and its muscles are vital to maintain equilibrium with precise muscle activity coordination in order to position one's head in space (Bogduk 2005).

This part of the spine has a great deal of flexibility. Its movements are usually three-dimensional: the range of motion is up to 90° of rotation to both sides, about 80° to 90° of flexion, 70° of extension and 20° to 45° of lateral flexion (Windle 1980). However, motion of the cervical spine does not follow a simple mechanism; it is complex. Motion in one segment at the cervical spine involves other individual vertebrae and requires complementary motion between cervical levels (Van Mameren et al 1989). This confounds the kinematics of the cervical segment and the resulting mechanisms.

The cervical spine involves a complex system of ligaments, tendons and muscles to support and stabilize the neck and spinal column, as well as for facilitating normal joint motion. It relies heavily on ligaments for the stability of the spine as well as for movement; for example, the craniocervical junction requires many ligaments for stabilization because it accommodates a wide variety of motions (Steilen et al 2014). The ligaments in the cervical spine are usually divided into two columns: anterior and posterior. The anterior column provides stability during extension, and the posterior column provides stability during flexion (Austin et al 2014). This over-reliance on ligamentous tissues predisposes the cervical spine to a number of serious injuries, including the odontoid fracture, hangman's fracture (acute spondylolysis of C2), C1 ring fractures, atlanto-occipital dislocation (AOD), paralysis of the arms, legs and diaphragm to name a few.

Types of cervical spine

The cervical vertebrae consist of two functionally and anatomically different segments, namely the superior or suboccipital cervical (C0–C2) segment and the inferior cervical (C3–C7) segment.

Superior cervical segment (C0–C2)

The superior cervical segment has unique anatomical features; it is quite different from the rest of the cervical spine. It consists of the occiput (C0) and the first two cervical vertebrae: the atlas (first vertebra or C1) and the axis (second vertebra or C2). These two cervical vertebrae are more specialized than other cervical vertebrae as they support the weight and movement of the head (Steilen et al 2014).

The atlas is ring-shaped and does not contain a vertebral body. It articulates superiorly with the occipital condyles and forms the atlanto-occipital joint. The primary motions of the atlas are flexion and extension. The axis has a prominent vertebral body, known as the odontoid process (dens), which works as a pivot point for the atlas. The axis articulates with the atlas via its superior articular facets and forms the atlanto-axial joint (Driscoll 1987).

The range of motion of the superior cervical spine is shown in Table 5.1.

The atlanto-axial joint (C1–C2) is responsible for 50% of all cervical rotation (White & Panjabi 1990).

Inferior cervical segment (C3–C7)

The inferior cervical segment is from the inferior axis surface to the superior surface of vertebra T1.

Superior cervical joint	Movement type	Range of motion (°)
Atlanto-occipital / C0–C1	Flexion and extension	25
	Axial rotation	5
	Lateral bending	7
Atlanto-axial / C1–C2	Flexion and extension	15
	Axial rotation	30
	Lateral bending	≤ 4

Table 5.1

Superior cervical range of motion

Data from Tubbs et al (2010, 2011)

It consists of five cervical vertebrae, C3–C7, which are quite similar to each other but very different from the first two cervical vertebrae, C1 and C2. Each of these vertebrae has a vertebral body that is convex on its lower surface and concave on its upper surface.

An intervertebral disc – a piece of fibrocartilage that resists spinal compression – lies between adjacent vertebrae. These discs provide more stability in the lower cervical vertebrae. They are more fibrous in the cervical segment than other segments of the spine and, as a result, they herniate less often compared to those in the lumbar spine (Frobin et al 2002).

The degree of cervical range of motion is proportional to the height of the intervertebral disc: a greater degree of cervical range of motion will result from a greater height of intervertebral disc. Degeneration of the discs consequently leads to decline in range of motion (Muhle et al 1998).

The inferior cervical segment's range of motion is greatest at C4–C5 and C5–C6 (see Table 5.2). The extension and flexion primarily take place in the central cervical vertebrae, with most of the flexion taking place around C4–C6 and extension at C5–C7. Lateral bending takes place at close proximity to the head, particularly at C2–C3 and C3–C4. According to Steilen et al (2014), 50% of total neck flexion, extension and rotation takes place at the upper cervical segment (C0–C2), and the remaining 50% takes place at the inferior cervical segment, especially at C2–C3, C3–C4 and C4–C5.

The facet joints

The facet joints of the cervical vertebrae, also known as zygapophyseal joints, are complex biomechanical structures located in the spine. They join the inferior articular process of the upper vertebra, with the exception of C0–C1, and the superior articular process of the lower vertebra (Steilen et al 2014).

At each vertebra, there are two sets of joint surfaces – a superior and an inferior articulating surface. One pair faces upwards and one downwards. The lower vertebra's superior facet is relatively flat in the cervical and thoracic segments and more convex in the lumbar segment. In contrast, the upper vertebra's

Motion unit	Movement type	Range of motion (°)
C2–C3	Flexion and extension	8
	Rotation	9
	Lateral bending	10
C3–C4	Flexion and extension	13
	Rotation	12
	Lateral bending	10
C4–C5	Flexion and extension	19
	Rotation	12
	Lateral bending	10
C5–C6	Flexion and extension	17
	Rotation	14
	Lateral bending	8
C6–C7	Flexion and extension	16
	Rotation	10
	Lateral bending	7

Table 5.2

Inferior cervical range of motion

Data from Schafer & Faye (1990)

inferior facet is concave and makes an arch with its apex directing towards the vertebral body (Jaumard et al 2011).

Anatomically, the cervical facet joints are diarthrodial synovial joints with fibrous capsules, and they function in a way similar to the knee joint. These joint capsules hold adjacent vertebrae to one another. In addition, the capsular joints in the inferior cervical segment are relatively more lax than in other segments of the spine; thus, they facilitate mobility and allow more gliding movements of the facets (Milligram & Rand 2000).

The cervical facet joints play a significant role in the overall stability and behavior of the spine. They guide vertebral motion and facilitate transmission of loads applied to the spine (Kalichman & Hunter 2007). Their mechanical behavior has an influence on the spinal response through their relationship with the intervertebral discs and via their anatomical orientation. However, their behavior is also reliant on the overall spine responses (Jaumard et al 2011). Moreover, they resist torsion relatively less than the lumbar spine, and they are involved in a certain amount of weight bearing. Since the facet joints help to integrate the essential structure of the spine, injury to their mechanical integrity can cause cervical spine instability. Lee and Sung (2009) suggest that injury or trauma to the facet joints can have a direct impact on a motion segment's mechanical behavior and even on the overall spine.

Epidemiology

Chronic neck pain

Chronic neck pain often pinpoints cervical spine instability and has been identified as a common symptom of a variety of conditions, such as cervical spondylosis, post-concussion syndrome, disc herniation, whiplash injury and associated disorders, Barré–Liéou syndrome and vertebrobasilar insufficiency.

Numerous epidemiological studies have shown that the incidence of chronic neck pain in the overall population is high and could be a common source of disability. The prevalence has been reported to be in the range of 30–50%, with women of 50 years of age and above identified as the larger portion (Hogg-Johnson et al 2008). Croft et al (2001) estimated that about one in every five persons in the United Kingdom had suffered from a new neck pain episode within the previous year.

Cases of chronic neck pain usually require minimal intervention, and they often resolve with time, but the recurrence rate is high. In a population-based cohort study of 1100 adults, Côté et al (2004) found around 22.8% of participants with recurrent episodes of pain. An epidemiological study reported that only 6.3% of participants with mechanical neck disorders in the previous year were free of recurrent episodes (Picavet & Schouten 2003).

Cervical spine injury

A fracture of the cervical vertebrae caused by trauma or injury – for example, from a fall, a car or diving accident that causes trauma, a blow to the head or any other serious cervical injury – may lead to damage to the spinal cord. Spinal cord damage leads to cervical pain and poor functioning of the spine depending on which vertebra of the cervical spine has been affected (Torretti & Sengupta 2007).

Injury	Anatomical changes and severity of the injury
Hyperextension	Distracts the anterior column
	Includes the unstable compressing injuries, such as Jefferson fracture and diving injury, and the unstable but decompressed injury, such as hangman's fracture
Hyperflexion	Distracts or overstretches the anterior column
	Accounts for up to 46% of overall cervical spinal injuries
	Ranges from mild stable injuries, such as clay-shoveler's fracture and wedge fractures, to severe unstable injuries, such as facet joint fractures
Compression	Forms small spinal canal, and commonly manifests as a cervical burst fracture
	Relatively stable injury but can impair the spine with disc fragments
Clinically minor injuries	Include injuries that are clinically insignificant or do not considerably affect the cervical spine

Table 5.3
Cervical spine injuries
Data from Austin et al (2014)

Cervical spine injury can affect between 2% and 5% of blunt trauma victims (Crosby & Lui 1990); this risk increases dramatically if there is a focal neurological deficit, decreased level of consciousness, or head or facial injury (Hackl et al 2001). Certain demographic factors are also found to influence blunt cervical spine injury. These include age over 65 years, male sex and white ethnicity (Lowery et al 2001).

Types of cervical spine injury include hyperextension, hyperflexion, compression and clinically minor injuries (see Table 5.3).

In the upper cervical region, the atlanto-axial joints have been identified as the most common site of injury; in the subaxial cervical spine, C6–C7 has been found to be the most commonly injured level (Goldberg et al 2001). Impairment depends on the cervical vertebra(e) injured (see Table 5.4).

Cervical spine examination

Medical history

A detailed patient history is vital for cervical spine examination. The healthcare provider must listen to the patient's past medical history and history of present illness very carefully. In most cases, the narrative provided by the patient will consist of information critical to determine red flags and facilitate the cervical examination. In addition, the healthcare provider must ask the patient whether they have pain or other symptoms in other parts of the body, such as the shoulder or thoracic spine, to inform the cervical examination. The completion of medical screening forms is useful.

Red flags

While questioning patients, be on the lookout for red flags in their narrative (see Table 5.5). Review completed medical screening forms.

Investigation

Radiological considerations are as follows:

* A referral for imaging is needed if the patient is positive on the Canadian C-spine rule.

* A cervical spine radiograph or cervical CT (more sensitive) should be performed to rule out fractures.

* A referral for cervical multiplanar reformatting (MPR) should be considered if the patient shows rapidly worsening neurological signs and symptoms.

* A referral for diagnostic imaging procedures should be given if the patient is with certain red flags, such as possible instability or having a history of cancer.

Physical examination

Observation

The therapist should observe the patient's posture when he or she sits and stands. Postural deviations can be

Cervical vertebra	Type of impairment
C1, C2 or C3	Functional loss of the diaphragm (a ventilator is required to facilitate breathing)
C4	Functional loss of control of the shoulders and biceps
C5	Functional loss of the wrists and hands
	Partial functional loss of the shoulders and biceps
C6	Complete functional loss of the hand
	Partial functional loss of the wrist
C7	Reduced use of the hands and fingers
	Limited arm use

Table 5.4
Type of impairment from cervical vertebra injury

Condition	Signs and symptoms
Cervical myelopathy	Hands show sensory disturbances
	Intrinsic muscle wasting of hand
	Clonus
	Babinski
	Hoffman's reflex
	Unsteady gait
	Bladder and bowel disturbances
	Inverted supinator sign
	Hyperreflexia
	Multisegmental sensory changes
	Multisegmental weakness
Inflammatory or systemic disease	Temperature above 100 °F (37.8 °C)
	Blood pressure above 160/95 mmHg
	Resting pulse above 100 bpm
	Fatigue
	Resting respiration above 25 bpm
Neoplastic conditions	Over 50 years of age
	Patient has a previous history of cancer
	Constant pain that does not subside even with rest
	Unexplained weight loss
	Night pain
Upper cervical ligamentous instability	Post trauma
	Occipital numbness and headache
	Severe limitation during the neck's active range of motion (AROM) in every direction
	Down's syndrome, rheumatoid arthritis (RA)
	Signs of cervical myelopathy
Vertebral artery insufficiency	Dizziness
	Drop attacks
	Ataxia
	Nausea
	Dysphasia
	Dysarthria
	Positive cranial nerve signs
	Diplopia

Table 5.5
Red flags for neck pain during cervical spine examination

rectified in order to note the effect on signs and symptoms. Common deviations of posture may include:

- rounded shoulders or protracted shoulder girdle
- forward head posture or protracted cervical spine
- upper thoracic spine
  - flexed or kyphotic
  - extended or lordotic
- middle thoracic spine.

Test	Procedure	Positive sign	Interpretation
Cervical AROM	Using an inclinometer, the practitioner measures neck flexion, extension and rotation. The practitioner uses a universal goniometer to assess cervical motion while sitting. The practitioner may apply passive overpressure at the end of the motion assessment for end feel and pain response.	Decreased range of motion and weakness	Foraminal encroachment
Cervical and thoracic segmental mobility	With the patient positioned in prone, the practitioner uses his or her thumb to contact each spinal process by applying oscillatory posterior to anterior force.	Pain and hypermobility or hypomobility	Upper cervical joint dysfunction in patients suffering from headaches
Passive OA joint testing (flexion/extension)	The patient lies supine and the practitioner stands at the head of the patient. The practitioner rotates the patient's head 20–30° to the right. The occiput is translated anteriorly to the superior facet C1 and then posteriorly. The procedure is repeated on the left side.	Pain and reproduction of symptoms	Foraminal encroachment
AA mobility testing	The practitioner cradles the patient's head with both hands and contacts the posterior aspect of C1 using his or her fingertips. The practitioner then flexes the cervical spine, maintaining the flexion during passive rotation.	Pain	C1 or C2 dysfunction

Table 5.6
Movement patterns in cervical spine examination

Activity limitations or movement related to the patient's neck pain can be used to evaluate how an episode of care affects his or her level of function. Activities should be reproducible and measurable, such as looking over the shoulder as if to check the blind spot while driving to note the point at which motion symptoms arise. These activities can be used again to see if intervention improves symptoms and enhances range of motion, thus eliciting improvement in function.

Movement patterns

See Table 5.6.

Palpation

With the patient lying supine, the practitioner palpates the bilateral sternoclavicular joints, the acromioclavicular joint and suboccipital muscles, upper trapezius, levator scapula and pectoralis minor in order to assess tenderness. An increase in tenderness/fluid accumulation, fibrosis or reproduction of symptoms will indicate inflammatory disease.

Special tests

Special tests for the cervical spine are summarized in Table 5.7.

Test	Procedure	Positive sign	Interpretation
Cranial cervical flexion (CCF) test	The patient lies supine. Towels may be required to be placed under the occiput for a neutral position. With the occiput kept stationary, the patient is instructed to perform CCF in five increments in a graded manner while attempting to hold each position for 10 seconds with 10 seconds' rest between stages. The practitioner palpates the neck while the patient performs CCF to monitor unrequired activation of the more superficial cervical muscles.	Inability to increase pressure to at least 6 mmHg Inability to hold the generated pressure for a period of 10 seconds Using sudden chin movements of forceful pushing of the neck against the pressure device Using superficial neck muscles for CCF	Inflammatory disease
Upper limb tension test	The patient lies supine and the practitioner tests the patient's response to pressure applied in the median nerve. The practitioner introduces scapular depression, shoulder abduction to 90° with the patient's elbow flexed, forearm supination, wrist and finger extension, shoulder lateral rotation, elbow extension and contralateral and ipsilateral cervical side bending.	Reproduction of symptoms Radicular pain Increase of patient's symptoms with contralateral side bending Decrease in patient's symptoms with ipsilateral side bending	Dural or meningeal irritation or nerve root compression
Spurling's test	With the patient seated, the practitioner stands behind the patient with his or her hands interlocked on the crown of the patient's head. The patient laterally flexes the cervical spine and the practitioner applies a compressive force along the cervical spine.	Pain and reproduction of symptoms radiating down the patient's arm	Foraminal encroachment
Valsalva test	The patient is seated and the practitioner asks the patient to take a deep breath and hold the breath while trying to exhale for 2–3 seconds.	Reproduction of symptoms	Presence of lesion, herniated disc, osteophyte or tumor in the cervical canal
Distraction test	The patient is positioned in supine to relax the cervical spine postural muscles. The practitioner stands at the head of the patient and places one hand on the occiput and the other on top of the forehead to stabilize the head. The practitioner then flexes the patient's cervical spine to a position of comfort. Force is applied to the skull to produce distraction of the cervical spine.	Pain decreases or disappears	Nerve root compression may exist during normal posture/positioning

Table 5.7
Special tests for cervical spine examination

Cervical spine muscles

Name	Origin	Insertion	Action	Nerve supply
Platysma	Subcutaneous fascia of chest	Subcutaneous fascia and mandible	Draws the corners of the mouth inferiorly; draws the skin of the neck superiorly	Cervical branch of the facial nerve (CN VII)
Sternocleidomastoid	Sternal head: manubrium of sternum Clavicular head: medial portion of the clavicle	Mastoid process of the temporal bone, superior nuchal line of occipital bone	Singly, tilts the head to its own side and rotates it towards the opposite side Acting as a pair, flex the neck, raise the sternum and are a secondary muscle of respiration	Motor: accessory nerve Sensory: cervical plexus (C2–C3)
Digastric	Anterior belly: digastric fossa (inner side of mandible) Posterior belly: mastoid process of temporal bone	Intermediate tendon (hyoid bone)	Opens the jaw, raises the hyoid bone	Anterior belly: mandibular division of the trigeminal (CN V) via the mylohyoid nerve Posterior belly: facial nerve (CN VII)
Stylohyoid	Styloid process (temporal)	Greater cornu of hyoid bone	Elevates the hyoid during swallowing, elevates tongue	Facial nerve (CN VII)
Mylohyoid	Mylohyoid line (mandible)	Median raphé	Raises the oral cavity floor, elevates the hyoid, depresses the mandible	Mandibular division of the trigeminal nerve
Geniohyoid	Symphysis menti (medial surface of mandible)	Hyoid bone	Protrudes the hyoid bone and tongue	C1 via the hypoglossal nerve
Sternohyoid	Manubrium of sternum	Hyoid bone	Depresses the hyoid bone	Ansa cervicalis (C1–C3)
Sternothyroid	Manubrium	Thyroid cartilage	Elevates the larynx, may slightly depress the hyoid bone	Ansa cervicalis (C1–C3)
Thyrohyoid	Thyroid cartilage	Hyoid bone	Depresses the hyoid bone	C1 via the hypoglossal nerve

(Continued)

Name	Origin	Insertion	Action	Nerve supply
Omohyoid	Superior notch of scapular	Inferior belly: clavicle via central tendon Superior belly: hyoid bone	Depresses the hyoid bone	Ansa cervicalis (C2–C3)
Longus colli (superior oblique part)	Transverse processes of C3–C5	Anterior arch of atlas	Flexes the neck and head	C2–C7
Longus colli (inferior oblique part)	Anterior surface of T1–T3	Transverse process of C5–C6	Flexes the neck and head	C2–C7
Longus colli (vertical part)	Anterior surface of C5–C7 and T1–T3	Anterior surface of C2–C4	Flexes the neck and head	C2–C7
Longus capitis	Anterior tubercles of the transverse processes of C3–C6	Occipital bone	Flexion of the neck/head	C1–C3
Scalenus anterior	Transverse process of C3–C6	First rib (scalene tubercle)	When the neck is fixed, elevates the first rib to aid in breathing; when the rib is fixed, bends the neck forward and sideways and rotates it to the opposite side	Ventral ramus of C5, C6
Scalenus posterior	Transverse processes of C4–C7	Second rib	Elevate the second rib, tilt the neck to the same side	C6–C8
Scalenus medius	Transverse process of C2–C7	First rib	Elevate the first rib, rotate the neck to the opposite side	Ventral rami of C3–C8
Levator scapulae	Posterior tubercles of transverse processes of C1–C4	Superior part of medial border of scapula	Elevates and rotates the scapula	Cervical nerve (C3–C4) and dorsal scapular nerve (C5)
Trapezius	Medial third of superior nuchal line, external occipital protuberance, ligamentum nuchae, spinous processes and supraspinous ligaments of C1 –T12	Lateral third of clavicle, acromion and crest of spine of scapula, medial portion of spine of scapula	Elevates, retracts and depresses the scapula Rotation of the scapula during arm elevation	Accessory nerve C3–C4
Rectus capitis anterior	Transverse process of atlas (C1)	Occipital bone	Flexion of the neck at the atlanto-occipital joint	C2–C3

(Continued)

Name	Origin	Insertion	Action	Nerve supply
Rectus capitis lateralis	Upper surface of the transverse process of the atlas (C1)	Jugular process of the occipital bone	Bends the head laterally	C2–C3
Rectus capitis posterior major	Spinous process of the axis (C2)	Inferior nuchal line of the occipital bone	Extends and rotates the head	Suboccipital nerve
Rectus capitis posterior minor	Tubercle on the posterior arch of the atlas (C1)	Medial part of the inferior nuchal line of the occipital bone	Extends the head	Suboccipital nerve
Obliquus capitis superior	Transverse process of atlas	Occipital bone between inferior and superior nuchal line	Extends and bends the head laterally	Suboccipital nerve
Splenius capitis	Ligamentum nuchae, spinous processes of C7–T6	Mastoid process and superior nuchal line	Extend, rotate, and laterally flex the head	Lateral branches of the dorsal primary division of the middle and lower cervical nerves
Splenius cervicis	Spinous process of T3–T6	Transverse processes of C1–C3	As a pair, extend the head and neck Singly, laterally flex and rotate the neck	Lateral branches of the dorsal primary divisions of the middle and lower cervical nerves
Iliocostalis cervicis	Angles of third to sixth ribs	Transverse processes of C4–C6	Extension and lateral flexion of the neck	Dorsal primary division of spinal nerves
Longissimus cervicis	Transverse processes of T1–T5	Transverse processes of C2–C6	Extension and lateral flexion of the neck	Dorsal primary division of the spinal nerves
Longissimus capitis	Transverse processes of T1–T5, articular processes of C5–C7	Posterior part of mastoid process of temporal bone	Extends and rotates the head	Dorsal primary division of the middle and lower cervical nerves
Spinalis cervicis	Ligamentum nuchae, spinous process of C7	Spinous process of axis	Extends the vertebral column	Dorsal primary division of the spinal nerves
Semispinalis thoracis	Transverse processes of T6–T10	Spinous processes of C6–C7 and T1–T4	Extends and rotates the vertebral column	Dorsal primary division of the spinal nerves
Semispinalis cervicis	Transverse process of T1–T6	Spinous processes of C2–C5	Extends and rotates the vertebral column	Dorsal primary division of the spinal nerves

(Continued)

Name	Origin	Insertion	Action	Nerve supply
Semispinalis capitis (and spinalis capitis, medial part of semispinalis capitis)	Transverse processes of C4–C7 and T1–T7	Between superior and inferior nuchal lines of occipital bone	Extends and rotates the neck	Dorsal primary division of the spinal nerves
Multifidus (cervical division)	Articular processes of C4–C7	Spinous process two vertebrae superior to origin	Extends and rotates the neck	Dorsal primary division of the spinal nerves
Rotatores (cervical division)	Transverse process of each vertebra	Base of spinous process of next vertebra above	Extends and rotates the neck	Dorsal primary division of the spinal nerves
Interspinales (cervical division)	Spinous processes of C3–C7	Spinous process of next superior vertebra	Extends the neck	Dorsal primary division of the spinal nerves
Intertransversarii anteriores	Anterior tubercle of transverse processes of vertebrae C1–T1	Anterior tubercle of next superior vertebra	Lateral flexion of the spine	Ventral primary division of the spinal nerves
Intertransversarii posteriores	Posterior tubercle of transverse processes of vertebrae C1–T1	Posterior tubercle of next superior vertebra	Lateral flexion of the spine	Ventral primary division of the spinal nerves

Table 5.8
Cervical spine muscles

Techniques: cervical spine

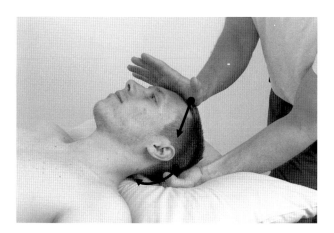

T5.1 Upper cervical spine extension

- With the patient supine, place your left hand under the occiput with your fingers under the mastoid processes.
- Place the palm of your right hand gently over the patient's forehead and, as you push down towards the pillow, pull your left hand up, inducing extension of the upper occiput.

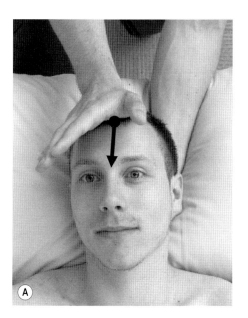

T5.2 Upper cervical spine flexion

- With the patient supine, place your left hand under the occiput with your fingers under the mastoid processes.
- With your right hand place palm gently over patient's forehead and as you push down towards the nose the left hand pulls up inducing flexion of the upper occiput.

A

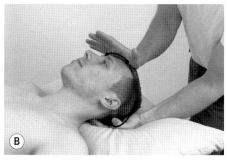

B

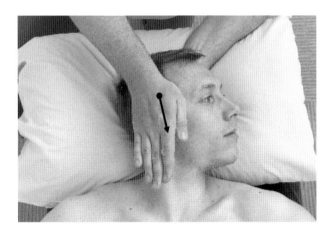

T5.3 Upper cervical side bending

- With the patient supine, stand by the patient's head.
- Place one hand under the side of patient's neck and temporal area with your fingers under the mastoid process.
- With the top hand, place your thenar and hypothenar eminence above the patient's ears (over the zygomatic and temporal area) and push down, inducing right upper cervical side bending.

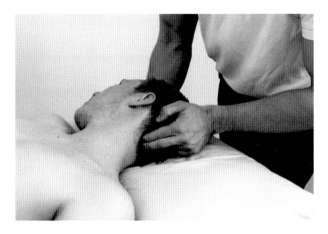

T5.4 Side-bending hand position

- Note two fingers under the patient's right mastoid process with the side of the patient's head resting on the palm of your opposite hand.

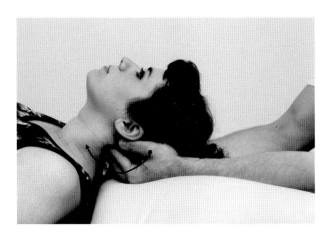

T5.5 Cervical spine extension

- With the patient supine, place your finger pads on the cervical spinal processes with the patient's head resting on your palms.
- Apply a posterior–anterior push, taking the cervical spine into extension.

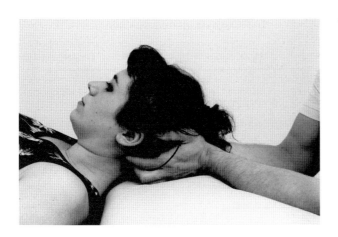

T5.6 Cervical spine flexion

- With the patient supine, place your finger pads on the cervical spinal processes with the patient's head resting on your palms.
- Pull towards and up with your fingers, inducing flexion.

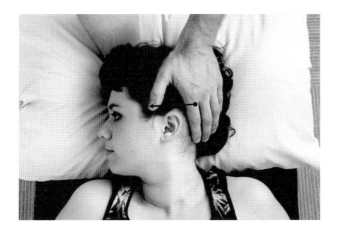

T5.7 Cervical spine rotation

- With the patient supine, stand behind the patient and place your right hand under the head.
- Place your left hand over the temporal occipital area and pull gently into rotation.

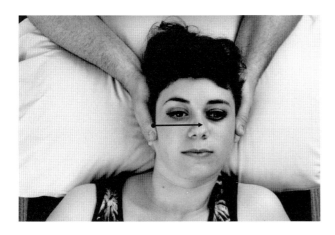

T5.8 Cervical spine side shift left

- With the patient supine, hold the head with your palms, placing your fingers on the lateral aspect of the articular pillars.
- Move the patient's head laterally to the left, creating a lateral side shift/translation.

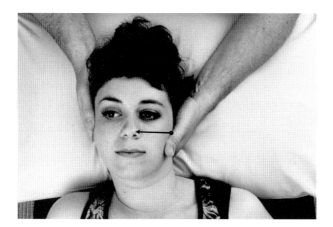

T5.9 Cervical spine side shift

- With the patient supine, hold the patient's head with your palms, placing your fingers on the lateral aspect of the articular pillars.
- Move the patient's head laterally to the right, creating a lateral side shift/translation.

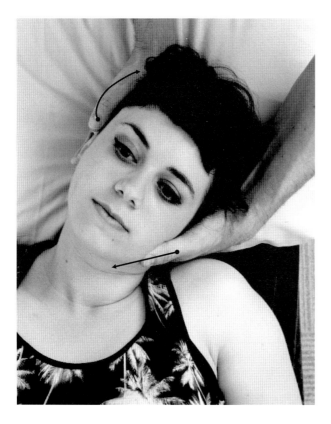

T5.10 Cervical spine side bending

- With the patient supine, hold the patient's head with your palms, placing your fingers on the lateral aspect of the articular pillars.
- Place the metacarpophalangeal joint of your left hand over the transverse processes and push, with your opposite hand holding the patient's temporal-occiput.
- Push gently in the same direction to induce side bending.

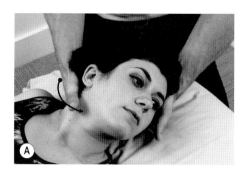

T5.11 Articulation of the cervical spine using 'wind up' technique (short angle)

- With the patient supine, stand at the angle of the plinth with your knees slightly bent.
- Holding the patient's occiput with your left palm, rotate the neck to the left.
- Place the index finger (metacarpophalangeal joint) of your right hand on the cervical lateral masses (articular pillar).
- Using a combination of side-bending and rotation to the neck, gently articulate the desired level you are contacting.

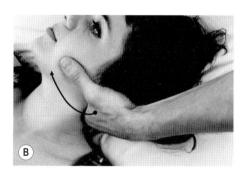

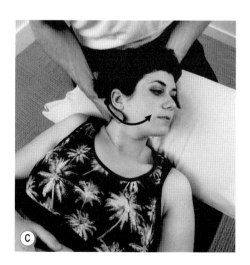

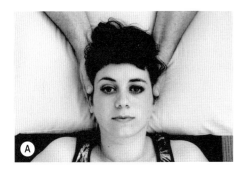

T5.12 'Figure of eight' articulation of the cervical spine

a Figure of eight, starting position

- Starting position for the 'figure of eight' technique.
- With the patient supine, stand at the head of the couch and gently stabilize your fingers on a segment in the cervical spine, C2–C7, applying light compression to focus force around that specific segment.
- The patient is slightly in flexion with the use of a pillow supporting the head.
- The patient will start and end in this position after the targeted segment has been taken through all ranges of movement (see below).

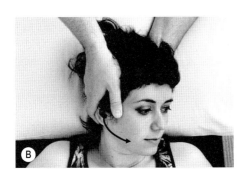

b Figure of eight, lower left

- With the patient supine, stand at the head of the couch and gently stabilize your fingers on a segment in the cervical spine, C2–C7, applying light compression to focus force around that specific segment.
- The patient is slightly in flexion with the use of a pillow supporting the head.
- The picture shows a rotation to the left-hand side of the couch.
- The technique is a figure of eight. The therapist will take the segment through that movement, articulating the segment in all vectors.

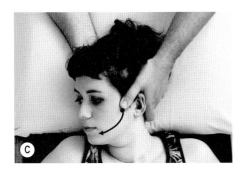

c Figure of eight, lower right

- With the patient supine, stand at the head of the couch and gently stabilize your fingers on a segment in the cervical spine, C2–C7, applying light compression to focus force around that specific segment.
- The patient is slightly in flexion with the use of a pillow supporting the head.
- The picture shows a rotation to the right-hand side of the couch.
- The technique is a figure of eight. The therapist will take the segment through that movement, articulating the segment in all vectors.

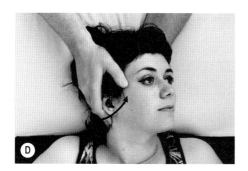

d Figure of eight, upper left

- With the patient supine, stand at the head of the couch and gently stabilize your fingers on a segment in the cervical spine, C2–C7, applying light compression to focus force around that specific segment.
- The patient is slightly in flexion with the use of a pillow supporting the head.
- The picture shows an extension to the left-hand side of the couch.
- The technique is a figure of eight. The therapist will take the segment through that movement, articulating the segment in all vectors.

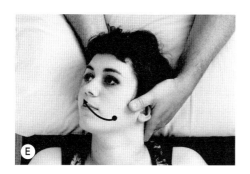

e Figure of eight, upper right

- With the patient supine, stand at the head of the couch and gently stabilize your fingers on a segment in the cervical spine, C2–C7, applying light compression to focus force around that specific segment.
- The patient is slightly in flexion with the use of a pillow supporting the head.
- The picture shows a extension to the right-hand side of the couch.
- The technique is a figure of eight. The therapist will take the segment through that movement, articulating the segment in all vectors.

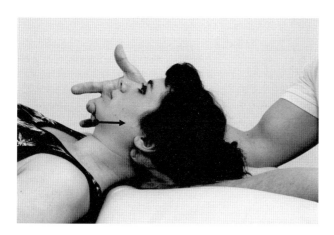

T5.13 Cervical spine traction supine

- With the patient supine, stand at the head of the couch, your left hand under the patient's occiput with their head resting on your forearm.
- With the third and fourth fingers of your opposite hand, lightly clasp the patient's chin.
- Apply a gentle traction force, articulating the cervical spine.

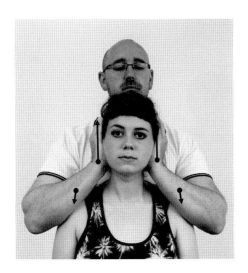

T5.14 Cervical spine sitting traction

- With the patient seated, stand behind the patient, rest your forearms over the patient's shoulders and cup under the mastoids and inferior occiput with your thenar and hypothenar, with fingers resting gently on the side of the head.
- Apply an upward traction.

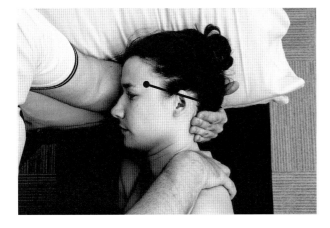

T5.15 Side-lying cervical–thoracic extension

- With the patient side-lying (picture shows the patient lying on her right side), support the patient's head and neck with your left hand, the patient's forehead coming into contact with your bicep to allow you to lock out the upper cervical spine and avoid excessive movement during the technique.
- Place your opposite hand over the patient's left shoulder/upper trapezius, applying pressure against the C7/T1 vertebrae. This will allow your hand to act as the fulcrum to articulate the C7/T1.
- With your left hand, apply a posterior to anterior push, bending the head backwards to induce extension.

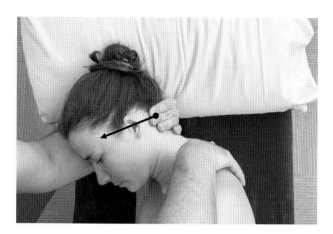

T5.16 Side-lying cervical–thoracic flexion

- With the patient side-lying (picture shows the patient lying on her right side), support the patient's head and neck with your left hand, the patient's forehead coming into contact with your bicep to allow you to lock out the upper cervical spine and avoid excessive movement during the technique.

- Place your opposite hand over the patient's left shoulder/upper trapezius, applying pressure against the C7/T1 vertebrae. This will allow your hand to act as the fulcrum to articulate the C7/T1.

- With your left hand, bend the patient's head forwards to induce flexion.

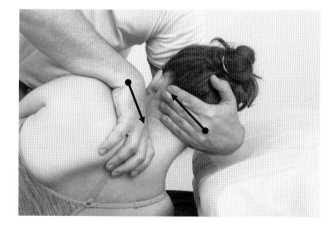

T5.17 Side-lying cervical–thoracic side bending

- With the patient side-lying (picture shows the patient lying on her right side), support the patient's head and neck with your left hand, the patient's forehead coming into contact with your bicep to allow you to lock out the upper cervical spine and avoid excessive movement during the technique.

- Place your opposite hand over the patient's left shoulder/upper trapezius, applying pressure against the C7/T1 vertebrae. This will allow your hand to act as the fulcrum to articulate the C7/T1.

- With the supporting hand, side bend the neck to the left.

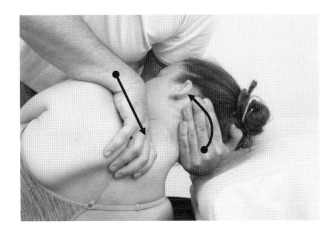

T5.18 Side-lying cervical–thoracic rotation

- With the patient side-lying (picture shows the patient lying on her right side), support the patient's head and neck with your left hand, the patient's forehead coming into contact with your bicep to allow you to lock out the upper cervical spine and avoid excessive movement during the technique.

- Place your opposite hand over patient's left shoulder/upper trapezius, applying pressure against the C7/T1 vertebrae. This will allow your hand to act as the fulcrum to articulate the C7/T1.

- With your supporting hand, rotate the neck to the left.

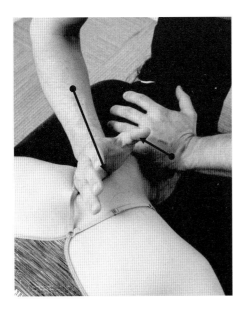

T5.19 Prone cervical–thoracic articulation

- With the patient prone, gently side bend and slightly rotate the neck and head with your left hand so that the patient's face is resting at a slight angle in the face hole of the couch.

- The side bending and rotation will allow you to wind the cervical spine down to the level of C7–T1 and lock out the cervical spine above, reducing excessive movement.

- Place the hypothenar of your other hand on the lateral aspect to the spinous process of C6/C7, ensuring continued contact.

- Start to push the spinous process gently laterally, articulating the cervico-thoracic junction. Repeat on the opposite side if needed.

- Ensure that there is not much compression, as this can be uncomfortable for the patient. Be aware that articulation into this junction can sometimes result in a spontaneous cavitation of the C7–T1.

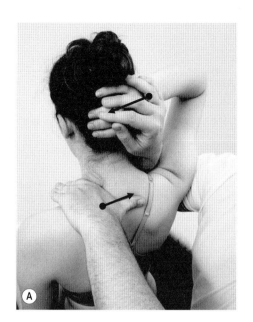

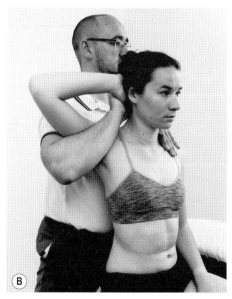

T5.20 Seated cervical–thoracic articulation

- With the patient seated, the patient places one hand behind their neck, holding on to the base of their head.
- Stand behind the patient and place your stabilizing hand on top of the patient's hand, supporting the head and neck. Ensure that you do not add too much flexion because this can be uncomfortable for the patient.
- With your free hand, place your thumb laterally against the spinous process of C7/T1, applying a gently lateral pressure.
- The thumb forms a fulcrum for side-bending movement, allowing you to articulate that spinal segment.
- Rest your finger pads over the patient's shoulder to add stability and support as you move through the technique.

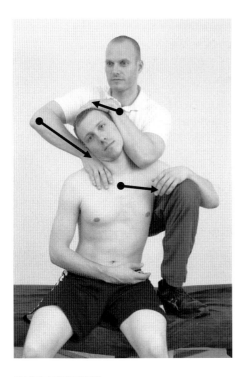

T5.21 Cervical–thoracic articulation

- Seat the patient as far back as possible on the plinth.
- Stand behind the patient with your foot on the plinth to the side you wish to articulate, allowing the patient's arm and hand to rest over your thigh.
- Rest your arm on the patient's shoulder, placing your hand on the patient's forehead, level with their hairline.
- Place your other hand on the base of the cervical spine. The objective is to place your metacarpophalangeal joint of the little finger on the side of the cervical–thoracic joint.
- Raise your elbow so as to direct the movement towards the patient's opposite axilla.
- To articulate, shift your body towards the foot that is on the plinth and, with your hand, side bend the patient's neck, thus opening the same side as the arm that is over your leg.
- Please note that this is very similar to the seated technique T7.3 First rib articulation given in Chapter 7.

REFERENCES

Allison GT, Nagy BM, Hall T (2002). A randomized clinical trial of manual therapy for cervico-brachial pain syndrome – a pilot study. Manual Therapy 7(2):95-102.

Austin N, Krishnamoorthy V, Dagal A (2014). Airway management in cervical spine injury. International Journal of Critical Illness and Injury Science 4(1):50.

Bassols A, Bosch F, Banos JE (2002). How does the general population treat their pain? A survey in Catalonia, Spain. Journal of Pain Symptom Management 23:318-28.

Bogduk N (2005). Clinical Anatomy of the Lumbar Spine and Sacrum. Oxford: Elsevier Health Sciences.

Bronfort G, Haas M, Evans R et al (2010). Effectiveness of manual therapies: the UK evidence report. Chiropractic & Manual Therapies 18(1):3.

Carlesso LC, Gross AR, Santaguida PL et al (2010). Adverse events associated with the use of cervical manipulation and mobilization for the treatment of neck pain in adults: a systematic review. Manual Therapy 15:434-444.

Cassidy JD, Boyle E, Cote P, et al (2008). Risk of vertebrobasilar stroke and chiropractic care: results of a population-based case-control and case-crossover study. Spine (Phila Pa 1976) 33:S176-183.

Childs JD, Cleland JA, Elliott JM et al (2008). Neck pain: clinical practice guidelines linked to the International Classification of Functioning, Disability, and Health from the Orthopaedic Section of the American Physical Therapy Association. Journal of Orthopaedic and Sports Physical Therapy 38(9):A1-A34.

Côté P, Cassidy JD, Carroll LJ et al (2004). The annual incidence and course of neck pain in the general population: a population-based cohort study. Pain 112(3):267-273.

Croft PR, Lewis M, Papageorgiou AC et al (2001). Risk factors for neck pain: a longitudinal study in the general population. Pain 93(3):317-325.

Crosby ET, Lui A (1990). The adult cervical spine: implications for airway management. Canadian Journal of Anaesthesia 37(1):77-93.

Di Fabio RP (1999). Manipulation of the cervical spine: risks and benefits. Physical Therapy 79:50-65.

Driscoll DR (1987). Anatomical and biomechanical characteristics of upper cervical ligamentous structures: a review. Journal of Manipulative and Physiological Therapeutics 10(3):107-110.

Dunning JR, Cleland JA, Waldrop MA et al (2012). Upper cervical and upper thoracic thrust manipulation versus non-thrust mobilization in patients with mechanical neck pain: a multicenter randomized clinical trial. Journal of Orthopaedic and Sports Physical Therapy 42(1):5-18.

Frobin W, Leivseth G, Biggemann M et al (2002). Sagittal plane segmental motion of the cervical spine. A new precision measurement protocol and normal motion data of healthy adults. Clinical Biomechanics 17(1):21-31.

Goldberg W, Mueller C, Panacek E et al (2001). Distribution and patterns of blunt traumatic cervical spine injury. Annals of Emergency Medicine 38(1):17-21.

Gross AR, Goldsmith C, Hoving JL et al (2007). Conservative management of mechanical neck disorders: a systematic review. The Journal of Rheumatology 34(5):1083-1102.

Hackl W, Hausberger K, Sailer R et al (2001). Prevalence of cervical spine injuries in patients with facial trauma. Oral Surgery, Oral Medicine, Oral Pathology, Oral Radiology, and Endodontology 92 (4):370-376.

Haldeman S, Kohlbeck FJ, McGregor M (1999). Risk factors and precipitating neck movements causing vertebrobasilar artery dissection after cervical trauma and spinal manipulation. Spine 24:785-794.

Hall T, Robinson K (2004). The flexion–rotation test and active cervical mobility – a comparative measurement study in cervicogenic headache. Manual Therapy 9:197-202.

Hall TM, Briffa K, Hopper D et al (2010). Comparative analysis and diagnostic accuracy of the cervical flexion-rotation test. The Journal of Headache and Pain 11:391-397.

Hogg-Johnson S, van der Velde G, Carroll LJ et al (2008). The burden and determinants of neck pain in the general population. European Spine Journal 17(1):39-51.

Hoving JL, de Vet HC, Koes BW et al. (2006). Manual therapy, physical therapy, or continued care by the general practitioner for patients with neck pain: long-term results from a pragmatic randomized trial. Clinical Journal of Pain 22(4):370-377.

Hoving JL, Koes BW, de Vet HC, et al (2002). Manual therapy, physical therapy, or continued care by a general practitioner for patients with neck pain. A randomized, controlled trial. Annals of Internal Medicine 136(10):713-722.

Hurwitz EL, Mortgenstern H, Vassilaki M et al (2005). Frequency and clinical predictors of adverse reactions to chiropractic care in the UCLA neck pain study. Spine 30:1477-1484.

Jaumard NV, Welch WC, Winkelstein BA (2011). Spinal facet joint biomechanics and mechanotransduction in normal, injury and degenerative conditions. Journal of Biomechanical Engineering 133(7):071010.

Jull G, Trott P, Potter H et al (2002). A randomized controlled trial of exercise and manipulative therapy for cervicogenic headache. Spine 27:1835-1843.

Kalichman L, Hunter DJ (2007). Lumbar facet joint osteoarthritis: a review. Seminars in Arthritis and Rheumatism 37(2):69-80.

Korthals-de Bos IBC, Hoving JL, van Tulder MW et al (2003). Cost-effectiveness of physiotherapy, manual therapy, and general practitioner care for neck pain: economic evaluation alongside a randomized controlled trial. British Medical Journal 326:1-6.

Lee SH, Sung JK (2009). Unilateral lateral mass-facet fractures with rotational instability: new classification and a review of 39 cases treated conservatively and with single segment anterior fusion. Journal of Trauma and Acute Care Surgery 66(3):758-767.

Lowery DW, Wald MM, Browne BJ et al (2001). Epidemiology of cervical spine injury victims. Annals of Emergency Medicine 38(1):12-16.

Milligram MA, Rand N (2000). Cervical spine anatomy. Spine State of the Art Reviews 14 (3):521-532.

Muhle C, Bischoff L, Weinert D et al (1998). Exacerbated pain in cervical radiculopathy at axial rotation, flexion, extension, and coupled motions of the cervical spine: evaluation by kinematic magnetic resonance imaging. Investigative Radiology 33(5):279-288.

 Ogince M, Hall T, Robinson K et al (2007). The diagnostic validity of the cervical flexion-rotation test in C1/2-related cervicogenic headache. Manual Therapy 12:256-262.

Persson LCG, Lilja A (2001). Pain, coping, emotional state and physical function in patients with chronic radicular neck pain. A comparison between patients treated with surgery, physiotherapy or neck collar – a blinded, prospective randomized study. Disability and Rehabilitation 23:325-35.

Picavet HSJ, Schouten JSAG (2003). Musculoskeletal pain in the Netherlands: prevalences, consequences and risk groups, the DMC 3-study. Pain 102(1):167-178.

Schafer RC, Faye LJ (1990). The cervical spine. In: RC Schafer, LJ Faye eds. Motion Palpation and Chiropractic Technique: Principles of Dynamic Chiropractic. Huntington Beach, CA: Motion Palpation Institute; 93.

Steilen D, Hauser R, Woldin B et al (2014). Chronic neck pain: making the connection between capsular ligament laxity and cervical instability. The Open Orthopaedics Journal 8:326.

Torretti JA, Sengupta DK (2007). Cervical spine trauma. Indian Journal of Orthopaedics 41(4):255.

Tubbs RS, Dixon J, Loukas M et al (2010). Ligament of Barkow of the craniocervical junction: its anatomy and potential clinical and functional significance: Laboratory investigation. Journal of Neurosurgery: Spine 12(6):619-622.

Tubbs RS, Hallock JD, Radcliff V et al (2011). Ligaments of the craniocervical junction: A review. Journal of Neurosurgery: Spine 14(6):697-709.

Van Mameren H, Drukker J, Sanches H et al (1989). Cervical spine motion in the sagittal plane (I) range of motion of actually performed movements, an X-ray cinematographic study. European Journal of Morphology 28(1):47-68.

Vernon H, Humphreys K, Hagino C (2007). Chronic mechanical neck pain in adults treated by manual therapy: a systematic review of change scores in randomized clinical trials. Journal of Manipulative and Physiological Therapeutics 30(3):215-227.

White AA, Panjabi MM (1990). Kinematics of the spine. In: Clinical Biomechanics of the Spine, 2nd ed. Philadelphia: Lippincott Williams & Wilkins; 85-125.

Windle WF ed (1980). The Spinal Cord and its Reaction to Traumatic Injury: Anatomy, Physiology, Pharmacology, Therapeutics (vol 18). New York: M Dekker.

Wolsko PM, Eisenberg DM, Davis RB et al. (2003). Patterns and perceptions of care for treatment of back and neck pain: results of a national survey. Spine 28:292-297.

Zito G, Jull G, Story I (2006). Clinical tests of musculoskeletal dysfunction in the diagnosis of cervicogenic headache. Manual Therapy 11:118-129.

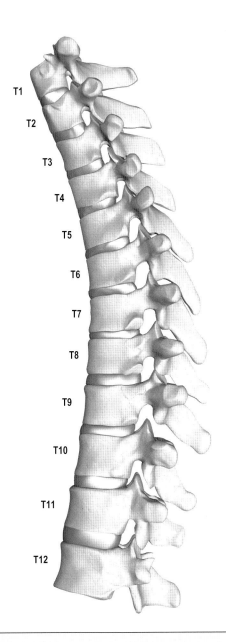

T1
T2
T3
T4
T5
T6
T7
T8
T9
T10
T11
T12

Figure 6.1
The thoracic spine

The thoracic spine 6

Introduction

The thoracic spine is a common site for dysfunction, including rheumatological (e.g. ankylosing spondylitis), infective (e.g. tuberculosis), metabolic (e.g. Paget's disease) and degenerative (e.g. osteoporosis) problems, to name a few. In comparison to the lumbar and cervical spine, the thoracic spine has received less focus in epidemiological, clinical and occupational research (Briggs et al 2009a). One explanation for this is that researchers investigating back pain have often grouped lumbar and thoracic spine pain into one category (Briggs et al 2009a). In a study by Dionne et al (2007), thoracic spine pain was found to be a major factor in working hours lost and reported work disability. Many occupations are at risk of developing thoracic spine pain, among them manual laborers, office workers, health professionals and drivers (Briggs et al 2009b), with some groups experiencing up to 50% incidence. Briggs et al (2009b) also found that females experienced a higher occurrence of thoracic spine pain than males.

Recent studies have found an increasing incidence of thoracic pain in adolescents (Wedderkopp et al 2001, Grimmer et al 2006, Trevelyan & Legg 2006, Jeffries et al 2007, Briggs et al 2009b). Some of this has been linked to poor posture or ergonomics within the classroom (Murphy et al 2004, Lafond et al 2007) or to the use of heavy school bags and backpacks for transporting books to and from school (Sheir-Neiss et al 2003, Skaggs et al 2006, Papadopoulou et al 2013). Links have also been made between thoracic spine pain and poor posture, inactivity and prolonged sitting when playing computer games (Zapata et al 2006, Hakala et al 2012). Back problems in adolescence could potentially cause further issues and problems as these young people progress into adulthood (Hakala et al 2002, Ståhl et al 2014). Kujala and colleagues (1999) found that up 10% of adolescents suffered thoracic spine pain to the point that it restricted their participation in activities. Thoracic spine pain is one of the factors that have been associated with an increase in painkiller consumption among adolescents participating in sports (Selanne et al 2014). Education about posture, ergonomics and training is therefore an important component when treating adolescent patients within the clinical environment.

Interestingly, Imagama et al (2014) found that an increase in thoracic kyphosis, increased spinal inclination and weak posterior musculature are factors associated with shoulder injuries and limitation of shoulder movement. Therefore good maintenance of the thoracic spine not only leads to decreased thoracic spine symptoms, but is also associated with healthy shoulder mechanics.

Articulation of the thoracic spine has been shown to be beneficial in decreasing pressure pain thresholds in that section of the spine. Fryer et al (2004) found that passive rhythmical repetitive articulation of the thoracic spine caused a greater decrease in the pain threshold of participants with thoracic spine symptoms than manipulation of the spine on a short-term basis. Furthermore, Cleland et al (2007) found that thoracic spine articulation caused a reduction in pain and disability in patients experiencing cervical spine pain, although significant reduction and relief were only short term and, like most research, these findings require further investigation to validate them and to investigate long-term effects.

Anatomy

The thoracic spine is one of three regions of the spinal column and is located in the middle segment of the spine, between the cervical spine in the neck and the lumbar spine in the lower back. It comprises 12 vertebrae (labelled T1 to T12) that caudally increase in size, reflecting the caudal increase in body load. However, although it is not common, the number of thoracic vertebrae in the spine can vary from 11 to

13 because they are usually defined by paired rib-bearing elements. Early recognition of the precise number of thoracic vertebrae in a patient is important so that the discrepancy does not lead to inappropriate surgical planning, which may endanger the patient's site of pathology (Wigh 1980).

The thoracic vertebrae are intermediate in size compared with vertebrae of other segments. The size and shape of the superior thoracic segment closely resembles the cervical vertebrae, whereas the inferior thoracic vertebrae are more similar to the lumbar (White & Panjabi 1978). These vertebrae curve inward and outward to give support and stability for the ribs and sternum. They play a significant protective role for the lungs, heart and major blood vessels and provide structure and flexibility for the body, while guarding the vertebral column (McKenzie & May 2006). The intervertebral discs from T1 to T12 also vary considerably in their size and shape.

The thoracic spine is more rigid than other spinal segments, due to the structural integrity provided by the ribcage and its articulations, facet orientations and vertebral body configurations. For this reason, unlike the cervical or lumbar spine, the thoracic spine is presumed to build for load transfer and stability. White (1969) suggested that the compressive load at the first thoracic vertebra (T1) was approximately 9% of the participant's body weight, which increased up to 33% at T8 and 47% at T12. The vertebral bodies are thought to withstand and distribute the majority of this load. Edmondston and Singer (1997) state that, in order to accommodate this load, the vertebral body's height, end-plate cross-sectional area and bone mass increase caudally, mainly in the middle and lower parts.

Its articulations to the ribcage mean that the thoracic spine is the least mobile segment of the vertebral column. Thin intervertebral discs also contribute to the lower mobility of the thoracic vertebrae, as they comprise only 1/7 of the vertebral body's height. According to McKenzie and May (2006), the additional vertebral–rib joints (costovertebral and costotransverse joints) and the configuration of the zygapophyseal joints and the spinous processes are all factors that restrict the movement of the thoracic spine.

Bony anatomy

Vertebral bodies

The vertebral bodies of the thoracic spine are wedge-shaped, round blocks of bones that are larger posteriorly than anteriorly. They are concave on their cranial and caudal end-plate surfaces, flat above and below, deeper dorsally than ventrally, and slightly constricted laterally and in front. They vary substantially in their size and shape from T1 to T12, increasing considerably in more inferior segments. The vertebral bodies function primarily to support and transfer the weight of the trunk, because of the anterior concavity of the thoracic kyphosis (Singer & Goh 2000). The thoracic vertebral bodies also support two demifacets on each of their lateral posterior surfaces, superiorly and inferiorly adjacent to the end-plate surfaces. These are present for the articulation of the head of each respective rib bilaterally.

Vertebral arches

The vertebral arch is a thin, bony ring attachment at the posterior portion of each vertebral body. Each vertebral arch encloses the vertebral foramen and provides space for the spinal cord. It acts to protect the spinal cord and the roots of the spinal nerves (McKenzie & May 2006).

Pedicles

Pedicles are short bones that extend posteriorly from the vertebral body to form the vertebral arch. They act as a connector between the vertebral body and its posterior elements.

Laminae

Laminae are broad, thick bones that connect with the pedicles to complete the vertebral arch. They are the outer rim of the bony ring and form the posterior border of the vertebral foramen.

Transverse processes

The bony knobs that project from the lateral sides of each vertebral arch, one on the left and one on the right, are called transverse processes. They articulate with a pair of ribs, forming the costotransverse joints and provide attachment sites for muscles and ligaments.

Spinous processes

The spinous process is a long bony structure that is directed obliquely downward especially in the mid thoracic area. The spinous process extends so far downward that, in the mid thoracic area (T4–T8), it is level with the vertebral body of the vertebra below. It arises from the junction of the laminae and ends at a tuberculated extremity. It serves to attach several muscles of the back.

Articular processes

Articular processes are projections of the vertebra that spring from the junctions of the pedicles and laminae, and extend superiorly and inferiorly toward the adjacent vertebrae. There are four articular processes, two superior and two inferior, that project from a vertebra. They serve to stabilize the spine, forming a facet joint where they join with an adjacent vertebra (Moore et al 2013).

Ligaments

The thoracic spine has the same ligaments as elsewhere in the vertebral column. These include the anterior and posterior longitudinal ligaments, supraspinous and interspinous ligaments, intertransverse ligaments and the ligamentum flavum. However, the ligamentous support provided for the ribs by the thoracic spine also involves the costotransverse and radiate ligaments and the ligaments of the costovertebral joint capsule (Putz & Muller-Gerbil 2000).

Lang et al (2013) found that ossification of the ligamentum flavum was relatively common in the patients they examined, with a predictive occurrence of 63.9%. The peak occurrence of this was in patients between 50 and 59 years of age, but they did find some evidence of it occurring in adolescents between 10 and 19 years of age. The main area where this occurred was the lower thoracic spine between T10 and T12, and more commonly in males, which led Lang et al to suggest that it is triggered by higher mechanical stresses to the tissue.

Joints

Costovertebral joints

The costovertebral joints are formed when the head of the rib articulates with the costal facets of adjacent vertebral bodies and the intervertebral disc between. The heads of ribs 2 to 9 articulate with two vertebral bodies; the heads of ribs 1 and 10 to 12 connect with only one vertebra each. Each costovertebral joint is composed of a fibrous capsule, the fan-shaped radiate ligament and the interarticular ligament (Macdonald 1986).

Costotransverse joints

The costotransverse joints are formed when the tubercle of the rib articulates with the transverse process of the corresponding vertebra. These joints include the neck and tubercle ligaments, a capsule and the costotransverse ligaments. They are absent in T11 and T12 (Duprey et al 2010).

Zygapophyseal joints

The zygapophyseal joints, also known as the facet joints, are synovial, plane joints formed joining the articular processes of two neighboring vertebrae. They primarily serve to guide and constrain the motion of the vertebrae (Pal et al 2001). Manchikanti (2004) found that 42% of chronic thoracic spine pain originated from the facet joint.

Range of motion

Unlike the other spinal segments, where a considerable number of movement analyses have been performed, serious studies to evaluate the movement of the thoracic spine are very limited. Although there are reports of range of motion, they are based largely on an early cadaver study (White 1969). The study of thoracic movements presents significant methodological difficulties because it includes studying the ribcage and the complex interaction between the vertebrae and the ribs, and Valencia (1994) stated that the measurement of thoracic movements is technically difficult. However, a few in vivo and in vitro studies have been done that suggest some possible range of movements, but these give different measurements (see Table 6.1).

Epidemiology

The epidemiology of thoracic spine pain is hindered by two major drawbacks: the difficulty in defining the thoracic pain and the lack of high-quality literature. Moreover, there are very limited epidemiological

Movement type	Motion unit	Range of motion (°)
Flexion	C7–T1	≈ 9
	T1–T6	4
	T6–T7	4–8
	T12–L1	8–12
Lateral bending	T1–T10	≈ 6
	T11–L1	≈ 8
Sagittal	T1–T10	< 5
	T10–T12	≈ 5
Rotation	T1–T4	8–12
	T5–T8	≈ 8
	T9–T12	< 3

Table 6.1

Possible range of movement of the thoracic spine

Data from McKenzie & May (2006), Leahy & Rahm (2007)

data in relation to thoracic pain. Reviewers of the available data suggest that the clinical pain syndromes associated with the thoracic spine are less common than those associated with the cervical and lumbar regions (Lemole et al 2002). According to Singer and Edmondston (2000), the percentage of patients in the chronic pain clinic environment is only 2–3%.

Although limited literature is available on the epidemiology of thoracic spine pain, there are a few notable population-based studies. In one such study of age group 35–45 years, Linton et al (1998) reported that the annual prevalence of spinal pain in the general population was 66%. Only 15% of individuals with spinal pain symptoms reported pain in the thoracic spine region compared to 56% in the lumbar spine and 44% in the cervical spine. This equates to an annual prevalence of approximately 3% in the general population for thoracic pain. However, the percentage of thoracic pain prevalence varies between studies. According to the majority of reports, including surveys by osteopath clinics, chiropractors and physiotherapists, the thoracic pain prevalence range is between 2.6% and 14%. Considering these data, McKenzie and May (2006) stated that about 5–17% of all spinal problems are thoracic in origin (see Table 6.2).

Condition	Description	Reference
Spinal canal stenosis	May result from either hypertrophy of the posterior elements of the thoracic spine or congenital deformation	Barnett et al (1987), McRae (2010)
	Often occurs in relation with generalized rheumatological, metabolic or orthopaedic conditions, such as osteofluorosis, achondroplasia, acromegaly, Paget's disease or previous fracture	
	Average age of presentation: 65 years	
Vertebral body fractures	Most common in the thoracolumbar spine	Kostuik et al (1991), Jansson et al (2010)
	Usually result from a high-energy accident or osteoporosis	
	May also occur because of an underlying disorder, such as ankylosing spondylitis, a vertebral tumor or infection	
	Symptoms include pain or the development of neural deficits such as numbness, weakness, tingling, spinal shock and neurogenic shock	
	Predominant in men	
	Age of presentation: 2nd to 4th decades	

(Continued)

Condition	Description	Reference
Juvenile kyphosis	A form of juvenile osteochondrosis of the spine, which leads to wedge-shaped vertebrae Commonly affects the T7 and T10 vertebrae Usually occurs in adolescence, between 14 and 18 years of age Slightly predominant in women Results in lower and mid-level back pain, poor posture and increased kyphosis	Scheuermann (1934), Bullough & Boachie-Adjei (1988)
Thoracic neurofibroma	One of the most common tumors of the spine Also known as neurilemmoma, neurinoma or schwannoma Accounts for 1/3 of the spine tumors Often originates from the dorsal root of the spine Usually arises from proliferating nerve fibers, Schwann cells and fibroblasts Often appears at the lower thoracic segment and the thoracolumbar junction Peak incidence: between 4th and 5th decade	Gautier-Smith (1967), Borenstein & Wiesel (1989), Conti et al (2004)
Paget's disease	A chronic metabolically active bone disease, characterized by thickening and deformation of the disturbed bone Often caused by hyperactive osteoclasts and osteoblasts Mainly affects flat bones and the ends of the long bones Approximately 45% of patients with this disease have thoracic spine involvement Affects around 3% of the population over 40 years of age Slightly predominant in males Overall prevalence: 3–3.7%	Altman et al (1987), Dell'Atti et al (2007)
Tuberculosis (TB) of the spine	Usually involves the thoracolumbar region, particularly the lower thoracic and upper lumbar spines May cause anterior and sometimes lateral wedging of the spine May compromise the spinal cord extrinsically and intrinsically and may produce angular kyphotic or scoliotic deformities Accounts for about 50% of all cases of musculoskeletal TB Occurs in less than 1% of patients with TB	Turgut (2001), McRae (2010), Garg & Somvanshi (2011)

Table 6.2
Common disorders of the thoracic spine

Thoracic spine examination

Medical history

Taking a detailed medical history of the patient is essential for the thoracic spine examination. In most cases, the narrative provided by the patient helps determine the red flags and facilitate the physical examination. The examiner must approach the patient in a friendly and respectful manner. They should collect the necessary information in a logical format and must listen to the patient's responses very carefully. Apart from questioning about pain, swelling, numbness, tingling or any other issues over the thoracic region, they must inquire about the onset of the problem, behavior since onset, symptom pattern, and exacerbating and relieving factors.

Red flags

Red flags are used to provide clues to the existence of serious spinal pathology in patients with back problems (Honet & Ellenberg 2003). While questioning the patient, the examiner must look out for the presence of the red flags listed in Table 6.3 in their narrative. The screening process should begin with a detailed medical history and the use of a medical screening form.

Physical examination

After taking a detailed medical history of the patient, the clinician will have sufficient information to make tentative decisions about certain aspects of the case. Based on the findings from the initial interview, the clinician should then proceed to the physical examination. This involves a variety of observations and movements, so that the clinician can confirm initial findings, fully explore the nature and extent of the problem, and make judgments.

Observation

The physical examination process should start with a careful observation of the patient's posture. Posture is best observed when the patient is unaware that the clinician

Table 6.3
Red flags for serious pathology in patients with thoracic spine pain
Data from Nachemson & Vingard (2000), Ombregt (2003), McKenzie & May (2006)

Condition	Signs and symptoms
Spinal tumors	Over 50 years of age
	Past history of cancer
	Unintentional loss of weight, about 10 kg within 6 months
	Constant, severe and progressive back pain at night
	Pain lasting for more than a month
	No improvement after a month of conventional treatment
Spinal infection	Over 50 years of age
	Recent bacterial infection such as respiratory, urinary tract or skin infection, tuberculosis
	History of intravenous drug abuse
	Persistent fever or systemic illness
Fracture	Over 70 years of age
	Recent history of major trauma
	Prolonged use of corticosteroids
	History of osteoporosis
Inflammatory arthropathy	Gradual onset: less than 40 years of age
	Family history
	Morning stiffness > 1 hour
	Persisting limitation of movement
	Involvement of peripheral joint
	Iritis, colitis, skin rashes or urethral discharge
Vascular/neurological	Excessive dizziness
	Blackouts or falls
	Positive cranial nerve signs

is doing so, such as during the history taking. The clinician should note how the patient sits and stands. When the patient is standing, it should be noted whether the thoracic curvature appears regular or increased. While the patient is seated unsupported on a treatment table or examination couch, the clinician should note the curve of the spine. Obliteration of an abnormal curve during unsupported sitting suggests presence of scoliosis. It also suggests that scoliosis is mobile and may be secondary to shortening of a leg.

Movement patterns

Movements in flexion, extension and rotation should be examined in erect sitting. The clinician should initially perform the single movements to check the patient's ability to move, and then repeated movements to determine the range and quality of movement and pain response to movement. The symptoms and mechanical responses should be noted carefully. The clinician should instruct the patient to repeat the movements that eliminate or reduce symptoms, and temporarily avoid movements that peripheralize or increase symptoms. Any deviations or discrepancies between sides must be recorded properly.

Special tests

See Table 6.4.

Test	Procedure	Positive sign	Interpretation
Slump test	The patient sits on the edge of a treatment table, with legs supported, hands behind the back and hips in neutral. The examiner instructs the patient to slump forward at full thoracic and lumbar flex. The patient flexes the neck by placing the chin on the chest and the examiner maintains overpressure. The patient actively extends one knee as much as possible and the examiner then dorsiflexes the ankle.	Reproduction of symptoms in back and radicular symptoms	Increased tension in dura or meninges neural tissue sensitivity
Brudzinski's sign	The patient lies in the supine position. One of the examiner's hands is behind the patient's head and the other hand is on the patient's chest. The examiner then passively flexes the patient's neck by pulling the head to the chest, while restraining the body from rising.	Reproduction of pain in the back, and the patient involuntarily flexes the knees and hips to relieve the back pain	Dural or meningeal irritation Nerve root involvement
Beevor's sign	The patient lies in supine position and crosses the arms in front of the chest. The examiner then asks the patient to raise the trunk slightly off the couch and carefully observes the umbilicus.	Movement in a cranial or caudal direction or to the side	Denervation of the contralateral muscles

Table 6.4

Special tests for thoracic spine examination

Data from Saberi & Syed (1999), Baxter (2003), Ombregt (2013)

Thoracic spine muscles

Name	Origin	Insertion	Action	Nerve supply
Trapezius	Medial third of superior nuchal line, external occipital protuberance, ligamentum nuchae, spinous processes and supraspinous ligaments of C1–T12	Lateral third of clavicle, acromion and crest of spine of scapula, medial portion of spine of scapula	Elevates, retracts, depresses the scapula Rotation of scapula during arm elevation	Accessory nerve (C3–C4)
Latissimus dorsi	Spinous processes of thoracic T6–T12, thoracolumbar fascia, iliac crest and inferior 3 or 4 ribs	Floor of bicipital groove of humerus	Extends, adducts and medially rotates the arm. Draws the shoulder downward and backward. Keeps the inferior angle of the scapula against the ribcage; accessory muscle of respiration	Thoracodorsal nerve
Rhomboid major	Spinous processes of T2–T5 vertebrae	Medial border of scapula, inferior to insertion of rhomboid minor muscle	Retracts the scapula and rotates it to depress the glenoid cavity. Also fixes the scapula to the thoracic wall	Dorsal scapular nerve (C4–C5)
Rhomboid minor	Nuchal ligaments and spinous processes of C7–T1 vertebrae	Medial border of scapula, superior to insertion of rhomboid major muscle	Retracts the scapula and rotates it to depress the glenoid cavity. Also fixes the scapula to the thoracic wall	Dorsal scapular nerve (C4–C5)
Splenius cervicis	Spinous processes of T3–T6	Transverse processes of C1–C3	As a pair, they extend the head and neck Singly, they laterally flex and rotate the neck	Lateral branches of dorsal primary divisions of middle and lower cervical nerves
Splenius capitis	Ligamentum nuchae, spinous processes of C7–T6	Mastoid process and superior nuchal line	Extend, rotate and laterally flex the head	Lateral branches of dorsal primary division of middle and lower cervical nerves
Iliocostalis cervicis	Angles of third to sixth ribs	Transverse processes of C4–C6	Extension and lateral flexion of the neck	Dorsal primary division of spinal nerves

(Continued)

Name	Origin	Insertion	Action	Nerve supply
Iliocostalis thoracis	Angles of ribs 7–12	Angles of ribs 1–6 and transverse process of C7	Extension and lateral flexion of the spine Rotates the ribs for inspiration	Dorsal primary division of spinal nerves
Longissimus cervicis	Transverse processes of T1–T5	Transverse processes of C2–C6	Extension and lateral flexion of the neck	Dorsal primary division of spinal nerves
Longissimus capitis	Transverse processes of T1–T5, articular processes of C5–C7	Posterior part of mastoid process of temporal bone	Extends and rotates the head	Dorsal primary division of middle and lower cervical nerves
Longissimus thoracis	Lateral and medial crests of sacrum, medial portion of iliac crest, spinous processes of L1–L5 and T11–T12	Transverse process of T1–T12	Extension and lateral flexion of the spine Inspiration	Dorsal primary division of spinal nerves
Semispinalis thoracis	Transverse processes of T6–T10	Spinous processes of C6–C7 and T1–T4	Extends and rotates the vertebral column	Dorsal primary division of spinal nerves
Semispinalis cervicis	Transverse processes of T1–T6	Spinous processes of C2–C5	Extends and rotates the vertebral column	Dorsal primary division of spinal nerves
Semispinalis capitis (& spinalis capitis, medial part of semispinalis capitis)	Transverse processes of C4–C7 and T1–T7	Between the superior and inferior nuchal lines of occipital bone	Extends and rotates the neck	Dorsal primary division of spinal nerves
Spinalis thoracis	Spinous processes of T11–T12 and L1–L2	Spinous process of T1–T8	Extends the spine	Dorsal primary division of spinal nerves
Multifidus (thoracic division)	Transverse processes of T1–T12	Spinous process two to four vertebrae superior to origin	Extends and rotates the spine	Dorsal primary division of spinal nerves
Rotatores (thoracic division)	Transverse processes of T1–T12	Base of spinous process of next vertebra above	Extends and rotates the spine	Dorsal primary division of spinal nerves
Interspinales (thoracic division)	Spinous processes of T1–T3 and vertebrae of T11–T12	Spinous process of next vertebra above	Extends the spine	Dorsal primary division of spinal nerves

(Continued)

Name	Origin	Insertion	Action	Nerve supply
Intertranscersarii posterior (thoracic division)	Transverse process of T11–L1	Transverse process of next vertebra above	Laterally flexes the spine	Ventral primary division of spinal nerves
Levatores costarum	Transverse process of C7 and T1–T11	Laterally to superior surface of next rib below	Raises the ribs in inspiration and extends, laterally flexes and rotates the spine	Intercostal nerves

Table 6.5
Thoracic spine muscles

Techniques: thoracic spine

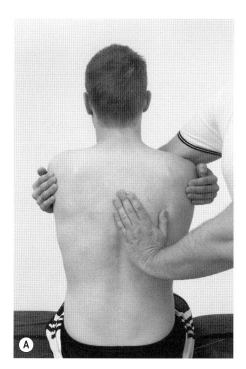

T6.1 Seated hand position

- Ask the patient to sit on the side of the plinth, as far back as possible.
- Ask the patient to hold their shoulders with one arm under the other, forming a V rather than crossing and forming a W with their arms (see photograph **a**).
- Standing behind the patient, assume a split side stance with your knees slightly flexed.
- To ensure close contact with the patient, position your axilla over the patient's shoulder and hold on to the patient's elbow (as shown in photograph **b**).
- Have your chest in close contact with the hip of the patient.
- Palpate over the spinous process of the desired segment you are examining.

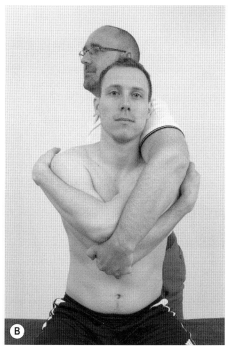

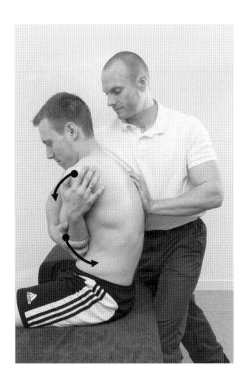

T6.2 Seated flexion of the thoracic spine

- Ask the patient to sit on the side of the plinth, as far back as possible.
- Please refer to technique T6.1 Seated hand position, photographs **a** and **b**, for the starting position.
- While supporting the patient, ask them to relax into you.
- From the starting position, apply pressure on to the lower elbow in an inferior direction towards the patient, causing the patient to slump, thus inducing flexion in the thoracic spine.

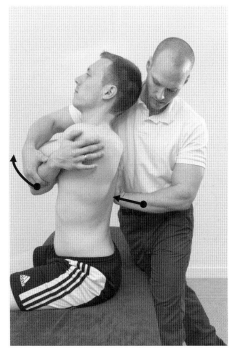

T6.3 Seated extension of the thoracic spine

- Ask the patient to sit on the side of the plinth, as far back as possible.
- Please refer to technique T6.1 Seated hand position, photographs **a** and **b**, for the starting position.
- While supporting the patient, ask them to relax into you.
- From the starting position, lift through the elbows by lifting and straightening up through your body, thus inducing extension in the thoracic spine (as shown in the photograph).
- To aid local extension, apply segmental pressure over or slightly to the side of the spinous process of the segment you wish to influence.

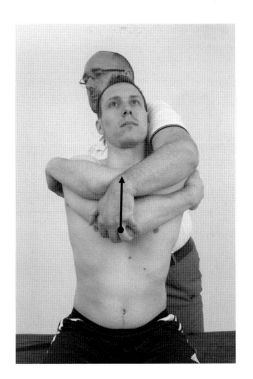

T6.4 Seated extension of the thoracic spine

- Ask the patient to sit on the side of the plinth, as far back as possible.
- Please refer to technique T6.1 Seated hand position, photographs **a** and **b**, for the starting position.
- While supporting the patient, ask them to relax into you.
- From the starting position, lift through the elbows by lifting and straightening up through your body, thus inducing extension in the thoracic spine (as shown in the photograph).
- To aid local extension, apply segmental pressure over or slightly to the side of the spinous process of the segment you wish to influence.

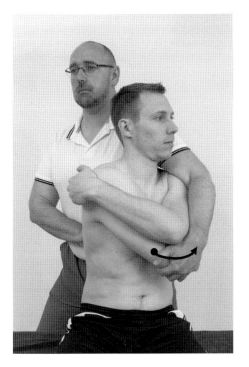

T6.5 Seated rotation of the thoracic spine

- Ask the patient to sit on the side of the plinth, as far back as possible.
- Please refer to technique T6.1 Seated hand position, photographs **a** and **b**, for the starting position.
- While supporting the patient, ask them to relax into you.
- Turn and rotate your body towards the plinth, keeping a close and positive contact with the patient, thus inducing thoracic rotation within the patient.
- In order to assess rotation bilaterally, this examination is repeated by alternating your hand and rotating from the alternate direction.

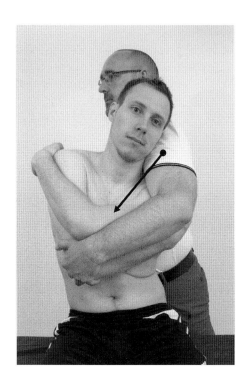

T6.6 Seated side bending of the thoracic spine

- Ask the patient to sit on the side of the plinth, as far back as possible.
- Please refer to technique T6.1 Seated hand position, photographs **a** and **b**, for the starting position.
- While supporting the patient, ask them to relax into you.
- Apply force in an oblique downward direction towards the patient's opposite anterior superior iliac spine, using the axilla on your opposite side while flexing your knees to introduce thoracic side bending.
- In order to assess rotation bilaterally, this examination is repeated by alternating your hand and rotating from the alternate direction.

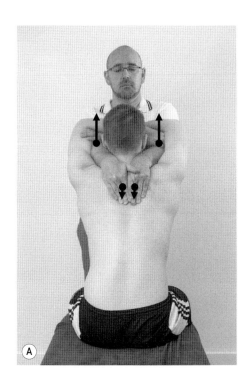

T6.7 Reinforced seated extension of the upper thoracic spine

- Seat the patient facing you.
- Ask the patient to fold their arms and rest their forehead on their forearms.
- Stand with a split stance.
- Reach through and under the patient's folded arms.
- Locate the segment of interest with your finger pads and contact either side of the spinous process.
- Using your own body weight to assist the movement, gently lean back and straighten your legs, directing the force up and posteriorly through your body to encourage extension (refer to photograph **b**).
- To focalize the extension, apply positive pressure through your finger pads either side of the patient's spine.

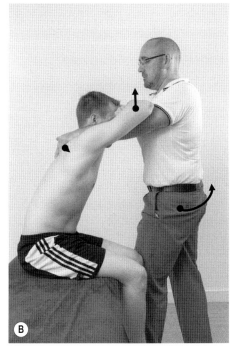

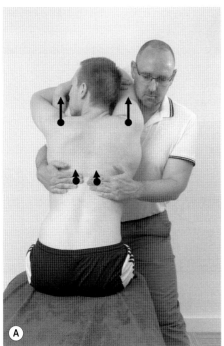

T6.8 Seated reinforced extension of the lower thoracic spine

- Seat the patient facing you.
- Stand with a split stance.
- Ask the patient to fold their arms and rest their head on their forearms with their head turned away from you.
- Rest the patient's folded arms on your shoulder (you may wish to place a towel or pillow over your shoulder for the patient to rest on).
- Locate the segment of interest with your finger pads and contact either side of the spinous process.
- Using your own body weight to assist the movement, gently lean back and straighten your legs, directing the force up and posteriorly through your body to encourage extension (refer to photograph **b**).
- To focalize the extension, apply positive pressure through your finger pads either side of the patient's spine.

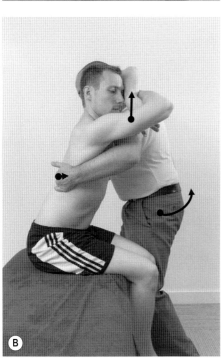

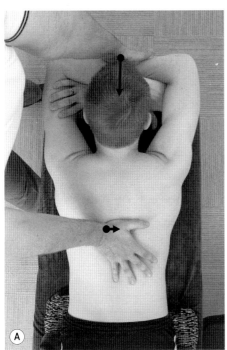

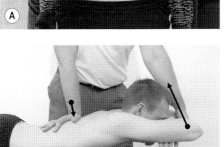

T6.9 Prone extension of the thoracic spine

- Lay the patient in the prone position.
- Ask the patient to fold their arms and rest their forehead on their uppermost forearm.
- Stand to the side of the plinth, level with the patient's head.
- Grasp the patient's forearm in the middle where the patient's forearms cross.
- To enable thoracic extension, lift up through the forearms by leaning back, thus raising the forearms off the plinth (refer to photograph **b**).
- To focalize the extension, apply positive pressure on to the patient through your lower hand that is palpating the spine.

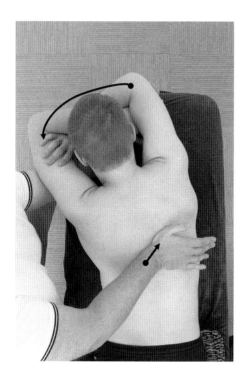

T6.10 Prone side bending of the thoracic spine

- Lay the patient in the prone position.
- Ask the patient to fold their arms and rest their forehead on their uppermost forearm.
- Stand to the side of the plinth, level with the patient's head.
- Place your forearm under the patient's forearms, grasping the furthest elbow.
- Pull and rotate through the forearms in an arcing movement to induce side bending through the thoracic spine.
- To focalize the side bending, apply positive pressure on to the patient through your lower hand that's palpating the spine on the area to the side of the spinous process, thus blocking the movement of the lower vertebrae of the joint you wish to articulate.

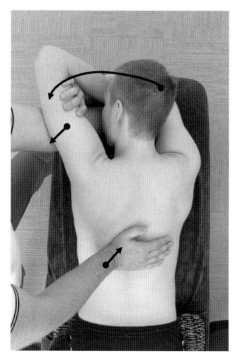

T6.11 Prone rotation of the thoracic spine

- Lay the patient in the prone position.
- Ask the patient to fold their arms and rest their forehead on their forearms.
- Stand to the side of the plinth, level with the patient's head.
- Place your forearm under the patient's forearms, grasping the furthest elbow.
- To generate rotation, lift the elbow closest to you via straightening your own posture, while pulling through the opposite elbow.
- To focalize the rotation, apply positive pressure through your lower hand on the area of the transverse process of the upper vertebrae of the joint you wish to articulate.

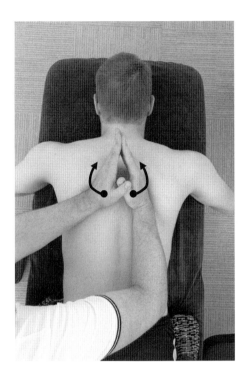

T6.12 Prone anterior/posterior articulation of the thoracic spine

- Ask the patient to lie face down.
- Using the contact of the hypothenar (ulnar border of your hand), contact over the area of the transverse processes, either side of the spinous process.
- Initially compress down on to the patient with your hands.
- While radially deviating your hands, apply a superior/anterior force (direction in relation to the patient) to compress through the thoracic spine, thus causing an anterior/posterior shift through the segment you wish to articulate.

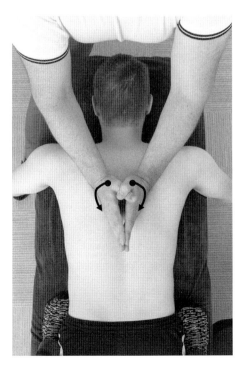

T6.13 Prone extension articulation of the thoracic spine

- Ask the patient to lie face down.
- Using the contact of the hypothenar (ulnar border of your hand), contact over the area of the transverse processes, either side of the spinous process.
- Initially compress down on to the patient with your hands.
- While radially deviating your hands, apply an inferior/anterior force (direction in relation to the patient) to compress through the thoracic spine, thus causing an extension shift through the segment you wish to mobilize.

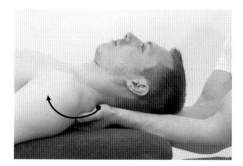

T6.14 Supine articulation of the upper thoracic spine

- Lay the patient supine.
- Place one hand under either side of the shoulder.
- With your finger pads, palpate either side of the spinous process of the upper thoracic spine.
- Using an inferior anterior movement with your hands creates local extension to the upper thoracic spine.
- Try variations of local rotation and side bending to help aid the articulation at the segmental level and to help focalize to either the left or right side.

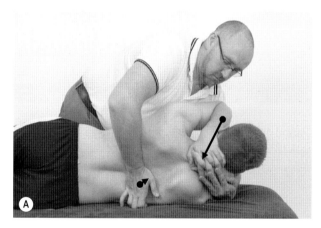

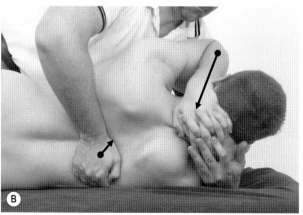

T6.15 Side-lying thoracic extension

- Lay the patient on their side.
- Ask the patient to interlace their fingers behind their neck.
- Place your hand around the patient's interlaced fingers while supporting under the patient's forearm and elbow.
- Using your lower hand as a fulcrum, apply positive compression to the inferior spinous process of the segment you wish to articulate.
- A forward movement of your body will create a backward movement of the patient's upper body, thus creating an extension in the patient's thoracic spine.

REFERENCES

Altman RD, Brown M, Gargano F (1987). Low back pain in Paget's disease of bone. Clinical Orthopaedics and Related Research 217:152-161.

Barnett GH, Hardy RW Jr, Little JR et al (1987). Thoracic spinal canal stenosis. Journal of Neurosurgery 66(3):338-344.

Baxter RE (2003). Pocket Guide to Musculoskeletal Assessment. Philadelphia: WB Saunders.

Borenstein D, Wiesel S (1989). Low Back Pain. Philadelphia: Saunders.

Briggs AM, Bragge P, Smith AJ et al (2009a). Prevalence and associated factors for thoracic spine pain in the adult working population: a literature review. Journal of Occupational Health 51(3):177-192.

Briggs AM, Smith AJ, Straker LM et al (2009b). Thoracic spine pain in the general population: prevalence, incidence and associated factors in children, adolescents and adults. A systematic review. BMC Musculoskeletal Disorders 10(1):77.

Bullough PG, Boachie-Adjei O (1988). Atlas of Spinal Diseases. Philadelphia: Lippincott.

Cleland JA, Glynn P, Whitman JM et al (2007). Short-term effects of thrust versus nonthrust mobilization/manipulation directed at the thoracic spine in patients with neck pain: a randomized clinical trial. Physical Therapy 87(4):431-440.

Conti P, Pansini G, Mouchaty H et al (2004). Spinal neurinomas: retrospective analysis and long-term outcome of 179 consecutively operated cases and review of the literature. Surgical Neurology 61(1):34-43.

Dell'Atti C, Cassar-Pullicino VN, Lalam RK et al (2007). The spine in Paget's disease. Skeletal Radiology 36 (7):609-626.

Dionne CE, Bourbonnnais R, Frémont P et al (2007). Determinants of 'return to work in good health' among workers with back pain who consult in primary care settings: a 2-year prospective study. European Spine Journal 16(5):641-655.

Duprey S, Subit D, Guillemot H et al (2010). Biomechanical properties of the costovertebral joint. Medical Engineering and Physics 32(2):222-227.

Edmondston SJ, Singer KP (1997). Thoracic spine: anatomical and biomechanical considerations for manual therapy. Manual Therapy 2(3):132-143.

Fryer G, Carub J, McIver S. (2004). The effect of manipulation and mobilization on pressure pain thresholds in the thoracic spine. Journal of Osteopathic Medicine 7(1):8-14.

Garg RK, Somvanshi DS (2011). Spinal tuberculosis: a review. The Journal of Spinal Cord Medicine 34(5):440-454.

Gautier-Smith PC (1967). Clinical aspects of spinal neurofibromas. Brain 90(2):359-394.

Grimmer K, Nyland L, Milanese S (2006). Repeated measures of recent headache, neck and upper back pain in Australian adolescents. Cephalalgia 26(7):843-851.

Hakala, P, Rimpelä A, Salminen JJ et al (2002). Back, neck, and shoulder pain in Finnish adolescents: national cross sectional surveys. British Medical Journal 325(7367):743.

Hakala PT, Saarni LA, Punamäki RL et al (2012). Musculoskeletal symptoms and computer use among Finnish adolescents – pain intensity and inconvenience to everyday life: a cross-sectional study. BMC Musculoskeletal Disorders 13(1):41.

Honet JC, Ellenberg MR (2003). What you always wanted to know about the history and physical examination of neck pain but were afraid to ask. Physical Medicine and Rehabilitation Clinics of North America 14(3):473-491.

Imagama S, Hasegawa Y, Wakao N et al (2014). Impact of spinal alignment and back muscle strength on shoulder range of motion in middle-aged and elderly people in a prospective cohort study. European Spine Journal 23(7):1414-1419.

Jansson KÅ, Blomqvist P, Svedmark P et al (2010). Thoracolumbar vertebral fractures in Sweden: an analysis of 13,496 patients admitted to hospital. European Journal of Epidemiology 25(6):431-437.

Jeffries LJ, Milanese SF, Grimmer-Somers KA (2007). Epidemiology of adolescent spinal pain: a systematic overview of the research literature. Spine 32(23):2630-2637.

Kostuik J, Huler R, Esses S et al (1991). Thoracolumbar spine fracture. In: The Adult Spine: Principles and Practice. Raven Press.

Kujala UM, Taimela S, Viljanen T (1999). Leisure physical activity and various pain symptoms among adolescents. British Journal of Sports Medicine 33(5):325-328.

Lafond D, Descarreaux M, Normand MC et al (2007). Postural development in school children: a cross-sectional study. Chiropractic and Manual Therapies 15(1):1.

Lang N, Yuan HS, Wang HL et al (2013). Epidemiological survey of ossification of the ligamentum flavum in thoracic spine: CT imaging observation of 993 cases. European Spine Journal 22(4):857-862.

Leahy M, Rahm M (2007). Thoracic spine fractures and dislocations. eMedicine 12. Available from: http://emedicine.medscape.com/article/1267029-overview#a04 [Accessed 31 January 2016].

Lemole GM Jr, Bartolomei J, Henn JS et al (2002). Thoracic Fractures. In: AR Vaccaro ed. Fractures of the Cervical, Thoracic, and Lumbar Spine. New York: CRC Press.

Linton SJ, Hellsing AL, Halldén K (1998). A population-based study of spinal pain among 35–45-year-old individuals: prevalence, sick leave, and health care use. Spine 23(13):1457-1463.

Macdonald AJR (1986). An Introduction to Medical Manipulation: JK Paterson and L Burn, MTP Press, Lancaster. (A review.)

McKenzie R, May S (2006). The Cervical and Thoracic Spine: Mechanical Diagnosis and Therapy, 2nd ed. Two-volume set. Orthopedic Physical Therapy Products.

McRae R (2010). Clinical Orthopaedic Examination. Oxford: Elsevier Health Sciences; 89-120.

Manchikanti L, Boswell MV, Singh V et al (2004). Prevalence of facet joint pain in chronic spinal pain of cervical, thoracic, and lumbar regions. BMC Musculoskeletal Disorders 5(1):15.

Moore K, Dalley AF, Agur AM (2013). Clinically Oriented Anatomy. Philadelphia: Lippincott Williams & Wilkins.

Murphy S, Buckle P, Stubbs D (2004). Classroom posture and self-reported back and neck pain in schoolchildren. Applied Ergonomics 35(2):113-120.

Nachemson A, Vingard E (2000). Assessment of patients with neck and back pain: a best-evidence synthesis. In: A Nachemson, E Jonsson eds. Neck and Back Pain: The Scientific Evidence of Causes, Diagnosis, and Treatment. Philadelphia: Lippincott Williams & Wilkins.

Ombregt L (2003). The thoracic spine – disorders of the thoracic spine: non-disc lesions. In: L Ombregt, P Bisschop, HJ ter Veer eds. A System of Orthopaedic Medicine, 2nd ed. Edinburgh: Churchill Livingstone.

Ombregt L. (2013). Clinical examination of the thoracic spine. In: A System of Orthopaedic Medicine. Edinburgh: Elsevier Health Sciences.

Pal GP, Routal RV, Saggu SK (2001). The orientation of the articular facets of the zygapophyseal joints at the cervical and upper thoracic region. Journal of Anatomy 198(04):431-441.

Papadopoulou D, Malliou P, Kofotolis N et al (2013). The association between grade, gender, physical activity, and back pain among children carrying schoolbags. Archives of Exercise in Health and Disease 4(1):234-242.

Putz RV, Muller-Gerbil M (2000). Ligaments of the human vertebral column. In: KP Singer, LGF Giles eds. The Clinical Anatomy and Management of Thoracic Spine Pain. London: Butterworth–Heinemann.

Saberi A, Syed SA (1999). Meningeal signs: Kernig's sign and Brudzinski's sign. Hospital Physician 35:23-26.

Scheuermann H (1934). Roentgenologic studies of the origin and development of juvenile kyphosis, together with some investigations concerning the vertebral epiphyses in man and in animals. Acta Orthopaedica 5(1-4):161-220.

Selanne H, Ryba TV, Siekkinen K et al (2014). The prevalence of musculoskeletal pain and use of painkillers among adolescent male ice hockey players in Finland. Health Psychology and Behavioral Medicine: an Open Access Journal 2(1):448-454.

Sheir-Neiss GI, Kruse RW, Rahman T et al (2003). The association of backpack use and back pain in adolescents. Spine 28(9):922-930.

Singer KP, Edmondston SJ (2000). Introduction: the enigma of thoracic spine. In: KP Singer, LGF Giles eds. The Clinical Anatomy and Management of Thoracic Spine Pain. London: Butterworth–Heinemann.

Singer KP, Goh S (2000). Anatomy of the thoracic spine. In: KP Singer, LGF Giles eds. The Clinical Anatomy and Management of Thoracic Spine Pain. London: Butterworth–Heinemann.

Skaggs DL, Early SD, D'Ambra P et al (2006). Back pain and backpacks in school children. Journal of Pediatric Orthopaedics 26(3):358-363.

Ståhl MK, El-Metwally AA, Rimpelä AH (2014). Time trends in single versus concomitant neck and back pain in Finnish adolescents: results from national cross-sectional surveys from 1991 to 2011. BMC Musculoskeletal Disorders 15(1):296.

Trevelyan FC, Legg SJ (2006). Back pain in school children–where to from here? Applied Ergonomics 37(1):45-54.

Turgut M (2001). Spinal tuberculosis (Pott's disease): its clinical presentation, surgical management, and outcome. A survey study on 694 patients. Neurosurgical Review 24(1):8-13.

Valencia F (1994). Clinical anatomy and biomechanics of the thoracic spine. In: JD Boyling, N Palastanga eds. Grieve's Modem Manual Therapy. Edinburgh: Churchill Livingstone.

Wedderkopp N, Leboeuf-Yde C, Andersen LB et al (2001). Back pain reporting pattern in a Danish population-based sample of children and adolescents. Spine 26(17):1879-1883.

White AA III (1969). Analysis of the mechanics of the thoracic spine in man: an experimental study of autopsy specimens. Acta Orthopaedica 40(127):1-105.

White AA, Panjabi MM (1978). Clinical Biomechanics of the Spine. Philadelphia: JB Lippincott Company.

Wigh RE (1980). Classification of the human vertebral column: phylogenetic departures and junctional anomalies. Medical Radiography and Photography 56(1):2-11.

Zapata AL, Moraes AJP, Leone C et al (2006). Pain and musculoskeletal pain syndromes related to computer and video game use in adolescents. European Journal of Pediatrics 165(6):408-414.

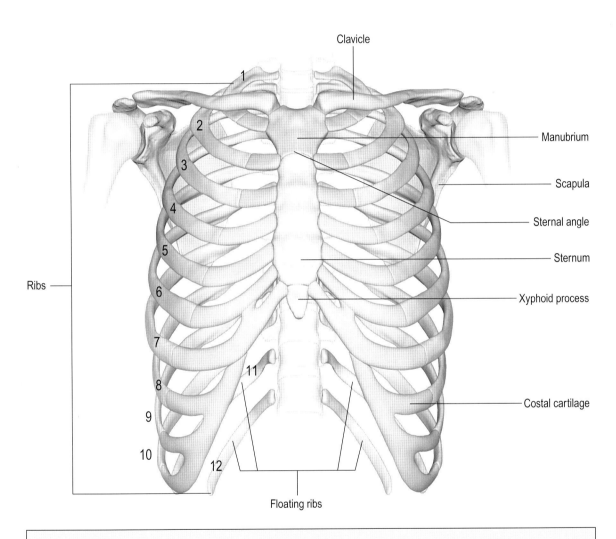

Clavicle

Manubrium

Scapula

Sternal angle

Sternum

Xyphoid process

Ribs

Costal cartilage

Floating ribs

1
2
3
4
5
6
7
8
9
10
11
12

Figure 7.1
Bones of the human thorax, showing the ribcage

The ribcage

Introduction

Along with injuries to the thoracic spine, rib musculoskeletal injuries have been researched in less depth than injuries to other areas. But injuries to the ribs are not uncommon, particularly in athletes, where they can be caused by repetitive and extreme forces put through the ribcage during exercise. Rowers, for example, are at risk of rib fractures, and it is interesting that the incidence in elite rowers is higher than in amateur rowers (McDonnell et al 2011). Rib fractures are not restricted among sports players to rowers, however, and they can occur in golfers (Bugbee 2010), lacrosse players (Wild et al 2011), weightlifters (Eng et al 2008, Miller 2015), individuals involved in martial arts, and boxers (Gartland et al 2001, Zazryn et al 2006), and in any sport that has an impact component, such as rugby and American football (Feeley et al 2008, Brooks & Kemp 2011). Although less common, rib fractures have also been reported in swimmers (Chaudhury et al 2012, Heincelman et al 2014), possibly caused by high repetitive strains placed upon the ribcage during overhand swimming motions. Not caused exclusively by repetitive loading during sporting activities, fractures of the ribs can also be caused by occupational stresses, such as in manual labor (Miller et al 2013).

Fractures are not the only ribcage injury that can occur in athletes or individuals with manual occupations. Another is intercostal muscle strain, again frequently seen as a result of sporting activities, including baseball (Stevens et al 2010, Conte et al 2012), cricket (Cam et al 2006, Milsom et al 2007), tennis (Maquirriain & Ghisi 2006, García & Ros 2011) and football (Durandt et al 2009). These sports all involve forced and repetitive rotation of the thorax, which predisposes a patient to suffer with costal and intercostal symptoms. For safety reasons, the therapist must always rule out the possibility of a fracture before proceeding with examination and treatment of any patient presenting with these symptoms.

Chest problems are extremely widespread. It has been projected that, by 2020, chronic obstructive pulmonary disease (COPD) will be the fourth-highest cause of death (Patel & Hurst 2011). The current cost to the NHS in the United Kingdom is estimated to be over £800 million a year, and this figure is set to rise as life expectancy increases (Fromer 2011). Manual therapy in the form of physiotherapy for pulmonary rehabilitation, physical exercise and hands-on treatment is a mainstay in respiratory wards in hospitals (Benzo et al 2000, Hondras et al 2005). The principal aims of this therapy are to encourage fluid dynamics (i.e. the movement of mucus within the lung and airways) and to increase lung capacity. This is attempted by the use of several different types of breathing technique (Thomas et al 2009, Bruton et al 2011). Although research seems to support the beneficial use of breathing exercises, studies into the effectiveness of manual therapy and treatment of COPD have so far proved inconclusive. There has been some research into the effects of osteopathic and chiropractic treatments on COPD, but most of this is based on manipulation of the thoracic spine and costotransverse joints rather than the ribcage. Some of the treatments may be effective in helping some of the conditions associated with COPD, but most of the evidence to date is anecdotal or not statistically significant (Noll et al 2000, Hondras et al 2005, Ernst 2009a, 2009b, Kaminskyj et al 2010, Heneghan et al 2012, Engel et al 2014).

Bony anatomy

The ribcage, also called the thoracic cage, is an osteocartilaginous frame in the thorax that forms a core portion of the human skeletal system. It shields the vital organs of the body, provides attachment sites for muscles, and forms a semi-rigid chamber that can expand and contract during respiration (White & Folkens 2005). Anatomically, the ribcage is an arrangement of bones and cartilages that encloses the chest cavity and supports the shoulder girdle and upper extremities. Structurally, it appears broad below, narrow above, longer behind and flattened anteroposteriorly (Datta 1994).

A ribcage is typically made up of 12 pairs of ribs with their costal cartilages, the sternum and the 12 thoracic vertebrae (Mader 2004). Men and women usually have the same number of ribs; a few reports have identified an anatomical variation in the number of ribs, but most of those were associated with a variation in the number of thoracic vertebrae. Each pair of ribs is symmetrically in articulation with a thoracic vertebra on the right and left side. The sternum consists of the manubrium (prosternum), an intermediate body (mesosternum or body) and xiphoid process (metasternum) (see Figure 7.1). At the chest, many of the ribs are connected to the sternum via costal cartilages (Joshua et al 2014).

The ribs

The ribs are long, curved bones with a rounded and a flattened end. The rounded ends (head of the rib) articulate posteriorly with the T1–T12 thoracic vertebrae via a synovial joint articulation; most of the flattened ends attach anteriorly to the sternum via costal cartilages. These cartilages are hyaline in type and can extend for a few inches/centimeters (Open-Stax 2013).

The ribs are divided into two groups based on their anterior and posterior attachments. Anteriorly, the ribs are classified into two further groups: **true and false ribs**. The first seven pairs of ribs (1–7) are called the true ribs, or the vertebrosternal ribs, because they attach directly via their costal cartilages to the sternum. The next five pairs of ribs (8–12) are called the false ribs, or vertebrochondral ribs, because they do not attach directly to the sternum. Ribs 8–10 are attached indirectly to the sternum, as their costal cartilages ventrally attach to the cartilage of the ribs above. The last two pairs of false ribs (11–12) are known as floating ribs, or vertebral ribs, because they do not attach to the sternum at all (Mader 2004).

Posteriorly, the ribs are classified as **typical and atypical ribs**. Ribs 3–9 are classified as typical ribs, and ribs 1, 2 and 10–12 are atypical. The typical ribs have similarities in their structure. The head, or the posterior end, of a typical rib articulates with two costal facets on the bodies of two adjacent vertebrae and the intervertebral disc between them. The superior rib facet articulates with the costal demifacet on the body of the next higher vertebra, and the inferior rib facet attaches with the costal demifacet of the same numbered thoracic vertebra (Warwick 1973). The tubercle, a small bump on the posterior rib surface, attaches to the transverse process of the same vertebra. The neck of a typical rib is narrow and is between the head and tubercle. The remainder is the body, or shaft, of the rib. Just lateral to the tubercle is the angle of the rib, which is the point of greatest curvature (Cropper 1996).

The atypical ribs have structural features that are very different from the typical ribs. Apart from rib 2, all of the atypical ribs have only one demifacet on their head for articulation. Rib 2 is considered atypical because it attaches to the junction of the manubrium and the body of the sternum (Bourdillon et al 1992).

The sternum

The sternum, or breastbone, is an elongated bony structure that is slightly concave posteriorly and convex anteriorly. It is composed of three bones: the **manubrium**, the **body**, and the **xiphoid process**. Structurally, the sternum bears a resemblance to a sword, with the manubrium forming the superior portion (the handle), the body forming the central portion (the blade), and the xiphoid process forming the inferior and smallest portion (the tip) (Tate 2009).

At the top of the manubrium, there is a shallow depression, a U-shaped border, called the jugular (suprasternal) notch. This can easily be found at the anterior base of the neck, between the medial ends of the clavicles where they attach to the sternum (Open-Stax 2013). At the junction of the manubrium and the body, there is a slight ridge, called the sternal angle. This joint is a vital anatomical landmark because rib 2 articulates with the sternum at the sternal angle; as a result, it allows the ribs to be counted (Mader 2004).

The body is the middle and longest region of the sternum. It is wider inferiorly than superiorly and is flatter than the manubrium. The xiphoid process is the most inferior region of the sternum. It is cartilaginous early in life, but gradually becomes ossified in adulthood. The xiphoid process functions as a site of attachment for the diaphragm (Cropper 1996).

The manubrium attaches to the costal cartilages of ribs 1 and 2; the body connects the costal cartilages of ribs 2 to 10; the xiphoid process has no attachment with any ribs (Mader 2004).

Range of motion

The ribcage provides the thoracic mobility required for breathing. This mobility is attributable to the sternal and vertebral joints and the costal cartilages at either end of the rib structure. More precisely, movements of ribs primarily rely on the orientation of costovertebral and costotransverse joints, which are subjected to continual movement. Apart from its contribution during respiration, the ribcage can undergo movement if a misfit occurs at the costovertebral joint surfaces or external forces are applied to the chest, such as traumatic loading of the chest and cardiopulmonary resuscitation (Yoganandan & Pintar 1998).

The movements of the ribs are normally around two axes. The upper rib motion resembles a 'pump handle' and the lower rib motion resembles a 'bucket handle'. The axis for rib motion is represented as a line running between the costovertebral joint and the costotransverse joint via the rib neck. The axis for upper rib rotation (ribs 2–6) orients toward the frontal plane, whereas the lower ribs (excluding ribs 11 and 12) lie more toward the sagittal plane. Movement at the upper ribs about a side-to-side axis therefore results in elevation and depression of the sternal end of the rib. Conversely, motion of the lower ribs about an anteroposterior axis raises and lowers the middle of the rib (Cropper 1996).

Epidemiology

Rib fractures are one of the most common injuries to the chest, occurring in approximately 10% of all patients admitted after blunt trauma (Liman et al 2003). Melendez and Doty (2015) suggest that rib fractures account for over 50% of all thoracic injuries from non-penetrating trauma. They are usually uncommon in children of all ages, accounting for only 1% of all fractures in children (Hedström et al 2010). In ex-preterm infants, the prevalence of rib fractures in contemporary tertiary neonatal centers is approximately 2% (Lucas-Herald et al 2012).

The rate of multiple rib fractures is higher in adults than children. In a retrospective cohort study, Kessel et al (2014) found 11% of adults suffered from isolated rib fractures without associated injuries compared to 5.8% of children. More adults had four or more rib fractures than children did. However, the study reported a slightly higher mortality rate in children compared with adults (5.18% in children and 4.93% in adults).

The overall incidence of associated injuries, including brain and solid organ injuries, pneumothorax or hemothorax and lung contusion, in children is significantly higher than in adults. In adults, motor vehicle accidents were found to be the most common mechanism of injury; in children the most common mechanisms of injuries were pedestrian hit by car, bicycle accidents and child abuse (Bergeron et al 2003, Sirmali et al 2003).

In elderly people (age 65 or over), rib fractures are the most common non-spine fractures. Barrett-Connor and colleagues (2010) reported that the annual incidence of rib fracture was 3.5 per 1000 individuals, accounting for 24% of all non-spine fractures. Nearly 50% of the fractures reported resulted from falling from standing height or lower. The study also suggested a number of independent risk factors for rib fractures. These include a baseline history of rib or chest fracture, low bone density, difficulty in activities of daily living with instruments, and age 80 or above.

Common pathological conditions of the ribcage are shown in Table 7.1.

Ribcage examination
Medical history

While examining the ribcage of the patient, taking a detailed medical history of the patient's past and present problems is as essential as the physical examination itself. In most cases, the narrative provided by the patient consists of information critical to narrowing the differential diagnosis and facilitating the physical examination.

Condition	Description	Reference
Costochondritis	An acute and often temporary inflammation of the cartilage that attaches a rib to the sternum May result in sharp chest pain and tenderness More than one site is affected in 90% of cases May affect any of the seven costochondral junctions Occurs most frequently in females and in people over age 40	Jindal & Singhi (2011), Flowers (2015)
Rib fracture	Often results from a direct blow to the chest, but may also occur because of coughing or forceful muscular activity of the upper limb or trunk Most frequently affects ribs 7 and 10 Occurs more predominantly in older people than in younger adults Symptoms include severe well-localized pain, pain during deep inspiration or with movement, and grating sound with breathing or movement	Ombregt (2003), Melendez & Doty (2015)
Tietze syndrome	A rare, inflammatory disorder of one or more of the costal cartilages in the superior ribs Characterized by a sudden or a gradual onset of unilateral pain and swelling of one of the costosternal synchondroses Often occurs at the second rib pair Equally prevalent in men and women Affects people of all ages, including children	Kayser (1956), Proulx & Zryd (2009)
Manubriosternal arthritis	Affects the manubriosternal joint Can occur as a result of rheumatoid arthritis or ankylosing spondylitis One of the major symptoms is spontaneous pain at the angle of Louis May show subchondral cysts, narrowing of the joint space, erosion of the joint margin and sclerosis of bone close to the joint in radiographic analysis	Sebes & Salazar (1983), Ombregt (2003)
Intercostal neuralgia	Defined as an intense, sharp, shooting or burning pain Can be caused by a traumatic or iatrogenic neuroma, persistent nerve irritation or herpes zoster (shingles) Some association with post breast and abdominal surgery	Santos et al (2005), Ducic & Larson (2006), Williams et al (2008)

Table 7.1
Common pathological conditions of the ribcage

The clinician must approach the patient in a friendly and respectful manner. They should collect the necessary information in a logical format and must listen to the patient's responses very carefully. Apart from questioning about pain, swelling, tenderness or any other issues related to the ribcage, they must inquire about the onset of the problem, behavior since onset, symptom pattern(s), and exacerbating and relieving factors.

Red flags

See Table 7.2.

Physical examination

When the history taking is done, the clinician will have enough information to make tentative decisions about certain aspects of the condition. The clinician should then carry out the physical examination. This usually involves inspection, palpation and a variety of special tests for the chest.

Inspection

The physical examination process usually starts with a careful visual inspection of the patient's ribcage. It is helpful to inspect the posterior thorax while the patient is sitting and the anterior thorax with the patient supine. The patient's gown should be suitably arranged to allow complete inspection of the anterior and posterior thorax. During inspection of the thorax, the examiner should carefully observe the shape of the chest and the movement of the chest wall. If any asymmetry or deformities (e.g. thoracoplasty, pectus carinatum, pectus excavatum, gynecomastia, scoliosis, surgical or traumatic scars) are found, they should immediately be noted. The examiner should also note whether there is an impairment or unilateral lag (or delay) in respiratory movement. Any abnormal retraction of the interspaces during inspiration should also be noted (Bickley & Szilagyi 2012).

Condition	Signs and symptoms
Myocardial infarction	Chest pain or discomfort
	Pressure or tightness in the chest
	Shortness of breath, sweating, pallor, lightheadedness, nausea or tremors
	History of a sedentary lifestyle
	Previous history of ischemic heart disease, abnormally high blood pressure, diabetes, smoking, elevated triglyceride level and hypercholesterolemia
	Age: men over 40 years and women over 50 years
	Symptoms lasting for 30–60 minutes
Pericarditis	Sharp or stabbing pain over the center or left side of the chest
	Increased pain with deep breathing, swallowing, coughing or left side lying
	Relieved with forward leaning and sitting up
	Shortness of breath, heart palpitations, fatigue, nausea
Pneumothorax	Intensified pain the chest during inspiration, ventilation, or expanding of ribcage
	Abnormally rapid breathing
	Hypotension, dyspnea or hypoxia
	Distant or absent sounds of breath
Pneumonia	Sharp and piercing chest pain while breathing or coughing
	Fever, shaking chills, headache, sweating, fatigue or nausea
	Productive cough
Fracture	Greater than 70 years of age
	Recent history of major trauma
	Prolonged use of corticosteroids
	History of osteoporosis

Table 7.2

Red flags for serious pathology in the ribcage

Data from Dutton (2012), Magee (2014)

Palpation

While palpating the chest, the examiner should first place the palm of each hand on the upper portion of the thorax and then, softly but firmly, move the hand to the lower portion, just below the twelfth rib. The examiner repeats the same procedure, moving the hands laterally and subsequently anteriorly, feeling for rib deformities, areas of tenderness, respiratory expansion and abnormalities in the overlying skin. If a patient has a history of discomfort in the thorax, the examiner should carefully palpate the area(s) where pain has been reported. This should be done with increasing firmness to assess whether the pressure repeatedly elicits tenderness. If a patient is reporting anterior chest pain, particular attention should be given to the costochondral junctions, so that the possibility of costochondritis can be evaluated (Tuteur 1990).

Special tests

See Table 7.3.

Test	Procedure	Positive sign	Interpretation
Chest expansion test	**Posterior examination:** The therapist places their thumbs near to the 10th ribs. The fingers are in parallel to the lateral ribcage, loosely grasping the lower hemithorax on either side of the axilla. The clinician then slides their hands medially just sufficient to elevate a loose skin fold on each side between their thumb and the spine. The patient is requested to breathe and expire deeply. The therapist should then observe the space between their thumbs and feel for the symmetry of movement of the hemithorax. **Anterior examination:** The therapist places their thumbs laterally to each costal margin, with their hands along the lateral ribcage. The therapist then slides their hands medially to elevate loose skin folds between their thumbs. The patient is requested to breathe and expire deeply. The therapist should then observe how far their thumbs move while the thorax expands, and feel for the depth and symmetry of the hemithorax movement.	Asymmetrical chest expansion Abnormal side expands less and lags behind the normal side	Unilateral decrease or delay in chest expansion indicates pathology on that side, such as lobar pneumonia, pleural effusion and unilateral bronchial obstruction Bilateral decrease in chest expansion usually suggests COPD or asthma
Percussion	First, the therapist places the middle finger on the surface to be percussed. The distal phalanx of that finger should be pressed firmly, avoiding contact by any other fingers or part of the hand. With a quick but relaxed wrist motion, the therapist then strikes the finger placed directly on the thorax, using the other hand's tip of the middle finger. The aim of the strike should be focused at the distal interphalangeal joint. The striking finger should quickly be withdrawn to avoid damping the vibrations. However, if the sound and the vibrations created seem unsatisfactory, the therapist should check whether the middle finger in contact with the thorax is making firm contact with the chest wall. Using the same technique, the therapist percusses the posterior, lateral and anterior chest wall of the patient. The percussion is usually done on one side of the chest and then the other side at each level. When the percussion on both sides is done, the therapist finally compares one side to the other.	Flatness, dullness or hyperresonance percussion notes	Flatness may suggest either solid or fluid material in the pleural space (e.g. fibrothorax, pleural effusion, mesothelioma and empyema) Dullness is often associated with an interstitial pulmonary process, but it may also suggest a restrictive ventilatory defect (e.g. lobar pneumonia) Generalized hyperresonance indicates hyperinflated lungs – possibly emphysema or asthma. Unilateral hyperresonance suggests a large air-filled bulla in the lung, or maybe an acute pneumothorax

(Continued)

Test	Procedure	Positive sign	Interpretation
Anterior–posterior rib compression test	For this maneuver, the patient can be in either sitting or standing position. The therapist stands laterally to the patient and places one hand on the anterior and another on the posterior aspects of the ribcage. The therapist compresses the ribcage by pushing the hands together and then releases the pressure. Anterior–posterior compression is favoured over lateral compression due to risk of pneumothorax if fracture is present.	The rib shaft being prominent in the midaxillary line Pain or point tenderness with the ribcage compression Respiratory restrictions for both inhalation and exhalation	Possibly a rib fracture, contusion or separation
Ribcage respiratory test	**Ribs 1–10:** The patient lies in supine position. The therapist palpates directly over the ribs anteriorly, particularly on the intercostal spaces. The patient is then asked to make a full inspiratory and expiratory effort. The therapist should then assess the respiratory excursion for the superior and inferior ribs. **Ribs 11 and 12:** The patient lies in prone position. The therapist's hand is symmetrically placed over the 11th and 12th ribs posteriorly. The patient once again is asked to make a full inspiratory and expiratory effort. The therapist should then palpate the movement and assess the respiratory excursion.	One group of ribs stops moving first during either inhalation or exhalation	Rib dysfunction

Table 7.3

Special tests for ribcage examination

Data from Tuteur (1990), Bookhout (1996), Fedorowski (2000), Bickley & Szilagyi (2012)

Ribcage muscles

Name	Origin	Insertion	Action	Nerve supply
Primary muscles of respiration				
Diaphragm	Sternal portion: xiphoid process Costal portion: inner surfaces of ribs 7–12 and their associated cartilage Lumbar portion: L1–L2/3 vertebral body	Central tendon	Depression of the central tendon to encourage inspiration	Phrenic nerve (C3–C5)
Serratus posterior superior	Ligamentum nuchae, spinous process of C7, T1–T3	Superior surface of ribs 2–5	Elevates the ribs in inspiration	T1–T4
Serratus posterior inferior	Spinous process of T11–T12 and L1–L3	Inferior surfaces of ribs 8–12	Depresses the ribs while resisting the action of the diaphragm	T9–T12
External intercostals	Inferior surface of ribs 1–11	Superior surface of rib below (fibers travel obliquely towards costal cartilage)	Inspiration	Intercostal nerves
Internal intercostals	From costal cartilage towards costal angle of ribs 1–11	Superior surface of rib below (fibers travel obliquely away from costal cartilage)	Expiration	Intercostal nerves
Subcostals	Interior surface of each rib near costal angle	Medially to interior surface of second or third rib inferior	Expiration	Intercostal nerves
Transversus thoracis	Interior surface of lower sternum and adjacent costal cartilage	Interior surface of costal cartilage of ribs 2–6	Expiration	Intercostal nerves
Levatores costarum	Transverse process of C7 and T1–T11	Laterally to external surface of rib below	Inspiration, extends, laterally flexes and rotates the spine	Intercostal nerves
Secondary muscles of respiration				
Serratus anterior	Fleshy slips from outer surface of upper 8 or 9 ribs	Costal aspect of medial margin of scapula	Protracts and stabilizes the scapula, assists in upward rotation	Long thoracic nerve (C5–C7)

(Continued)

Name	Origin	Insertion	Action	Nerve supply
Pectoralis major	Anterior surface of medial half of clavicle Sternocostal head: anterior surface of sternum, the superior six costal cartilages	Lateral lip of bicipital groove of humerus	Clavicular head: flexes the humerus Sternocostal head: extends the humerus As a whole: adducts and medially rotates the humerus. Also draws the scapula anteriorly and inferiorly	Lateral pectoral nerve and medial pectoral nerve Clavicular head: C5 and C6 Sternocostal head: C7, C8 and T1
Pectoralis minor	Ribs 3–5	Medial border and superior surface of coracoid process of scapula	Stabilizes the scapula by drawing it inferiorly and anteriorly against the thoracic wall	Medial pectoral nerves (C8, T1)
Subclavius	First rib	Subclavian groove of clavicle	Depresses the clavicle	Subclavian nerve C5–C6
Scalenus anterior	Transverse process of C3–C6	First rib (scalene tubercle)	When the neck is fixed: elevates the first rib to aid in breathing When the rib is fixed: bends the neck forward and sideways and rotates it to the opposite side	Ventral ramus of C5, C6
Scalenus posterior	Transverse processes of C4–C7	Second rib	Elevates the second rib, tilts the neck to the same side	C6–C8
Scalenus medius	Transverse process of C2–C7	First rib	Elevates the first rib, rotates the neck to the opposite side	Ventral rami of C3–C8
Quadratus lumborum	Superior surface of iliac crest, ilio-lumbar ligament	Inferior surface of rib 12, transverse process of L1–L4	Lateral flexion of the spine, expiration	T12–L1

Table 7.4
Ribcage muscles

Techniques: ribcage

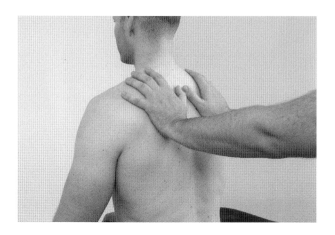

T7.1 Upper rib palpation

- With the patient seated on the plinth, stand behind the patient and identify the spinal level of the ribs you wish to palpate.
- Using both hands, place the finger pads of your thumbs adjacent to the transverse processes of the chosen segment and your hands spread over the upper ribcage.
- Ask your patient to inhale and exhale slowly and deeply. Note the quality and quantity of movement bilaterally, comparing elevation of the lateral aspects of both ribs.
- Note that the upper ribs move in a 'pump handle' movement.

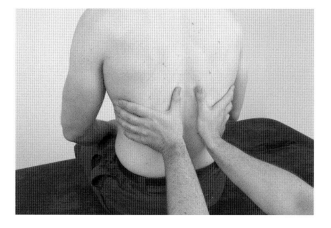

T7.2 Lower rib palpation

- With the patient seated on the plinth, stand behind the patient and identify the spinal level of the ribs you wish to palpate.
- Using both hands, place the finger pads of your thumbs adjacent to the transverse processes of the chosen segment with your fingers gently holding the thoracic cage.
- Ask your patient to inhale and exhale slowly and deeply. Note the quality and quantity of movement bilaterally, comparing elevation of the lateral aspects of both ribs.
- Note that the lower ribs move in a 'bucket handle' movement.

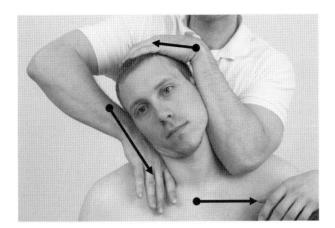

T7.3 First rib articulation

***Please also refer to technique T5.21 Cervical–
thoracic articulation in Chapter 5.***

- Position the patient seated as far back as possible on the plinth.
- Stand behind the patient with your foot on the plinth to the opposite side you wish to articulate, allowing the patient's arm and hand to rest over your thigh.
- Rest your arm on the patient's shoulder, placing your hand on the patient's forehead level with their hairline.
- Place your other hand on the base of the cervical spine. The objective is to place the side of the metacarpophalangeal joint of your little finger on the first rib to the side you are affecting.
- Raise your elbow in order to direct the movement towards the patient's opposite iliac crest.
- To articulate, shift your body towards the foot that is on the plinth and, with your hand, side-bend the patient's neck, thus articulating the first rib.
- Asking the patient to breathe out while doing the above can help enhance the technique.

T7.4 Prone lower rib articulation

- Lay the patient prone.
- With your lower hand, hold around the area of the anterior inferior iliac spine (AIIS). (If the patient finds this sensitive, a small towel can be used to 'pad' the area.)
- Using the hyperthenar (thenar) eminence to contact the posterior aspect of the rib you wish to articulate, place your upper hand just lateral to the costotransverse joint.
- Using a rotation of your body, lift and rotate the patient's pelvis towards you with an equal opposite force through your other arm on the posterior part of the ribcage.
- Asking the patient to breathe out while rotating and doing the above can help enhance the technique.

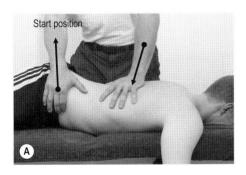

Start position

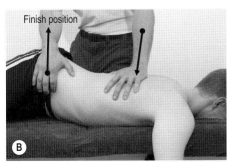

Finish position

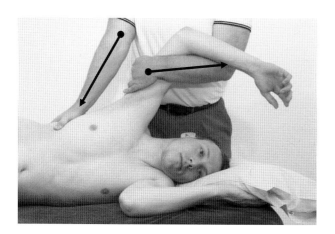

T7.5 Side-lying lower rib articulation

- With the patient lying on their side, stand behind the patient.
- Place the corresponding hand under the patient's arm, contacting above the axilla and supporting the patient's forearm.
- The opposite hand palpates over the rib angle. Palpate the rib and contact and fix on the rib.
- Maintain positive pressure with movement and stretch towards the direction of the patient's head.
- Asking the patient to breathe out while doing the above can help enhance the technique.

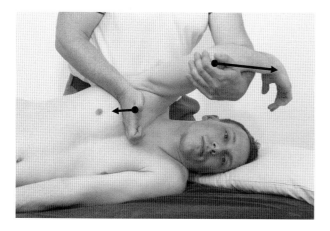

T7.6 Side-lying upper rib articulation

- Use the ulnar border of your hand as applicator, keeping your fingers into the palm.
- Place and fix the applicator hand on the upper ribs.
- Support the patient's elbow with your other hand and let their forearm rest on yours.
- The direction of the stretch is towards the patient's head, maintaining the fix on the rib.
- Reapply to stretch the intercostal muscles.
- Remember the angle of the upper ribs and its pump handle action.
- Asking the patient to breathe out while doing the above can help enhance the technique.

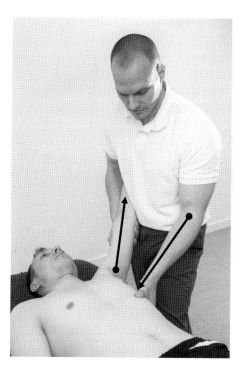

T7.7 Supine lower rib articulation

- Lie the patient on their back.
- Place the corresponding hand on the patient's forearm, which is held out straight.
- Place your other hand on the patients' ribcage.
- With the border of your index finger and thumb, palpate and fix.
- Create stretch by leaning on to your back foot and using the patient's straight arm as a lever to increase the stretch.
- Remember the angle of the ribs and the bucket handle action.
- Asking the patient to breathe out while doing the above can help enhance the technique.

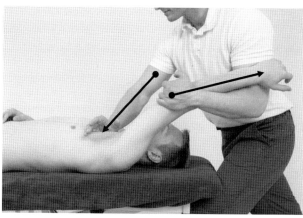

T7.8 Supine upper rib articulation

- Lie the patient on their back.
- Place one hand on the lateral aspect of the patient's elbow and allow their arm to be supported by your forearm. (In the photograph, you can see how the patient's arm is supported by the practitioner.)
- Use the ulnar border of your opposite hand as applicator. Place and fix. Take care where the hand is situated.
- The direction of the stretch is towards the patient's head, maintaining the fix on the rib.
- Provide traction and step back to create stretch while holding the position.
- Reapply to stretch the intercostal muscles.
- Asking the patient to breathe out while doing the above can help enhance the technique.

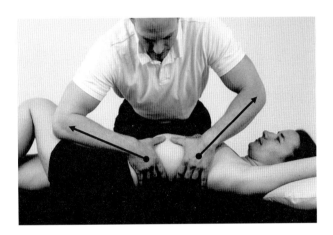

T7.9 Supine lower rib articulation 1

- Ask the patient to bend their knee on the desired side for the technique.
- On the side you are attempting to articulate, place the patient's arm above their head.
- Palpate the ribcage above and below the area you wish to articulate.
- Keep your elbows out at the sides (as demonstrated in the photograph by the practitioner).
- Use your body and stance so that, when bending your knees, the movement of your hands are away from each other as your elbows separate.
- To enhance the technique, with your elbow contacting the bent thigh, compress against the patient's side to induce rotation of the pelvis.
- Asking the patient to breathe out while doing the above can help enhance the technique.

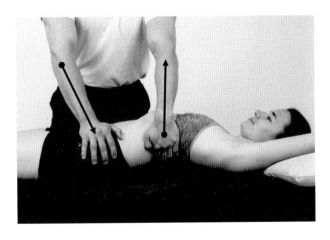

T7.10 Supine lower rib articulation 2

- Place your hand over the anterior superior iliac spine to stabilize innominate movements. (If the patient finds this area sensitive to touch, a small towel or pillow can be placed over the area before placing your hand.)
- On the side you are attempting to articulate, place the patient's arm above their head.
- Palpate the ribcage superior to the area you wish to articulate.
- Compress down with your lower hand on to the anterior superior iliac spine (ASIS) and fix down the pelvis. At the same time, rotate your body, lifting up through your other hand, thus rotating the patient's trunk and articulating the ribcage.
- Asking the patient to breathe out while doing the above can help enhance the technique.

REFERENCES

Barrett-Connor E, Nielson CM, Orwoll E et al (2010). Epidemiology of rib fractures in older men: Osteoporotic Fractures in Men (MrOS) prospective cohort study. British Medical Journal 340.

Benzo R, Flume PA, Turner D et al (2000). Effect of pulmonary rehabilitation on quality of life in patients with COPD: the use of SF-36 summary scores as outcomes measures. Journal of Cardiopulmonary Rehabilitation and Prevention 20(4):231-234.

Bergeron E, Lavoie A, Clas D et al (2003). Elderly trauma patients with rib fractures are at greater risk of death and pneumonia. Journal of Trauma and Acute Care Surgery 54(3):478-485.

Bickley L, Szilagyi PG (2012). Bates' Guide to Physical Examination and History-taking. Philadelphia: Lippincott Williams & Wilkins.

Bookhout MR (1996). Evaluation of the thoracic spine and rib cage. In: TW Flynn ed. The Thoracic Spine and Rib Cage: Musculoskeletal Evaluation and Treatment. Boston: Butterworth–Heinemann.

Bourdillon J, Day E, Bookhout M (1992). Spinal Manipulation. Oxford: Butterworth–Heinemann.

Brooks JH, Kemp SPT (2011). Injury-prevention priorities according to playing position in professional rugby union players. British Journal of Sports Medicine 45(10):765-775.

Bruton A, Garrod R, Thomas M (2011). Respiratory physiotherapy: towards a clearer definition of terminology. Physiotherapy 97(4):345-349.

Bugbee S (2010). Rib stress fracture in a golfer. Current Sports Medicine Reports 9(1):40-42.

Cam NB, Muthukumar N, Boyle S et al (2006). Rib impingement in first class cricketers: case reports of two patients who underwent rib resection. British Journal of Sports Medicine 40(8):732-733.

Chaudhury S, Hobart SJ, Rodeo SA (2012). Bilateral first rib stress fractures in a female swimmer: a case report. Journal of Shoulder and Elbow Surgery 21(3):e6-e10.

Conte SA, Thompson MM, Marks MA et al (2012). Abdominal muscle strains in professional baseball 1991–2010. The American Journal of Sports Medicine 40(3):650-656.

Cropper JR (1996). Regional anatomy and biomechanics. In: TW Flynn ed. The Thoracic Spine and Rib Cage: Musculoskeletal Evaluation and Treatment. Boston: Butterworth–Heinemann.

Datta AK (1994). Essentials of Human Anatomy. Thorax and Abdomen, 3rd ed. Calcutta: Current Books International; 80-86.

Ducic I, Larson EE (2006). Outcomes of surgical treatment for chronic postoperative breast and abdominal pain attributed to the intercostal nerve. Journal of the American College of Surgeons 203(3):304-310.

Durandt JJ, Evans JP, Revington P et al (2009). Physical profiles of elite male field hockey and soccer players – application to sport-specific tests. South African Journal of Sports Medicine 19(3):74-78.

Dutton M (2012). Dutton's Orthopaedic Examination Evaluation and Intervention. New York: McGraw Hill Professional.

Eng J, Westcott J, Better N (2008). Stress fracture of the first rib in a weightlifter. Clinical Nuclear Medicine 33(5):371-373.

Engel RM, Gonski P, Beath K et al (2014). Medium-term effects of including manual therapy in a pulmonary rehabilitation program for chronic obstructive pulmonary disease (COPD): a randomized controlled pilot trial. Journal of Manual and Manipulative Therapy 2042618614Y-0000000074.

Ernst E (2009a). Spinal manipulation for asthma: A systematic review of randomised clinical trials. Respiratory Medicine 103(12):1791-1795.

Ernst E (2009b). Chiropractic treatment for asthma? Journal of Asthma 46(3):211.

Fedorowski JJ (2000). Medical percussion. Hospital Physician 31.

Feeley BT, Kennelly S, Barnes RP et al (2008). Epidemiology of National Football League training camp injuries from 1998 to 2007. The American Journal of Sports Medicine 36(8):1597-1603.

Flowers KL (2015). Costochondritis. eMedicine. Available from: http://emedicine.medscape.com/article/808554-overview#showall [Accessed 1 February 2016].

Fromer L (2011). Diagnosing and treating COPD: understanding the challenges and finding solutions. International Journal of General Medicine 4:729.

García DG, Ros FE (2011). Lesiones en el tenis. Revisión bibliográfica. Apunts. Medicina de l'Esport 46(172):189-204.

Gartland S, Malik MHA, Lovell ME (2001). Injury and injury rates in Muay Thai kick boxing. British Journal of Sports Medicine 35(5):308-313.

Hedström EM, Svensson O, Bergström U et al (2010). Epidemiology of fractures in children and adolescents: increased incidence over the past decade: a population-based study from northern Sweden. Acta Orthopaedica 81(1):148-153.

Heincelman C, Brown S, England E et al (2014). Stress injury of the rib in a swimmer. Skeletal Radiology 43(9):1297-1299.

Heneghan NR, Adab P, Balanos GM et al (2012). Manual therapy for chronic obstructive airways disease: a systematic review of current evidence. Manual Therapy 17(6):507-518.

Hondras MA, Linde K, Jones AP (2005). Manual Therapy for Asthma. The Cochrane Library.

Jindal A, Singhi S (2011). Acute chest pain. The Indian Journal of Pediatrics 78(10):1262-1267.

Joshua A, Shetty L, Pare V (2014). Variations in dimensions and shape of thoracic cage with aging: an anatomical review. Anatomy Journal of Africa 3(2):346-355.

Kaminskyj A, Frazier M, Johnstone K et al (2010). Chiropractic care for patients with asthma: a systematic review of the literature. The Journal of the Canadian Chiropractic Association 54(1):24.

Kayser HL (1956). Tietze's syndrome: a review of the literature. The American Journal of Medicine 21(6):982-989.

Kessel B, Dagan J, Swaid F et al (2014). Rib fractures: comparison of associated injuries between pediatric and adult population. American Journal of Surgery 208(5):831-834. Epub 2014 Mar 26.

Liman ST, Kuzucu A, Tastepe AI et al (2003). Chest injury due to blunt trauma. European Journal of Cardio-thoracic Surgery 23(3):374-378.

Lucas-Herald A, Butler S, Mactier H et al (2012). Prevalence and characteristics of rib fractures in ex-preterm infants. Pediatrics 130(6):1116-1119.

McDonnell LK, Hume PA, Nolte V (2011). Rib stress fractures among rowers. Sports Medicine 41(11):883-901.

Mader SS (2004). Understanding Human Anatomy and Physiology, 5th ed. New York: McGraw-Hill.

Magee DJ (2014). Orthopedic Physical Assessment. Philadelphia: Elsevier Health Sciences.

Maquirriain J, Ghisi JP (2006). Uncommon abdominal muscle injury in a tennis player: internal oblique strain. British Journal of Sports Medicine 40(5):462-463.

Melendez LS, Doty IC (2015). Rib fractures. eMedicine. Available from: http://emedicine.medscape.com/article/825981-overview#showall [Accessed 1 February 2016].

Miller TL, Harris JD, Kaeding CC (2013). Stress fractures of the ribs and upper extremities: causation, evaluation, and management. Sports Medicine 43(8):665-674.

Miller TL (2015). Stress fractures of the ribs and girdle. In: TL Miller, CC Kaeding eds. Stress Fractures in Athletes: Diagnosis and Management. New York: Springer; 193-204.

Milsom NM, Barnard JG, Stretch RA (2007). Seasonal incidence and nature of cricket injuries among elite South African schoolboy cricketers: original research article. South African Journal of Sports Medicine 19(3):80-84.

Noll DR, Shores JH, Gamber RG et al (2000). Benefits of osteopathic manipulative treatment for hospitalized elderly patients with pneumonia. Journal of the American Osteopathic Association 100:776-782.

Ombregt L (2003). The thoracic spine: Disorders of the thoracic cage and abdomen. In: L Ombregt, P Bisschop, HJ ter Veer eds. A System of Orthopaedic Medicine, 2nd ed. Edinburgh: Churchill Livingstone.

OpenStax College (2013). Anatomy and Physiology. Available from: http://cnx.org/content/col11496/latest [Accessed 1 February 2016].

Patel AR, Hurst JR (2011). Extrapulmonary comorbidities in chronic obstructive pulmonary disease: state of the art. Expert Review of Respiratory Medicine 5(5):647-62.

Proulx AM, Zryd TW (2009). Costochondritis: diagnosis and treatment. American Family Physician 80(6):617-620.

Santos PSSD, Resende LAL, Fonseca RG et al (2005). Intercostal nerve mononeuropathy: study of 14 cases. Arquivos de Neuro-psiquiatria 63(3B):776-778.

Sebes JI, Salazar JE (1983). The manubriosternal joint in rheumatoid disease. American Journal of Roentgenology 140(1):117-121.

Sirmali M, Türüt H, Topçu S et al (2003). A comprehensive analysis of traumatic rib fractures: morbidity, mortality and management. European Journal of Cardio-thoracic Surgery 24(1):133-138.

Stevens KJ, Crain JM, Akizuki KH et al (2010). Imaging and ultrasound-guided steroid injection of internal oblique muscle strains in baseball pitchers. The American Journal of Sports Medicine 38(3):581-585.

Tate P (2009). Anatomy of Bones and Joints. Seeley's Principles of Anatomy and Physiology. Columbus, OH: McGraw-Hill; 149-196.

Thomas M, McKinley RK, Mellor S et al (2009). Breathing exercises for asthma: a randomised controlled trial. Thorax 64(1):55-61.

Tuteur PG (1990). Chest examination. In: HK Walker, WD Hall, JW Hurst eds. Clinical Methods: The History, Physical, and Laboratory Examinations. Butterworths. Available from: http://www.ncbi.nlm.nih.gov/books/NBK368/ [Accessed 1 February 2016].

Warwick R (1973). Gray's Anatomy (Vol. 424). PL Williams ed. Edinburgh: Longman.

White TD, Folkens PA (2005). The Human Bone Manual. Cambridge, Mass: Academic Press.

Wild AT, Begly JP, Garzon-Muvdi J et al (2011). First-rib stress fracture in a high-school lacrosse player: a case report and short clinical review. Sports Health: A Multidisciplinary Approach 3(6):547-549.

Williams EH, Williams CG, Rosson GD et al (2008). Neurectomy for treatment of intercostal neuralgia. The Annals of Thoracic Surgery 85(5):1766-1770.

Yoganandan N, Pintar FA (1998). Biomechanics of human thoracic ribs. Journal of Biomechanical Engineering 120(1):100-104.

Zazryn T, Cameron P, McCrory P (2006). A prospective cohort study of injury in amateur and professional boxing. British Journal of Sports Medicine 40(8):670-674.

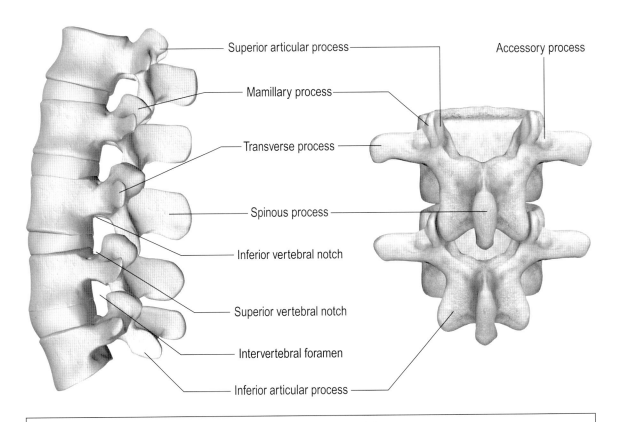

Superior articular process

Mamillary process

Transverse process

Spinous process

Inferior vertebral notch

Superior vertebral notch

Intervertebral foramen

Inferior articular process

Accessory process

Figure 8.1
The lumbar spine

The lumbar spine 8

Introduction

Lumbar spine (low back) pain is defined as pain between the costal margins and the gluteal folds, with or without pain radiating into the leg (Krismer & van Tulder 2007). It is one of the most common complaints presented to healthcare in the western world and, in the United States, it is the fifth commonest reason for any physician visit (Deyo et al 2006). Although most people who suffer with low back pain do not consult a healthcare practitioner – a report from the National Institute for Health and Care Excellence (NICE) found that only around 1 in 15 sufferers in the UK seeks treatment (NICE 2009) – low back pain is still one of the most draining conditions in terms of costs (Dagenais et al 2008, Lambeek et al 2011, Balagué et al 2012). The overall cost for treating patients with low back pain in the UK is estimated to exceed £500 million each year in the private sector and to be over £1000 million in the National Health Service (NHS) (NICE 2009). Moreover, in a recent analysis of the UK General Practice Research Database, it was reported that the annual healthcare costs of those with chronic low back pain were double the costs of those without (£1074 vs. £516) (Hong et al 2013). In the USA, the total spending for low back pain is estimated to be between $100 billion and $200 billion per year (World Health Organization 2013).

Studies have shown that the prevalence of low back pain increased over the second half of the 20th century, possibly linked to an increase in sedentary lifestyles and work (Louw et al 2007, El-Sayed et al 2010). What is interesting is that the incidence of low back pain is lower in countries with low- and middle-income economies than in high-income countries. Proposed reasons for this are that people in lower-income jobs are more active, have higher pain thresholds and have less contact with insurance companies than their higher-income counterparts (Volinn 1997).

Low back pain affects approximately 70–84% of people at some time in their lives (Hong et al 2013). It has been highlighted by the Global Burden of Disease study as the global leader in years lived with disability and the sixth highest with regard to disability-adjusted life years (Murray et al 2013, Vos et al 2013). Globally, the prevalence of low back pain limiting activity has been estimated at 39%. In the UK, it has been estimated that around one-third of the UK population experiences low back pain every year (NICE 2009). Symptoms in most of these patients (80–90%) resolve within a few weeks; the remaining 10–20% have an increased chance of developing chronic low back pain and experiencing disability connected to it (Hong et al 2013).

Both the NICE UK guidelines (NICE 2009) and the Joint Clinical Practice Guideline from the American College of Physicians / American Pain Society (Chou et al 2007) recommend manual therapy for low back pain. A systematic review by Bronfort et al (2004) demonstrated favorable results from articulation in the treatment of acute and chronic low back. Articulation has been shown to significantly decrease localized lower back pain on a short-term basis; it has also been observed to lead to a greater decrease in lower back pain in the long term when compared to no treatment (Hanrahan et al 2005). Studies have demonstrated that the treatment is most effective when directed to a specific joint level rather than a randomly selected vertebral level (Chiradejnant et al 2003).

A meta-analysis by Machado et al (2009) showed that articulation of the lumbar spine had a positive influence on the analgesic effects of treatments for non-specific low back pain, although the results were small for large study groups and larger in smaller groups. Pentelka (2012) also found that articulation of the lumbar spine decreased patients' pain thresholds but that at least four sets of articulation were needed over either 30 seconds or 60 seconds to achieve a change in threshold. McCollam and Benson (1993) used posterior–anterior articulation of the lower lumbar spine in 130 participants and found a significant increase in range of movement in lumbar extension post treatment. Powers et al (2008) also found increases in range of movement post articulation of the low back, although a later study by Stamos-Papastamos et al (2011) found no significant change in range of movement pre and post treatment.

Evidence suggests that different segments of the lumbar spine respond somewhat differently. For example, when a short-lever anterior–posterior compression is done on L3, L4 and L5, these segments are likely to move into extension; the three segments will move as a response to the anterior–posterior compression on the vertebra. However, with the upper segments, L1 and L2, the lower segments move into flexion (Powers et al 2008). The therapist therefore needs to be aware of the effect anterior–posterior articulation on the neighboring segments of the spine.

Beattie et al (2009) found that articulation of L5/S1 caused an increase in water diffusion of the associated intervertebral disc. Thus it was postulated that an increase in diffusion to the intervertebral disc would cause an elevation in intradiscal cells and activity, and an increase in oxygen levels thus increasing the formation of collagen and proteoglycans within the disc. Although these effects were noted to happen several hours after articulation of the joint, they would still contribute to the health and structural stability of the disc.

When assessing the effectiveness of articulation and the lumbar spine, there is conflicting evidence because some studies have looked at asymptomatic patients and others have looked at symptomatic, with varying numbers of participants and outcomes. There is also the question of what constitutes a good outcome. Is it an increase in range of movement, a decrease in perceived pain, or a decrease in pain threshold? There is clearly much more research to be done into lumbar spine pain and its management and treatment, especially given the extent of the problem.

Anatomy

The lumbar spine, also known as the lower back spine, is the third major segment of the vertebral column.

The word 'lumbar' has a Latin root and is derived from the word *lumbus*, which means loin (Arnold & Bryce 1987). The lumbar spine is designed to be incredibly strong, flexible and stable. It protects the spinal cord and spinal nerve roots, allows a wide range of motions, and serves to help support the weight of the body (Kishner et al 2014).

The anatomy of the lumbar spine is complex. It curves inward toward the abdomen, starting just below the thoracic spine and extending downward to the sacral region. It consists of five movable vertebrae, the intervertebral discs, large muscles, flexible ligament or tendons, and highly sensitive nerves (OpenStax 2013).

The lumbar vertebrae, designated L1 to L5, are irregular bones between the ribcage and the pelvis. They are characterized by their large, thick vertebral bodies, short spinous processes and thin transverse processes. They are distinguished from their counterparts by the absence of transverse foramina and costal facets. In addition, they have a horizontal diameter that is greater than their vertical height (Standring 2008).

The vertebral body of a lumbar vertebra is usually a large block of bone that is designed to carry most of the body's weight. It is wider transversely and is somewhat box-shaped, with essentially flat top and bottom surfaces (Bogduk 2005). It increases in size from L1 to L5. At the posterior end of the body, there is a thin, bony ring attachment called the vertebral arch. The arch encloses the hollow vertebral foramen and serves to protect the neural elements. Each vertebral arch is composed of two pedicles, two laminae and seven bony processes (Kishner et al 2014).

The vertebral foramen at lumbar levels is greater than at thoracic levels but smaller than at cervical levels. The pedicles change in morphology from the superior to the inferior. The laminae are broad and short, but they do not overlap like those of the thoracic vertebrae. The spinous process is more horizontal than in thoracic vertebrae. The transverse processes are typically thin and long; they increase in length from L1 to L3 but then shorten. The articular processes are large, with the superior processes bearing vertical concave articular facets and the inferior having vertical convex articular facets (Standring 2008).

The lumbar spine is normally made up of five vertebrae (L1–L5), but some people have genetic malformations of the lumbar spine that result in abnormalities classed as 'lumbosacral transitional vertebrae'. These transitional vertebrae can be subdivided into either sacralization or lumbarization. Sacralization is when the L5 is attached to the sacrum; lumbarization is when the first sacral vertebra is not fused (Dharati et al 2012). Research reports that, in most circumstances, the lumbosacral transitional vertebrae are asymptomatic and are most commonly unilateral (Singh et al 2014). Also there is some evidence that lumbosacral transitional vertebrae are racial variations. For example, 18% of Australian aboriginals (Mitchell 1936), 16% of Indians (Sharma et al 2011), 9.2% of Arabs (Hughes & Saifuddin 2006), and 5.8% of Japanese (Toyoda cited in Bergman, Afifi & Miyauchi 2008) have one of the forms of lumbosacral transitional vertebrae.

Intervertebral discs

Each lumbar vertebra is stacked vertically with another vertebra and between them is an intervertebral disc made of tough fibrocartilage. The structure of these discs is very similarly to those in other parts of the vertebral column. However, the discs in the lumbar spine are much thicker than between other vertebrae. Each disc consists of two distinct components: a central nucleus pulposus and a peripheral annulus fibrosus. The annulus fibrosus surrounds the nucleus pulposus by forming a retaining wall, but no clear boundary is observed between them within the disc (McKenzie 1981).

The intervertebral discs hold the vertebrae together, allow movement between them, and prevent them from grinding against each other. They also serve to absorb pressure and distribute stress during movement (Mader 2004).

Ligaments

The lumbar spine has similar ligaments to elsewhere in the vertebral column. These ligaments help to hold the vertebral bodies and the intervertebral discs together (Behrsin & Briggs 1988). The two named ligaments that attach to the lumbar bodies and discs are the anterior and posterior longitudinal ligaments. They cover the anterior and posterior aspects of the bodies and discs, respectively. However, these two ligaments are not restricted to the lumbar region only (Bogduk 2005); they can inferiorly extend into the sacrum and superiorly widen to cover the entire spinal column. The annuli fibrosi of the intervertebral discs are intimately attached to these ligaments (Kishner et al 2014).

The ligaments that join the posterior elements of the lumbar vertebrae are the supraspinous ligaments, the interspinous ligaments and the ligamentum flavum. The supraspinous ligament runs posteriorly to the posterior ends of the spinous processes and bridges the interspinous spaces. It attaches to the tips of the spinous processes of adjacent vertebrae from L1–L3 (Warwick & Williams 1980). The interspinous ligament connects adjacent spinous processes, from root to apex. The ligamentum flavum lies immediately behind the vertebral canal. It joins the laminae of consecutive vertebrae, connecting with the facet capsule laterally and the interspinous ligament medially (Bogduk 2005).

Another important ligament of the lumbar spine is the iliolumbar ligament. It is present bilaterally, and has five bands. It connects the transverse process of the fifth lumbar vertebra to the ilium. Briefly, each ligament arises from the tip of an L5 transverse process to the ilium's anteromedial surface and the iliac crest's inner lip (Shellshear & Macintosh 1949, Hughes and Saifuddin 2006).

Joints

All the vertebrae from L1 to L5 articulate by symphyseal joints between their vertebral bodies, synovial joints between their articular processes (zygapophyses), and fibrous joints between their laminae, transverse and spinous processes (Standring 2008). The symphyseal joints (also called the secondary cartilaginous joints) persist throughout the life of an individual and serve to provide mobility for the vertebral column. The articulations between the superior and inferior articular processes of two neighboring vertebrae are known as zygapophyseal joints. These protect the motion segment from anterior shear forces and allow simple gliding movements (Bogduk 2005).

Range of motion

The movements available at the lumbar spine and its individual joints are principally flexion, extension, lateral flexion and axial rotation. Flexion and extension usually occur because of a combination

Table 8.1

Ranges of segmental motion in the lumbar spine

Data adapted from White & Panjabi (1990)

Interspace	Combined flexion/extension (± x-axis rotation) (°)	Lateral flexion (z-axis rotation) (°)	Axial rotation (y-axis rotation) (°)
L1–L2	12	6	2
L2–L3	14	6	2
L3–L4	15	8	2
L4–L5	16	6	2
L5–S1	17	3	1

Table 8.2

Segmental range of motion in males aged 25 to 36 years (based on three-dimensional radiography technique)

Data from Pearcy et al (1984), Pearcy & Tibrewal (1984)

	Mean range of motion (°)						
				Lateral flexion		Axial rotation	
Interspace	Flexion	Extension	Flexion and extension	Left	Right	Left	Right
L1–L2	8	5	13	5	6	1	1
L2–L3	10	3	13	5	6	1	1
L3–L4	12	1	13	5	6	1	2
L4–L5	13	2	16	3	5	1	2
L5–S1	9	5	14	0	2	1	0

of rotation and translation in the sagittal plane between each vertebra (Hansen et al 2006). Horizontal translation has an involvement in the axial rotation of the spine, but is not available as an isolated or pure movement. Sagittal movement is considerably more available in the lumbar segment than rotation or lateral flexion, especially at the lowest regions (Bogduk 2005). The lumbosacral joint (L5–S1) undergoes the highest sagittal plane motion of the lumbar joints. This joint also offers a relatively small amount of lateral flexion and axial rotation (White & Panjabi 1990).

The range of motion of the lumbar spine is difficult to measure clinically, because it varies considerably from person to person. Moreover, a number of factors may also trigger it, including age, sex, genetics, pathology and ligamentous laxity (McKenzie & May 2003). For example, McGill et al (1999) found a decreased range of motion in full flexion and lateral flexion when comparing elderly participants

with younger. In addition, men are reported to have more mobility in flexion–extension, while women have more in lateral flexion (Biering-Sorensen 1984). Ranges of segmental motion are given in Table 8.1, and mean figures for range of motion in males are shown in Table 8.2.

Some research has demonstrated that in the majority of cases of lower back pain, flexion is commonly the first movement to become limited (Sullivan et al 2000, Neumann et al 2001).

Epidemiology

Low back pain is a very common spinal disorder that many people experience at some stage in their lives. It has variable etiologies. It can be due to lumbar arthritis, lumbar instability, spondylolisthesis, spinal deformity, spinal stenosis, disc herniation, disc degeneration, painful scoliosis, injury, arthritis or trapped nerves (Juniper et al 2009). However, the etiology of low back pain is unknown in the vast

Condition	Description	Reference
Lumbar spinal stenosis	A condition associated with extensive degenerative changes of the intervertebral disc and zygapophyseal joints at multiple levels in the spine Causes abnormal narrowing of the spinal canal and spinal nerve root Often occurs with generalized rheumatological, metabolic or orthopaedic conditions, such as osteofluorosis, achondroplasia, acromegaly, Paget's disease or previous fracture Accounts for 75% of all spinal stenosis Symptoms include age greater than 50 years, long history of low back pain, severe lower limb pain and the absence of pain when sitting	McKenzie & May (2003), McRae (2010), Eriator & Chambers (2014)
Lumbar dysfunction syndrome	Involves structural impairment of soft tissue Often develops following repair after derangement and limitation of flexion Usually affects peri-articular, contractile or neural structures Symptoms include movement loss, intermittent pain when loading at restricted end-range and pain when the abnormal tissue is loaded	McKenzie (1981), McKenzie & May (2003)
Derangement syndrome	Most common mechanical disorder of the spine Characterized by a varied clinical presentation and typical responses to loading strategies Causes an interruption in the normal resting position of the affected joint surfaces Can be associated with a constant pain in the lumbar region Symptoms include gradual or sudden onset of pain, diminished range of movement, centralization and/or peripheralization of pain, temporary deformity and deviation of normal movement pathways, and restoration of normal movement because of therapeutic loading strategies	McKenzie & May (2003), Clare et al (2007)
Postural syndrome	Characterized by intermittent pain due to persistent static loading of normal tissues Caused by mechanical deformation of normal soft tissues, arising from prolonged end-range positioning Especially common in schoolchildren and students Symptoms include no pain with movement or activity, no loss of normal range of motion, pain in slumped sitting posture and pain relief from postural correction	McKenzie (1981), McKenzie & May (2003)

Table 8.3

Common disorders of the lumbar spine

majority of cases: approximately 90% of cases have no recognizable cause and are defined as nonspecific (Manek & MacGregor 2005). In theory, any structure located in the lumbar spine that receives a neurological supply can be a source of lower back pain. Therefore pain can originate from any of the fascia, muscles, ligaments, joints or discs. Many therapists have postulated that articulation of the lower back has an effect on the nervous system (Knutson 2000, Pickar 2002, Clark et al 2009). Thus nonspecific low back pain may be defined as low back pain that is not connected with a specific pathology such as a tumor, infection, inflammatory disorder, fracture, osteoporosis or cauda equina.

Table 8.3 lists the common disorders of the lumbar spine.

Low back pain has an enormous social and economic impact. It causes difficulty in performing activities of daily living and can lead to activity limitation and work absence (Manchikanti et al 2008). Studies performed in the UK have suggested that low back pain has been the biggest single cause of work absence (Hoy et al 2014, Wynne-Jones et al 2014); it has been estimated that low back pain is responsible for 12.5% of all sick days (Bevan 2012). The financial burden from low back pain is also immense. In 1998, the annual total cost for low back pain in the UK was estimated at £12.3 billion (Maniadakis & Gray 2000).

The exact incidence and prevalence of low back pain in the UK are uncertain. Although a vast raft of literature is available on the subject, most of the epidemiological studies published on it are not only heterogeneous but also contradictory. The varying methodologies used in these studies often limit the ability to compare and pool data, and give rise to problems from clinical and policy perspectives (Friedly et al 2010). According to the systematic reviews carried out by Hoy et al (2010), the unadjusted point prevalence of low back pain in the UK ranges between 18% and 19% (data from Hillman et al 1996 and Harkness et al 2005), with an annual prevalence of 36.1% (data from Walsh et al 1992). The authors also mentioned that the estimated 1-year incidence of a first-ever episode of low back pain was 15.4%, while the estimated 1-year incidence of any or a recurrent episode of low back was 36% (data from Croft et al 1999).

Lumbar spine examination
Medical history

Taking an accurate medical history of the patient is the most important part for the lumbar spine examination, because it helps determine whether the conditions are mechanical or secondary. It also helps identify the red flags and facilitates the physical examination.

The clinician should ask the questions in a logical manner, so that they can draw a conclusion from the answers. The interview should include questions about osteoarthritis, osteoporosis and cancer, and a review of any previous imaging reports (Last & Hulbert 2009). Apart from questioning about pain and other issues related to the lumbar region, the clinician should also inquire about the onset of the problem, behavior since onset, symptom pattern, and exacerbating and relieving factors.

Red flags

While questioning the patient, the clinician should check for the presence of any red flags in their narrative (see Table 8.4). The screening process should begin with a detailed medical history and the use of a medical screening form.

Physical examination

The physical examination is important. It involves a variety of observations and movements, which help the clinician to confirm initial findings, fully explore the nature and extent of the problem, and make judgments.

Observation

Observation of the patient's overall movement and posture is recommended for all patients with low back pain. Posture is best observed when the patient is unaware that the clinician is doing so, such as during the history taking. The examiner should carefully observe how the patient sits, rises from sitting, stands and walks, and note any deformity that may be obvious.

Range of motion

The examiner should assess the patient's movement in flexion, extension, lateral bending and lateral rotation. The single movements should initially be performed to

Condition	Signs and symptoms
Cauda equina	Urinary incontinence or loss of bladder control Bowel incontinence or lack of control over defecation Saddle (perianal/perineal) anaesthesia or paraesthesia Progressive motor weakness in the lower extremities
Cancer	Over 55 years of age Past history of cancer Unintentional loss of weight (normally occurs in end stages) Constant, progressive back pain at night or at rest
Infection	Fever, chills Recent urinary tract or skin infection Penetrating wound near spine Unrelenting night pain or pain at rest Substance abuse, intravenous drug use No improvement after 6 weeks of conventional treatment
Inflammatory disorders	Gradual onset of symptoms Family history Morning stiffness > 45 minutes Persisting limitation of movements in all directions Involvement of peripheral joint Iritis, colitis, skin rashes, urethral discharge
Abdominal aneurysm	Abdominal pain (that may be constant or intermittent) Pain in the lower back that may radiate to the buttock, groin or thighs The feeling of a pulse or 'heartbeat' in the abdomen Greater risk in 65 years plus, male, smokers If the aneurysm bursts, symptoms include: • severe back or abdominal pain that begins suddenly • paleness • dry mouth/skin and excessive thirst • nausea and vomiting • signs of shock, such as shaking, dizziness, fainting, sweating, rapid heartbeat and sudden weakness
Other possible serious spinal pathology	Systemically unwell Widespread neuropathic pain History of significant trauma, such as a fall from a height History of trivial trauma and severe pain in potential osteoporotic individual Sudden onset of severe central pain causing patient to 'freeze'

Table 8.4

Red flags for serious spinal pathology in the lumbar region

Data from Nachemson & Vingard (2000); McKenzie & May (2003)

Test	Procedure	Positive sign	Interpretation
Lumbar quadrant test	The patient stands before the examiner and extends the spine. The examiner applies overpressure in extension while the patient laterally flexes and rotates to the side of pain.	Pain reproduced in the area of the back or lower extremities	Nerve root irritation
Femoral nerve tension test	The patient lies prone. The examiner hyperflexes the patient's knees bilaterally (heels to buttocks) and holds for 45–60 seconds. If no positive signs are detected in this position, the examiner extends the hip while maintaining knee flexion.	Decreased muscle stretch reflexes and muscle weakness when knees are in the range of 80–100° Unilateral pain in the lumbar region, buttocks or posterior thigh	L2–L3 or L3–L4 nerve root lesion
Straight leg raising test	The patient lies supine, raising each leg separately until pain occurs. The examiner notes the angle between the leg and the bed.	Pain occurs when the angle is in the range of 30–60°	Nerve root irritation
Slump test	The patient sits on the edge of a treatment table, with legs supported, hands behind back and hips in neutral. The patient slumps forward into full thoracic and lumbar flex. The patient then flexes the neck by placing the chin on the chest, and the examiner maintains overpressure. The patient actively extends one knee as much as possible and the examiner then dorsiflexes the ankle.	Reproduction of symptoms in back and radicular symptoms	Increased tension in dura or meninges Neural tissue sensitivity
Tripod sign test	The patient sits at the edge of a treatment table, with both knees flexed 90°. The examiner passively extends one knee while observing the patient's trunk.	Increased trunk extension to relieve tension	Dural/meningeal irritation

Table 8.5

Special tests for lumbar spine examination

Data from McKenzie (1981), Bratton (1999), Baxter (2003)

check the patient's ability to move, and then repeated movements performed to determine the range and quality of movement and pain response to movement. Pain with forward flexion often indicates mechanical causes, while pain with back extension usually points towards spinal stenosis. However, it is noteworthy to mention that, because of cutting-edge imaging technology, spinal movement has limited diagnostic use today.

Special tests

Special tests for lumbar spine examination are summarized in Table 8.5.

Lumbar spine muscles

Name	Origin	Insertion	Action	Nerve supply
Iliocostalis lumborum	Medial and lateral sacral crests and medial portion of iliac crest	Angles of ribs 7–12	Extension, lateral flexion of the lumbar spine, assists in inspiration	Dorsal primary divisions of spinal nerves
Longissimus thoracis	Medial and lateral sacral crests, medial portion of iliac crest, spinous process of T11–T12, L1–L5, thoracolumbar fascia	Transverse process of T1–T12, tubercles and angles of ribs 3–12	Extension, lateral flexion of the lumbar spine, assists in inspiration	Dorsal primary divisions of spinal nerves
Spinalis thoracis	Spinous process of T11–T12 and L1–L2	Spinous process of T1–T8	Extension of the spine	Dorsal primary divisions of spinal nerves
Multifidus (lumbar division)	Mammillary process of L1–L5	Spinous process two to four vertebrae superior to origin	Extends and rotates the spine	Dorsal primary division of spinal nerves
Rotatores (lumbar division)	Transverse process of L1–L5	Base of spinous process of next vertebra above	Extends and rotates the spine	Dorsal primary division of spinal nerves
Interspinales (lumbar division)	Spinous process of L2–L5	Spinous processs of next vertebra above	Extends the spine	Dorsal primary division of spinal nerves
Intertranscersarii laterales	Transverse process of L1–L5	Transverse process of next vertebra above	Laterally flexes the spine	Ventral primary division of spinal nerves
Intertranscersarii mediales	Mammillary process of L1–L5	Accessory process of next vertebra above	Laterally flexes the spine	Dorsal primary division of spinal nerves
Serratus posterior inferior	Spinous process of T11–T12 and L1–L3	Inferior surfaces of ribs 8–12	Depresses the ribs while resisting the action of the diaphragm	T9–T12
Quadratus lumborum	Superior surface of iliac crest, iliolumbar ligament	Inferior surface of rib 12, transverse process of L1–L4	Lateral flexion of the spine, expiration	T12–L1
Diaphragm	Sternal portion: xiphoid process Costal portion: inner surfaces of ribs 7–12 and their associated cartilage Lumbar portion: L1–L2/3 vertebral body	Central tendon	Depression of the central tendon to encourage inspiration	Phrenic nerve (C3–C5)

Table 8.6
Lumbar spine muscles

Techniques: lumbar spine

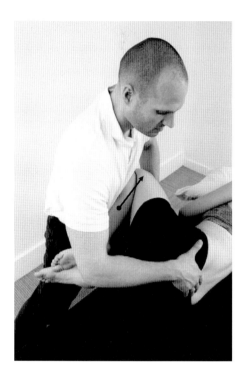

T8.1 Side-lying lumbar spine flexion

- Stand in front of side-lying patient.
- Face towards the patient's head. You should have a split stance with your leg closest to the plinth backward.
- With the arm closest to the patient, reach over the patient's body to the back of the pelvis.
- Your opposite hand is placed on the patient's knees.
- Lift the patient's legs and rest them on your outermost thigh.
- Place your palpating hand on the lumbar spine (LSP) between the spinous processes (SPs) to feel them open when flexed.
- Start with the patient's knees at 90° with the LSP in the neutral position.
- Gently compress on to the patient's femurs and rock from your front to back foot, slightly side to side, to create LSP flexion.
- Combined LSP flexion is approximately 70°–90°.

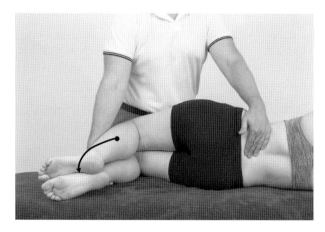

T8.2 Side-lying lumbar spine extension

- Stand in front of side-lying patient.
- Face towards the patient's feet. You should have a split stance with your leg closest to the plinth backward.
- Lift the patient's legs and rest them on your outermost thigh.
- With your outermost arm to the patient, hold under the stacked ankles for support, their shins against your anterior forearm.
- With the arm closest to the patient, reach over the patient's body to the back of the pelvis. This will be your palpating hand.
- Place your palpating hand on the LSP between the SPs to feel them close when extended.
- Start with the patient's knees at 90° with the LSP in the neutral position.
- Rock from front to back foot, curving across the plinth, to create LSP extension.
- Combined LSP extension is approximately 20°–30°.

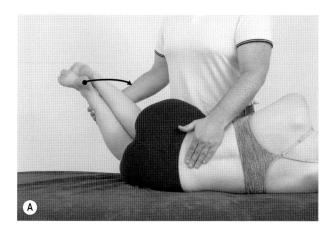

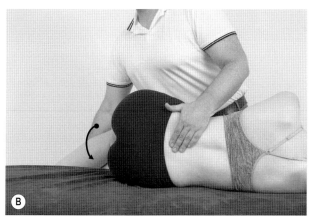

T8.3 Side-lying lumbar spine side bending

- With the patient lying on their side, face towards the patient's feet. You should have a split stance with your leg closest to the plinth backward.
- Lift the patient's legs and rest them on your outermost thigh.
- With your outermost arm to the patient, hold under the stacked ankles for support.
- With the arm closest to the patient, reach over the patient's body. This will be your palpating hand.
- Start with the patient's knees and hips at 90° with the LSP in the neutral position.
- Place your palpating hand on the LSP between the SPs to feel the side-bending motion.
- You may bend your front leg and lower the patient's legs or bend your back leg and raise the patient's legs to create a side-bending motion to either side.
- LSP side bending is approximately 25°–35° to either side.

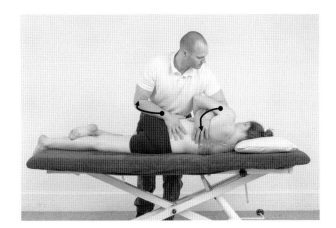

T8.4 Side-lying lumbar spine rotational articulation

- Straighten the side-lying patient's bottom leg along the plinth.
- Face towards the patient's head. You should have a split stance with your leg closest to the plinth backward.
- Stand approximately level to the superior part of the patient's pelvis.
- Ask the patient to rest their uppermost hand on the lateral border of their pelvis and to straighten their lower leg while keeping their upper leg bent.
- Hold on to the patient's lower arm and pull, thus rotating the spine down to the level you wish to work on. Then ask the patient to grasp their uppermost forearm.
- With pressure on the posterior part of the patient's pelvis and an opposing force through the anterior ribcage, you can thus apply a rotational force through these areas and the area you wish to articulate.

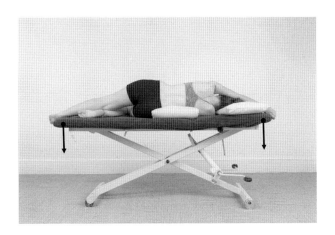

T8.5 Foraminal gapping position

- Ask the patient to lie on their side. (You may wish to place a pillow or towel on the plinth before, as shown in the photograph.)
- If you have a two- or three-part plinth, you can lower these sections to enhance the technique.

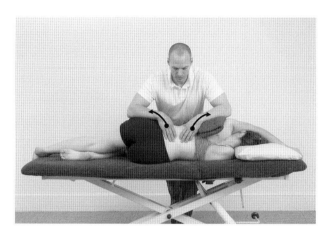

T8.6 Foraminal gapping 1

- Face towards the patient's head. You should have a split stance with your leg closest to the plinth backward.
- Straighten the patient's uppermost leg.
- Straighten the patient's uppermost arm.
- Place an inferior force through the pelvis and a superior force through the lower ribcage, thus causing a side-bending force through the LSP.

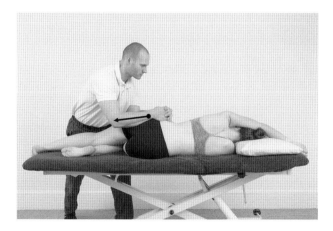

T8.7 Foraminal gapping 2

- You should have a split stance with your leg closest to the plinth backward.
- With the arm closest to the patient, reach over the patient's body to the back of the pelvis, cupping your hand around the iliac crest.
- Place your other hand around the front of the iliac crest with the heel of the hand against the patient's anterior superior iliac spine.
- Interlace your fingers together and compress the pelvis with your forearms.
- Bend your rear leg to initiate an arcing movement in the LSP, thereby creating LSP side bending.
- Gently take the pelvis inferiorly, towards the plinth, to encourage LSP side bending.

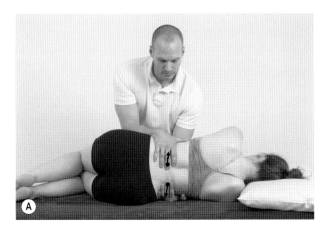

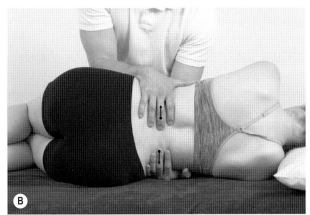

T8.8 Reinforced lumbar spine extension

- Face towards the patient's head. You should have a split stance with your leg closest to the plinth backward.
- Ask the patient to lift their abdomen up from the plinth and place your forearm through the gap as far as possible.
- With your other arm, reach over the patient's body to the other side of the low back.
- Gradually lean back, encouraging the LSP into extension.

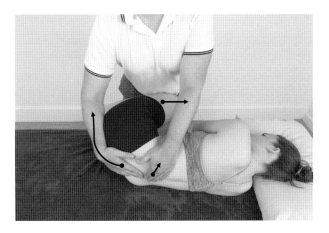

T8.9 Reinforced lumbar spine flexion side-lying

- Stand in front of the side-lying patient.
- Face towards the patient's head. You should have a split stance with your leg closest to the plinth backward.
- Rest the patient's legs across your thighs.
- With one hand, palpate for the spinous process of the joint below the one you wish to articulate, and use your forearm to compress along the posterior portion of the pelvis.
- Use your other hand to palpate and gently compress the spinous process of the vertebra above the joint you are targeting.
- With a shift of your body weight from the back foot to front foot, push the knees of the patient towards their head while compressing the posterior portion of the pelvis.

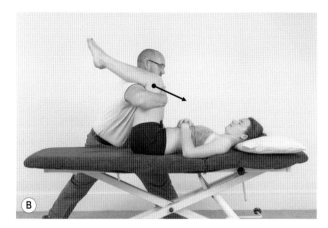

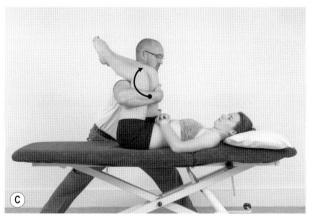

T8.10 Supine lumbar spine articulation/ examination

- The patient should be supine with their knees bent up.
- Stand to the side of the patient.
- Gently allow the patient's legs to drop away from you, creating space to put your palpating hand under their lumbar spine.
- The palpating hand is placed centrally under the patient, with finger pads palpating for the spinous processes of the lumbar spine (as shown in photograph **a**).
- Bring the patient back to the middle of the table.
- Place your shoulder under the patient's bent knees, trying to get the patient's legs as far as possible on to your shoulders, and gently lift their legs.
- With a staggered stance, flexion is induced by moving the patient's legs up toward their head (see photograph **b**).
- Create side bending by rotating around your front leg, inducing a rotation through the pelvis, with the patient's feet being moved towards your direction (see photograph **c**).
- Rotation is induced by rocking the patient's legs from the neutral position directly towards you.

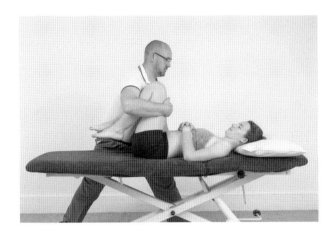

T8.11 Supine lumbar spine articulation/ examination – alternative hand position

- This hand hold is extremely effective, especially if the patient has particularly heavy legs, but be aware of the flexion compression in the knees.

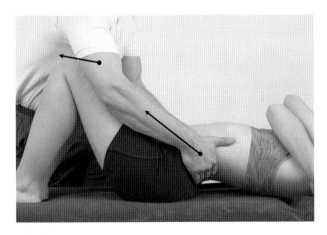

T8.12 Supine reinforced extension

- The patient lies supine, closer to the side you are standing, with their knees flexed.
- Ask the patient if you may sit on their toes and just cover them with your outer thigh.
- Reach your arms around either side of the patient's abdomen to either side of the spine.
- Compress your medial elbows against the patient's lateral thighs with their knees towards your axillae.
- Maintaining contact with the patient's thighs, create an arcing motion backward. This will gently tilt the patient's LSP into extension.
- Gradually lean back, hold, and then release slowly.

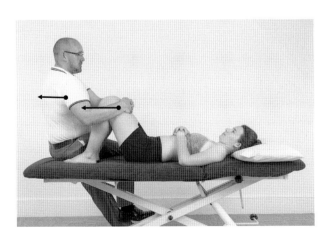

T8.13 Supine lumbar spine traction

- The patient lies supine, closer to the side where you are standing, with their knees flexed.
- Ask the patient if you may sit on their toes and just cover them with your outer thigh.
- Reach your arms around the patient's knees, interlocking your fingers if possible around their distal anterior thighs.
- Very slowly lean backward, hold, and then very slowly release.

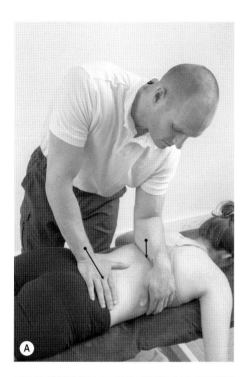

T8.14 Prone short-lever rotation articulation

- Stand to one side of the plinth. The patient should be lying prone, their arms either by their sides or in a comfortable position.
- Place your non-articulating hand over the mid-thoracic area of the spine, bracing it and resisting rotation moving further up the spine.
- Place your articular hand over the lumbar spine, with the heel of the hand behind the target segment.
- Push down in an arching movement to gain a rotation movement of the spine.

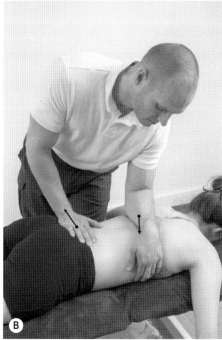

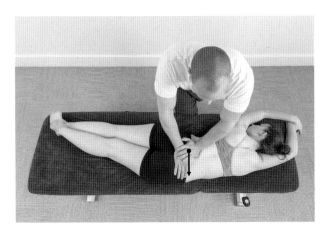

T8.15 Prone foraminal gripping

- With the patient lying prone, stand to one side and orient the patient into a side-bent position. Their arms and feet should be closer to your side of the table, with one foot crossed over the other, and the pelvis away from you (as shown).
- Place your non-articulating hand over the articulating hand, ideally behind the thumb, bracing it to minimize pressure through the thumb joint.
- Place your articular hand over the lumbar spine, with the thumb of that hand to the side of the spinous process of the target segment.

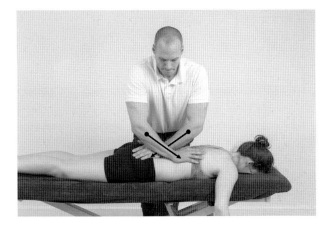

T8.16 Prone short-lever traction

- Stand to one side of the table. The patient should lie prone, with their arms either by their sides or in a comfortable position.
- In the example shown, the arms cross, the hand compressing the 12th rib pushing superiorly. The other hand compresses on top of the iliac crest, pushing inferiorly.
- Gently dropping your body weight down and allowing your arms to move in their respective ways induces movement.

REFERENCES

Arnold MA, Bryce D (1987). Arnold's Glossary of Anatomy. The University of Sydney – Anatomy & Histology Online Learning. Available from: http://www.anatomy.usyd.edu.au/glossary/glossary.cgi [Accessed 3 February 2016].

Balagué F, Mannion AF, Pellisé F et al (2012). Non-specific low back pain. The Lancet 379(9814):482-491.

Baxter RE (2003). Pocket Guide to Musculoskeletal Assessment. Philadelphia: WB Saunders.

Beattie PF, Donley JW, Arnot CF et al (2009). The change in the diffusion of water in normal and degenerative lumbar intervertebral discs following joint mobilization compared to prone lying. Journal of Orthopaedic and Sports Physical Therapy 39(1):4-11.

Behrsin JF, Briggs CA (1988). Ligaments of the lumbar spine: a review. Surgical and Radiologic Anatomy 10 (3):211-219.

Bergman RA, Afifi AK, Miyauchi R (2008). Illustrated Encyclopedia of Human Anatomic Variation. Available at http://www.anatomyatlases.org/AnatomicVariants/SkeletalSystem/Text/LumbarVertebrae.shtml [Accessed 6 May 2016].

Bevan S (2012). The Impact of Back Pain on Sickness Absence in Europe. Lancaster: The Work Foundation.

Biering-Sorensen F (1984). Physical measurements as risk indicators for low-back trouble over a one-year period. Spine 9(2):106-119.

Bogduk N (2005). Clinical Anatomy of the Lumbar Spine and Sacrum. Oxford: Elsevier Health Sciences.

Bratton RL (1999). Assessment and management of acute low back pain. American Family Physician 60(8):2299-2308.

Bronfort G, Haas M, Evans RL et al (2004). Efficacy of spinal manipulation and mobilization for low back pain and neck pain: a systematic review and best evidence synthesis. The Spine Journal 4(3):335-356.

Chiradejnant A, Maher CG, Latimer J et al (2003). Efficacy of 'therapist-selected' versus 'randomly selected' mobilisation techniques for the treatment of low back pain: a randomised controlled trial. Australian Journal of Physiotherapy 49(4):233-241.

Chou R, Qaseem A, Snow V et al (2007). Diagnosis and treatment of low back pain: a joint clinical practice guideline from the American College of Physicians and the American Pain Society. Annals of Internal Medicine 147(7):478-491.

Clare HA, Adams R, Maher CG (2007). Construct validity of lumbar extension measures in McKenzie's derangement syndrome. Manual Therapy 12 (4):328-334.

Clark BC, Walkowski S, Conatser RR et al (2009). Muscle function magnetic resonance imaging and acute low back pain: a pilot study to characterize lumbar muscle activity asymmetries and examine the effects of osteopathic manipulative treatment. Osteopathic Medicine and Primary Care 3:7.

Croft PR, Papageorgiou AC, Thomas E et al (1999). Short-term physical risk factors for new episodes of low back pain: prospective evidence from the South Manchester Back Pain Study. Spine 24(15):1556.

Dagenais S, Caro J, Haldeman S (2008). A systematic review of low back pain cost of illness studies in the United States and internationally. The Spine Journal 8(1):8–20.

Deyo RA, Mirza SK, Martin BI (2006). Back pain prevalence and visit rates: estimates from US national surveys, 2002. Spine 31(23):2724-2727.

Dharati K, Nagar SK, Ojaswini M et al (2012). A study of sacralization of fifth lumbar vertebra in Gujarat. National Journal of Medical Research 2(2).

El-Sayed AM, Hadley C, Tessema F et al (2010). Back and neck pain and psychopathology in rural Sub-Saharan Africa: evidence from the Gilgel Gibe Growth and Development Study, Ethiopia. Spine 35(6):684.

Eriator I, Chambers Z (2014). Lumbar spinal stenosis and neurogenic claudication. In: AD Kaye, RV Shah ed. Case Studies in Pain Management. Cambridge: Cambridge University Press.

Friedly J, Standaert C, Chan L (2010). Epidemiology of spine care: the back pain dilemma. Physical Medicine and Rehabilitation Clinics of North America 21(4):659-677.

Hanrahan S, Van Lunen BL, Tamburello M et al (2005). The short-term effects of joint mobilizations on acute mechanical low back dysfunction in collegiate athletes. Journal of Athletic Training 40(2):88.

Hansen L, De Zee M, Rasmussen J et al (2006). Anatomy and biomechanics of the back muscles in the lumbar spine with reference to biomechanical modelling. Spine 31(17):1888-1899.

Harkness EF, Macfarlane GJ, Silman AJ et al (2005). Is musculoskeletal pain more common now than 40 years ago? Two population-based cross-sectional studies. Rheumatology 44(7):890-895.

Hillman M, Wright A, Rajaratnam G et al (1996). Prevalence of low back pain in the community: implications for service provision in Bradford, UK. Journal of Epidemiology and Community Health 50(3):347-352.

Hong J, Reed C, Novick D et al (2013). Costs associated with treatment of chronic low back pain: an analysis of the UK General Practice Research Database. Spine 38(1):75-82.

Hoy D, Brooks P, Blyth F et al (2010). The epidemiology of low back pain. Best Practice and Research Clinical Rheumatology 24(6):769-781.

Hoy D, March L, Brooks P et al (2014). The global burden of low back pain: estimates from the Global Burden of Disease 2010 study. Annals of the Rheumatic Diseases 73(6):968-974.

Hughes RJ, Saifuddin, A (2006). Numbering of lumbosacral transitional vertebrae on MRI: role of the iliolumbar ligaments. American Journal of Roentgenology 187(1):W59-W65.

Juniper M, Le TK, Mladsi D (2009). The epidemiology, economic burden, and pharmacological treatment of chronic low back pain in France, Germany, Italy, Spain and the UK: a literature-based review. Expert Opinion on Pharmacotherapy 10(16):2581-2592.

Kishner S, Moradian M, Morello J K (2014). Lumbar spine anatomy. Medscape. Available from: http://emedicine.medscape.com/article/1899031-overview [Accessed 3 February 2016].

Knutson GA (2000). The role of the gamma-motor system in increasing muscle tone and muscle pain syndromes: a review of the Johnasson/Sojka hypothesis. Journal of Manipulative and Physiological Therapeutics 23(8):564-572.

Krismer M, Van Tulder M (2007). Low back pain (non-specific). Best Practice and Research Clinical Rheumatology 21(1):77-91.

Lambeek LC, van Tulder MW, Swinkels IC et al (2011). The trend in total cost of back pain in The Netherlands in the period 2002–2007. Spine 36(13):1050–1058.

Last AR, Hulbert K (2009). Chronic low back pain: evaluation and management. American Family Physician 79(12):1067-1074.

Louw QA, Morris LD, Grimmer-Somers K (2007). The prevalence of low back pain in Africa: a systematic review. BMC Musculoskeletal Disorders 8(1):105.

McCollam RL, Benson CJ (1993). Effects of postero-anterior mobilization on lumbar extension and flexion. Journal of Manual and Manipulative Therapy 1(4):134-141.

McGill SM, Yingling VR, Peach JP (1999). Three-dimensional kinematics and trunk muscle myoelectric activity in the elderly spine – a database compared to young people. Clinical Biomechanics 14(6):389-395.

Machado LAC, Kamper SJ, Herbert RD et al (2009). Analgesic effects of treatments for non-specific low back pain: a meta-analysis of placebo-controlled randomized trials. Rheumatology 48(5):520-527.

McKenzie R (1981). The Lumbar Spine: Mechanical Diagnosis and Therapy. Spinal Publications.

McKenzie R, May S (2003). The Lumbar Spine: Mechanical Diagnosis and Therapy, 2nd ed. Orthopedic Physical Therapy.

McRae R (2010). Clinical Orthopaedic Examination. Oxford: Elsevier Health Sciences; 89-120.

Mader SS (2004). Understanding Human Anatomy and Physiology, 5th ed. New York: McGraw-Hill.

Manchikanti L, Singh V, Datta S et al (2008). Comprehensive review of epidemiology, scope, and impact of spinal pain. Pain physician 12(4):E35-E70.

Manek NJ, MacGregor AJ (2005). Epidemiology of back disorders: prevalence, risk factors, and prognosis. Current Opinion in Rheumatology 17(2):134-140.

Maniadakis N, Gray A (2000). The economic burden of back pain in the UK. Pain 84(1):95-103.

Mitchell GAG (1936). The significance of lumbosacral transitional vertebrae. British Journal of Surgery 24(93):147-158.

Murray CJ, Vos T, Lozano R et al (2013). Disability-adjusted life years (DALYs) for 291 diseases and injuries in 21 regions, 1990–2010: a systematic analysis for the Global Burden of Disease Study 2010. Lancet 380(9859):2197–2223.

Nachemson A, Vingard E (2000). Assessment of patients with neck and back pain: a best-evidence synthesis. In: A Nachemson, E Jonsson eds. Neck and Back Pain: The Scientific Evidence of Causes, Diagnosis, and Treatment. Philadelphia: Lippincott Williams & Wilkins.

National Institute for Health and Clinical Excellence (NICE) (2009). Low back pain: Early management of persistent non-specific low back pain. NICE clinical guideline 88; developed by the National Collaborating Centre for Primary Care. Available from: http://guidance.nice.org.uk/CG88/NICE-Guidance/pdf/English [Accessed 3 February 2016].

Neumann WP, Wells RP, Norman RW et al (2001). Trunk posture: reliability, accuracy, and risk estimates for low back pain from a video-based assessment method. International Journal of Industrial Ergonomics 28(6):355-365.

OpenStax College (2013). Anatomy and physiology. Available from: http://cnx.org/content/col11496/latest [Accessed 3 February 2016].

Pearcy M, Portek IAN, Shepherd J (1984). Three-dimensional X-ray analysis of normal movement in the lumbar spine. Spine 9(3): 294-297.

Pearcy MJ, Tibrewal SB (1984). Axial rotation and lateral bending in the normal lumbar spine measured by three-dimensional radiography. Spine 9(6):582-587.

Pentelka L, Hebron C, Shapleski R et al (2012). The effect of increasing sets (within one treatment session) and different set durations (between treatment sessions) of lumbar spine posteroanterior mobilisations on pressure pain thresholds. Manual Therapy 17(6):526-530.

Pickar JG (2002). Neurophysiological effects of spinal manipulation. The Spine Journal 2(5):357-371.

Powers CM, Beneck GJ, Kulig K et al (2008). Effects of a single session of posterior-to-anterior spinal mobilization and press-up exercise on pain response and lumbar spine extension in people with nonspecific low back pain. Physical Therapy 88(4):485-493.

Sharma VA, Sharma DK, Shukla CK (2011). Oesteogenic study of lumbosacral transitional vertebra in central India region. Journal of Anatomical Society of India 60(2):212-217.

Shellshear JL, Macintosh NWG (1949). The transverse process of the fifth lumbar vertebra. In: JL Shellshear, NWG Macintosh eds. Surveys of Anatomical Fields. Sydney: Grahame; 21-32.

Singh AP, Sekhon J, Kaur N (2014). Sacralization: the structural complications and body biomechanics. Human Biology Review 3(1).

Stamos-Papastamos N, Petty NJ, Williams JM (2011). Changes in bending stiffness and lumbar spine range of movement following lumbar mobilization and manipulation. Journal of Manipulative and Physiological Therapeutics 34(1):46-53.

Standring S (2008). Gray's Anatomy: The Anatomical Basis of Clinical Practice. Edinburgh: Churchill Livingstone.

Sullivan MS, Shoaf LD, Riddle DL (2000). The relationship of lumbar flexion to disability in patients with low back pain. Physical Therapy 80(3):240-250.

Volinn E (1997). The epidemiology of low back pain in the rest of the world: A review of surveys in low-and middle-income countries. Spine 22(15):1747-1754.

Vos T, Flaxman AD, Naghavi M et al (2013). Years lived with disability (YLDs) for 1160 sequelae of 289 diseases and injuries 1990–2010: a systematic analysis for the Global Burden of Disease Study 2010. Lancet 380(9859):2163–2196.

Walsh K, Cruddas M, Coggon D (1992). Low back pain in eight areas of Britain. Journal of Epidemiology and Community Health 46(3):227-230.

Warwick R, Williams P (1980). Gray's Anatomy. Edinburgh: Longmans.

White AA, Panjabi MM (1990). Kinematics of the spine. In: AA White, MM Panjabi. Clinical Biomechanics of the Spine. Philadelphia: Lippincott Williams & Wilkins; 106-112.

World Health Organization (2013). Priority Medicine for Europe and the World Update Report, 2013. Chapter 6.24: Priority diseases and reasons for inclusion.

Wynne-Jones G, Cowen J, Jordan JL et al (2014). Absence from work and return to work in people with back pain: a systematic review and meta-analysis. Occupational and Environmental Medicine 71(6):448-456.

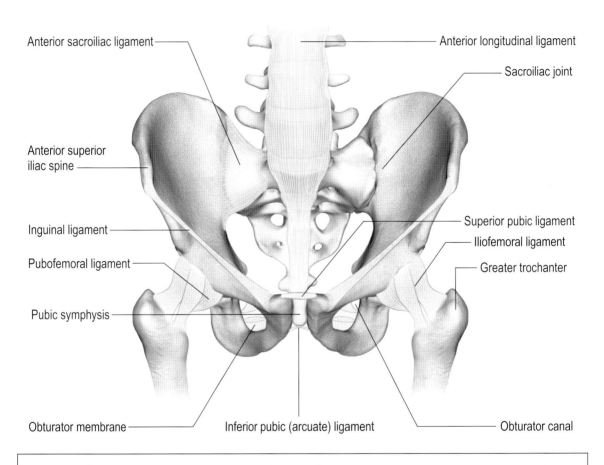

Anterior sacroiliac ligament

Anterior longitudinal ligament

Sacroiliac joint

Anterior superior iliac spine

Inguinal ligament

Superior pubic ligament

Pubofemoral ligament

Iliofemoral ligament

Greater trochanter

Pubic symphysis

Obturator membrane

Inferior pubic (arcuate) ligament

Obturator canal

Figure 9.1
The pelvis and hips

Introduction

Hip injury causing pain is common both in general and in sports, especially when there are elements of twisting and sharp movements. The definition of hip pain is soreness and/or restriction of range of movement in the hip joint. Differential diagnosis of hip and groin pain can be difficult because of the complex interactions of forces through the hip and pelvis, the wide-ranging pathological processes that can occur within this area, and the crossover of signs and symptoms presenting on physical examination (Omar et al 2008).

Manual therapy of the hip has been proven to be an effective treatment mode for hip pain; this can be in the form of either articulation or traction/distraction of the joint (Herding & Kessler 1990, Cibulka & Delitto 1993). Hoeksma et al (2004) and Brantingham et al (2009) found that articulation of the hip joint plus exercise advice was far more effective than exercise advice alone. The NICE *Osteoarthritis: National Clinical Guideline for Care and Management in Adults* (2008) recommends articulation and stretching for use as one of the core treatments in osteoarthritis of the hip. Similarly, the American Physical Therapy Association's (Orthopaedic Section) guidelines on hip pain and mobility deficits make the recommendation of manual therapy for pain relief and improvement of range of mobility within the hip for mild osteoarthritis (Cibulka et al 2009). In addition, manual therapy is recommended in the treatment of osteoarthritis focusing on addressing restriction of movement and the adaptations caused by this (Delarue et al 2007, Hunter & Lo 2008, Zhang et al 2008).

As discussed in Chapter 1 articulation of the hip joint is thought to help in the reduction of pain through the activation of large fiber afferent nerves or by assisting in the lubrication of the synovial joint (Yoder 1990, Makofsky et al 2007, Coelho 2008, Schmid et al 2008). It is also believed to improve the range of movement in the joint post treatment (Makofsky et al 2007, Schwellnus 2008).

Cibulka and Delitto (1993) found that treating the sacroiliac joint reduced pain levels in patients and that rhythmical articulation of the joint, initially with grade 2 and then with grade 4, caused an improvement in range of movement. They also observed that the changes after treatment were not immediate and postulated that this may be because of slower reaction changes to the synovial cartilage or capsule.

Although studies have found that articulation of the sacroiliac joint does not affect the position of the joint, it may still affect the muscular tension in the surrounding muscles (Cibulka et al 1986, Tullberg et al 1998, Foley & Buschbacher 2006). In a study by Kirkaldy-Willis and Cassidy (1985), 71% of patients reported a decrease in pain following articulation of the sacroiliac joint 2 weeks post treatment. However, there is still a great deal of contention about the effects of manual therapy and the sacroiliac joint, and more research into this is needed (Cohen et al 2013).

Bony anatomy

The hip is the name given to the anatomical region formed between the lateral parts of the pelvis and the superior part of the femur. The hipbones, also known as the coxal bones or os coxae, are two identical mirror-image bones that are strongly united to one another. They form a bony ring called the pelvic girdle (hip girdle), joining each other anteriorly and the sacrum posteriorly (Mader 2004). Each coxal bone results from the fusion of three bones – the ilium, the ischium and the pubis – and is firmly attached to the axial skeleton because of its articulation with the sacrum (McCann & Wise 2014). The coxal bones are largely immobile, weight-bearing structures. They also help transfer the weight of the body to the mobile lower limbs, thus providing more stability to the upper extremities (OpenStax 2013).

The bony pelvis is interposed between the lower spinal column and the lower extremities; it includes the pelvic girdle (the two coxal bones), the sacrum and the coccyx. It is divided into the false and true pelvis by an oblique line known as the pelvic brim (Gray 1958). The pelvis functions as the site of attachment for the lower limbs. It also protects the internal reproductive organs, the urinary bladder and a portion of the large intestine. In addition, a woman's pelvis helps protect the developing fetus during pregnancy and forms the pelvic ring through which the fetus passes during normal vaginal delivery (Tate 2009).

Ilium

The ilium is the largest part of the coxal bone that spreads slightly outward to provide the hip prominence. It is fan-shaped and forms the superior portion of the acetabulum. Each ilium attaches posteriorly to the sacrum at the largely immobile sacroiliac joint. The curved, top ridge of the ilium is known as the iliac crest (Mader 2004). The iliac crest terminates anteriorly as the anterior superior iliac spine (ASIS); inferior to this is a rounded protuberance called the anterior inferior iliac spine (AIIS). The crest ends posteriorly as the posterior superior iliac spine; more inferior to this is called the posterior inferior iliac spine (PIIS) (Tate 2009).

Medially, the upper ilium has a large, shallow depression on the internal surface known as the iliac fossa. The fossa is bounded below by the arcuate line and above by the iliac crest. Posteriorly, the ilium has an auricular surface on its medial aspect. This auricular surface is a large, roughened area that articulates with the sacrum's auricular surface to form the sacroiliac joint (OpenStax 2013).

Ischium

The ischium is the most inferior portion of each coxal bone. It forms the posteroinferior portion of a coxal bone and is located inferior to the ilium and behind the pubis. It is the strongest of the three bones that fuse to form the coxa and is itself made up of three portions: the superior ramus, the inferior ramus and the body (Moore & Dalley 1999).

The inferior ramus of the ischium unites with the inferior ramus of the pubis to form a compound structure known as the ischiopubic ramus. The body of the ischium joins with the ilium and pubis, and forms the posterolateral portion of the acetabulum. The posterior region of the inferior ischium has a large, roughened area called the ischial tuberosity, which bears the weight of the body while a person is sitting. Near the junction of the ilium and ischium is a bony projection known as the ischial spine, which projects into the pelvic cavity. The ischial spine separates the lesser sciatic notch and the greater sciatic notch; the space between the ischial spines thus helps determine the pelvic cavity size (OpenStax 2013).

Pubis

The pubis forms the anteromedial part of each coxal bone and constitutes the anterior portion of the acetabulum. The two pubic bones of the hip join with each other at a specialized joint known as the pubic symphysis. The pubic symphysis is a unique structure and is classed as a secondary cartilaginous joint (Standring 2008) because it has a fibrocartilaginous disc which separates the articular surfaces of the pubic bones (Li et al 2006). This allows a small quantity of movement through the joint to aid in the transmission of tensile, shearing and compressive forces placed through it mainly during locomotion and movement (Becker et al 2010). Similar to the ischium, the pubis is made up of three parts: the flat body and the two rami (superior and inferior) (Gray 1958).

The pubic body is the medial and flat portion of the pubis, which unite with the body of the opposite pubic bone at the pubic symphysis. The small bump located superiorly on the pubic body is the pubic tubercle. The superior ramus of the pubis is the portion of the pubic bone that extends laterally from the pubic body to unite with the ilium. The inferior ramus of the pubis is the segment of bone that passes laterally and downward from the medial end of the superior pubic ramus to articulate with the ischial ramus (Thompson 2002).

Acetabulum

The acetabulum is a shallow depression where the three parts – ilium, ischium, and pubis – of each coxal bone meet. It is a cup-shaped socket and is located on the lateral surface of the pelvis. The acetabulum serves as an articulation point between the lower limb and the pelvic girdle. It articulates with the femur head to make up the hip joint. Inferior to the acetabulum is the large obturator foramen (Mader 2004).

Range of motion

The hip muscles exert 3° of freedom on three mutually perpendicular axes. These include the transverse axis (flexion and extension), the longitudinal axis (lateral and medial rotation), and the sagittal axis (abduction and adduction) (Schünke et al 2006).

The normal range of motion of the hip has been estimated by a variety of studies (see Table 9.1). Although these have shown similar results in their estimates of normal hip flexion, abduction, and lateral and medial rotation, the estimates for hip extension varied widely (Roach & Miles 1991). It is known that the movement of the hip may vary with age, sex, race, and positioning during measurement, but there have been limited studies on the influence of these factors on range of motion. In addition, the active versus passive range of motion has still not been well documented (Prather et al 2010).

The amount of movement at the sacroiliac joint has been the subject of many arguments over the years among manual therapists, although it is basically agreed that some movement does occur at the joint as it transfers loading between the legs and torso (Vleeming et al 2013) and that the movement decreases from childhood to adulthood as our bodies

Movement type	Range of motion (°)
Flexion	115–125
Extension	15–30
Abduction	30–50
Adduction	30
Lateral (external) rotation	30–45
Medial (internal) rotation	40–60

Table 9.1

Estimated normal range of motion of the hip

Data from Daniels & Worthingharn 1972, Kendall et al 1973, Hoppenfeld 1976, Mohr 1989, Roach & Miles 1991, Seidenberg & Childress 2005

grow and increase in weight-bearing through the joint (Kampen & Tillmann 1998). Most of the current research on the sacroiliac joint suggests that there is between 1.3° and 3.6° of movement at the joint, with an average of 2° (Tullberg et al 1998, Sturesson et al 2000a, 2000b, Kibsgård et al 2012).

In the pubic symphysis there is also a small amount of movement that allows for forces to travel through the area. It is believed that, in normal physiological conditions, there is approximately 2 mm (approximately 1/12 inch) of movement at the pubic symphysis and approximately 1° of rotation (Becker et al 2010). During pregnancy this range of movement increases due to the effects of relaxin on collagen fibers within the pelvic ligaments (Samuel et al 1996). This increase in movement can be between 32–68% (Mens et al 2009).

Epidemiology

Hip and pelvis injuries are common in all populations, male and female, the young and the old, and athletes of numerous sports. However, the incidence and etiology of these injuries vary considerably depending on age, sex and sports type in which athletes participate (Larkin 2010). The sacroiliac joint is believed to be the source of pain in 15–30% of the population with low back pain (Dreyfuss et al 2004, Cohen et al 2013).

The prevalence of hip and pelvis injury and pain is highest in adolescents and older adults. Boyd et al (1997) suggest that 10–24% of injuries reported during recreational activities or athletics in children are associated with the hip. However, a significant acute injury to the hip and pelvis is very rare in young children. The most common hip disorder that affects children and adolescents is transient synovitis. Other notable disorders include developmental hip dysplasia, Legg–Calvé–Perthes disease (LCPD) and slipped capital femoral epiphysis (Spahn et al 2005).

In adults, the prevalence of hip and pelvis pain increases with age; the risk of pain from hip osteoarthritis also increases substantially (Larkin 2010). In addition, older adults are more prone to hip fractures. According to NICE (2011), hip fracture accounted for approximately 60,000 emergency hospital admissions in the UK in the year 2010–2011 in adults (age [3] 18 years). Among those patients, 54,000 were reported to have undergone a hip fracture procedure,

73% of whom were female and 92% were aged 65 or over. An estimated 103 per 100,000 standard population adults aged 18 or over undergo hip fracture procedures annually (NICE 2011).

The overall prevalence of sports injuries to the pelvis and hip is relatively low. According to Braly et al (2006), only 5–6% of sports injuries originate in this region. However, those who participate in explosive and contact sports have the maximum risk of developing a hip or pelvis problem (Watkins & Peabody 1996). Some studies have found that athletic hip injuries can relate to 2–8% of injuries and 13% in footballers (Ekstrand & Gillquist 1983, Ekstrand & Hilding 1999, Emery & Meeuwisse 2001). One study

Condition	Description	Reference
Hip dislocation	Usually results from a traumatic injury, a high energy directed along the axis of the femur Can be anterior, posterior or central May present with associated injuries, such as fractures of the femoral head or neck Often occurs because of motor vehicle accidents (about 70% of cases) Occurs predominantly in the posterior region (about 90% of cases)	Seidenberg (2010), Kovacevic et al (2011)
Osteitis pubis	A chronic inflammatory condition that affects the pubic symphysis and surrounding muscle insertions May occur as an inflammatory process in athletes Often reported in athletic sports requiring excessive side-to-side motion, cutting, twisting and pivoting on one leg, or multidirectional motions with frequent acceleration and deceleration Occurs most commonly in males aged 30–50 years	Sing et al (1995), Byrd (1996), Choi et al (2008)
Symphysis pubis dysfunction	During pregnancy Commonly associated with pain on weight-bearing activities such as walking and climbing stairs May hear or feel a grinding or clicking feeling in the joint Due to high levels of relaxin and increase in weight during pregnancy	Maclennan & Maclennan (1997), Jain et al (2006), Becker et al (2010)
Athletic pubalgia (sports hernia, Gilmore's groin)	Chronic groin pain Pain induced with sports, predominantly extension and twisting Pain can radiate into medial thigh and occasionally testicles in males Can be caused by tearing of external oblique aponeurosis, conjoint tendon (inguinal aponeurotic falx) or abdominal internal oblique, or by abnormality within the rectus abdominis	Larson et al (2011), Meyers et al (2012), Hegedus et al (2013)
Avascular necrosis of the femoral head (Perthes, Legg–Calvé–Perthes disease)	A pathological process that results from disturbance in blood supply to the bone This condition causes a softening and breaking down of the femoral head Results in bone death and osteophyte formation Causes progressive arthritis of the hip joint in relatively young adults Mean age of incidence: 38 years Possible causes include hip dislocation, fractures of the femoral neck, chronic corticosteroid use, heavy alcohol intake, blood clots and damage to the arteries	Steinberg (1997), Lavernia et al (1999)

(Continued)

Condition	Description	Reference
Osteoarthritis of the hip	Causes pain and swelling in the hip joint Results in anterior hip pain in most patients aged 50 years or over Often develops as people get older Symptoms include increased pain and stiffness, tenderness in joints, reduced range of movement in the joints, and weakness and muscle wasting	Idjadi & Meislin (2004), Seidenberg (2010)
Transient synovitis	A self-limited unilateral inflammatory synovitis in which an inflammation of the synovium occurs at the capsule of the hip joint The most common reason for hip pain in children aged 3–10 years Affects boys twice as often as girls	Illingworth (1978), Fabry (2010)

Table 9.2
Common disorders of the pelvis and hip

found that football (soccer) players had a historical presentation of 58% of hip/groin pain (Harris & Murray 1974). In other studies they found the incidence rate was on average 10–18 per hundred football patients (Hölmich & Amager 2014).

Hip and pelvis pain is more widespread in women than men. Regardless of age or sport, most studies note that women are twice as likely as men to suffer from hip pain (Tüchsen et al 2003).

The most common disorders of the pelvis and hip are summarized in Table 9.2.

Pelvis and hip examination

Medical history

Taking a detailed medical history of the patient is the most important part for the pelvis and hip examination. In most cases, the narrative provided by the patient presenting with hip pathology helps characterize the severity of the pain and facilitate the physical examination. Apart from characterizing the pain as constant or intermittent, sharp or dull, severe or mild, the examiner should ask the patient about the onset, behavior since onset, exacerbating and relieving factors, quality, radiation, severity, and timing (duration) of symptoms. The primary goal of the history taking should be to determine whether the injury or pain is acute, chronic, or acute-on-chronic in nature.

Red flags

Table 9.3 lists red flag conditions for the therapist to note.

Physical examination

Physical examinations of the pelvis and hip should be done in a systematic manner to confirm initial findings and fully explore the nature and extent of the problem. A general evaluation of the pelvis and hips usually involves inspection, palpation, range of motion and a variety of special tests.

Inspection

The physical examination process should start with a careful visual inspection of the how the patient is affected, and their posture and gait pattern. For this, the patient should be asked to sit and rise from the chair in a characteristic manner. While standing, the clinician should examine the patient from the anterior, posterior and lateral aspects. Any postural abnormalities observed, such as pelvic obliquity, muscular atrophy or weakness, and abnormal scoliotic or lordotic curves, should be noted carefully. It is also important to ascertain the presence or absence of shortening during visual inspection of the patient's hip and pelvis. In true shortening, the affected limb is shorter than the other; in apparent shortening, the limb is not shorter in length than the other, but appears shorter due to a contracture of the hip.

Condition	Signs and symptoms
Pathological fractures of the femoral neck	Older females over 70 years of age
	Severe, constant hip, groin or knee pain
	Past history of trauma, such as a fall from a standing position
Avascular necrosis (AVN) of the femoral head	Prolonged corticosteroid use
	History of excessive alcohol use
	History of slipped capital femoral epiphysis
	Gradual onset of pain
	Groin, thigh or medial knee pain – worse with weight-bearing
Cancer	Previous history of cancer (e.g. prostate, breast or any reproductive cancer)
	Unexpected loss of weight
	Constant, progressive pain unchanged by positions or movement
Colon cancer	Age > 50 years
	Family history of colon cancer
	Bowel disturbances (e.g. rectal bleeding, black stools)
Infection	Fever, chills
	Recent urinary tract or skin infection
	Burning sensation with urination
	Unrelenting night pain or pain at rest
	No improvement after 6 weeks of conventional treatment

Table 9.3
Red flags for serious pathology in the hip and pelvis region

Data from Meyers et al (2000), Henschke et al (2007), Gabbe et al (2009), Van den Bruel et al (2010), Reiman & Thorborg (2014)

Palpation

While examining the pelvis and hips, several important bony and soft-tissue structures need to be palpated to determine areas of pathology. Palpation should include the musculature, bony prominences, sacroiliac joint, pubic symphysis, tendinous origins and insertions, bursae and apophyses.

Range of motion

Range of motion of the hip should be assessed in three ways: active, passive and resisted isometric. The examiner may use a goniometer to assess the range of motion (McRae 2010). The movements to be tested include flexion, extension, abduction, adduction, lateral rotation and medial rotation. Special attention should be paid to abduction and internal rotation, as these two are the most frequently compromised motions, involved in many pathological conditions of the hip. After measuring the range of motion of the hip, the examiner should compare the collected data with a reliable standard (see Table 9.2).

Special tests

See Table 9.4.

Test	Procedure	Positive sign	Interpretation
Trendelenburg's sign	The patient stands on both feet. The examiner asks the patient to slowly raise one foot off the ground, without taking any additional support. The patient keeps an upright posture without significant tilt of the upper trunk.	A compensatory tilt of the torso or a drop of the contralateral iliac crest	Presence of a muscular dysfunction Subluxation or dislocation of the hip
Faber's test	The patient lies supine and the tested leg is placed in a flexed, abducted, externally rotated position.	Pain elicited on the ipsilateral side anteriorly Pain elicited on the contralateral side posteriorly	Hip joint disorder Sacroiliac joint dysfunction
Ober's test	The patient is placed in a lateral decubitus position. The affected knee is then flexed to 90° while the pelvis is stabilized. The examiner passively abducts and pulls the patient's upper leg posteriorly until the thigh is in line with the torso.	Leg remains abducted and does not fall to the table	Excessive tightness of the iliotibial band
Thomas test	The patient is placed in a supine position with their back flat on the table. The patient is then instructed to flex one leg and pull it to the chest with their hands.	Straight leg lifting off the exam table	Flexion contracture of the hip
Log roll test	The patient lies supine with both hip and knee extended. The examiner passively rotates both fully extended legs internally and externally.	Pain in the anterior hip or groin	Piriformis syndrome Slipped capital femoral epiphysis
Ely's test	The patient lies prone with their legs fully extended. The examiner passively flexes the knee, making the heel touch the buttock. The examiner then observes the ipsilateral hip for vertical separation from the exam table.	Hip is forced to lift off the exam table	Rectus femoris contracture

Table 9.4

Special tests for pelvis and hip examination

Data from Baxter (2003), McFadden & Seidenberg (2010), McRae (2010)

Pelvis and hip muscles

Name	Origin	Insertion	Action	Nerve supply
Ischiocavernosus	Ischial ramus and tuberosity	Crus of penis or clitoris	Maintains the erection of the penis or clitoris via vasocompression of the veins	Deep branch of perineal nerve (branch of pudendal nerve S2–S4)
Superficial transverse perineal	Ischial tuberosity	Perineal body	Reinforces the action of the deep transverse perineal muscle to stabilize the perineal body	Deep branch of perineal nerve (branch of pudendal nerve S2–S4)
Sphincter urethrae	Inferior aspect of pubic ramus and ischial tuberosity	Surrounds urethra; in females, some fibers also enclose vagina	Controls the flow of urine through the urethra; also compresses the vagina in females	Deep branch of perineal nerve (branch of pudendal nerve S2–S4)
Deep transverse perineal	Inner aspect of ischiopubic ramus	Median raphe (male), perineal body and external anal sphincter	Supports the function of the levator ani and sphincter urethra	Deep branch of perineal nerve (branch of pudendal nerve S2–S4)
Levator ani	Dorsal surface of pubis and fascia of obturator internus	Coccyx, opposite levator ani	Supports the pelvic viscera and structures that pass through it	Nerve to levator ani (branches of S4), inferior rectal nerve (from pudendal nerve S3–S4)
Coccygeus (ischiococcygeus)	Ischial spine	Lower two sacral and upper two coccygeal spinal segments, blends with sacrospinous ligament	Supports the pelvic viscera, flexion of the coccyx, stabilizes the sacroiliac joint	Anterior rami of S4–S5
Gluteus maximus	Outer surface of ilium, iliolumbar fascia, sacrum and sacrotuberous ligament	Gluteal tuberosity of femur and iliotibial tract	Abducts, laterally (externally rotates) and extends the thigh	Inferior gluteal nerve (L5–S2)
Gluteus medius	Outer surface of ilium	Lateral part of greater trochanter of femur	Abducts and medially rotates the thigh	Superior gluteal nerve (L4–S1)
Gluteus minimus	Outer surface of ilium	Anterior part of greater trochanter of femur	Abducts and medially rotates the thigh	Superior gluteal nerve (L4–S1)

(Continued)

Name	Origin	Insertion	Action	Nerve supply
Piriformis	Pelvic surface of sacrum, passes through greater sciatic foramen	Superior border of the greater trochanter of femur	Hip external rotation, assists with hip abduction if the hip is flexed	Anterior rami of S1–S2
Obturator internus	Internal obturator foramen	Medial part of the greater trochanter of femur	Hip external rotation, assists with hip abduction if the hip is flexed	Sacral plexus (L5–S2)
Obturator externus	Outer surface of inferior and superior rami of pubis and ramus of ischium	Trochanteric fossa of femur	Laterally (externally) rotates the femur	Obturator nerve (L3–L4)
Quadratus femoris	Lateral portion of ischial tuberosity	Inferior to intertrochanteric crest	Laterally (externally) rotates the femur	Sacral plexus (L5–S1)
Gemellus superior	Spine of ischium	Greater trochanter via tendon of obturator internus	Laterally (externally) rotates the femur	Sacral plexus (L5–S1)
Gemellus inferior	Superior surface of ischial tuberosity	Greater trochanter via tendon of obturator internus	Laterally (externally) rotates the femur	Sacral plexus (L5–S1)
Psoas major	Transverse processes and bodies of T12–L5	Lesser trochanter of femur	Flexion and laterally (externally) rotates the thigh	Lumbar plexus via anterior branches of L1–L4
Psoas minor	Body of T12–L1	Pectineal line and iliopectineal eminence	Weak trunk flexor	L1
Illiacus	Iliac fossa, ala of sacrum and anterior inferior iliac spine	Lesser trochanter of femur	Flexion of the hip	Femoral nerve (L2–L3)
Tensor fasciae latae	External anterior surface of iliac crest	Iliotibial tract (band)	Flexion and abduction of the hip	Superior gluteal nerve (L4–S1)
Sartorius	Anterior superior iliac spine	Superior medial surface of tibia (pes anserinus conjoined tendon of sartorius, gracilis and semitendinosus)	Flexion, abduction and laterally (externally) rotates the thigh	Femoral nerve (L2–L3)

(Continued)

Name	Origin	Insertion	Action	Nerve supply
Rectus femoris	Anterior head: anterior inferior iliac spine Posterior head: ilium superior to acetabulum	Quadriceps tendon to patella, via ligamentum patellae on to tubercle of tibia	Extension of the knee and flexion of the hip	Femoral nerve (L2–L4)
Gracilis	Ischiopubic ramus	Superior medial surface of tibia (pes anserinus conjoined tendon of sartorius, gracilis and semitendinosus)	Flexion, medially (internally) rotates, and adduction of the thigh	Obturator nerve (L3–L4)
Adductor magnus	Inferior pubic ramus, ramus and tuberosity of ischium	Linea aspera and adductor tubercle of femur	Adduction, extension and medial (internally) rotates the thigh	Obturator nerve (L3–L4)
Semimembranosus	Tuberosity of ischium	Medial condyle of tibia	Flexion of the knee and extension of the hip	Tibial portion of sciatic nerve (L5–S2)
Semitendinosus	Tuberosity of ischium	Superior medial surface of tibia (pes anserinus conjoined tendon of sartorius, gracilis and semitendinosus)	Flexion of the knee and extension of the hip	Tibial portion of sciatic nerve (L5–S2)
Biceps femoris	Long head: ischial tuberosity and sacrotuberous ligament Short head: linea aspera and lateral supracondylar ridge	Lateral (external) portion of fibular head and lateral condyle of tibia	Flexion of the knee and long head assists in extension of the thigh	Long head: tibial portion of sciatic nerve (S1–S3) Short head: common peroneal (fibula) portion of sciatic nerve (L5–S2)

Table 9.5
Pelvis and hip muscles

Techniques: pelvis and hip

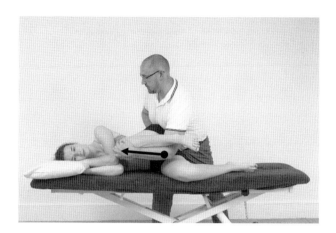

T9.1 Side-lying flexion of the hip joint

- With the patient lying on their side, stand behind the patient.
- Place your corresponding hand under the patient's knee, supporting the leg. Your forearm should be parallel with their leg.
- Use your opposite hand to support the pelvis from behind, stabilizing the patient.
- With a forward movement of your arm, bring the patient's leg forward and up in an arching motion.
- Hip joint flexion is approximately 120°.

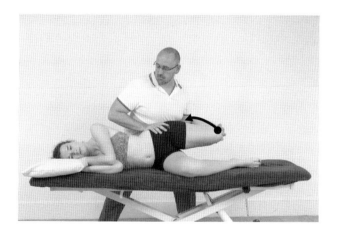

T9.2 Side-lying extension of the hip joint

- With the patient lying on their side, stand behind the patient.
- Place your corresponding hand under the patient's knee, supporting the leg.
- Use your opposite hand to support the pelvis from behind, stabilizing the patient.
- With a backward movement of your arm and body, bring the patient's leg backwards towards yourself.
- Hip joint extension is approximately 30°.

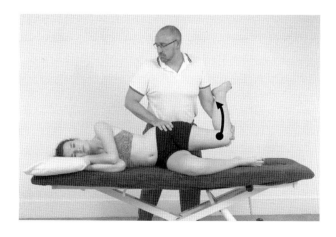

T9.3 Side-lying medial rotation of the hip joint

- With the patient lying on their side, stand behind the patient.
- Place your corresponding hand under the patient's knee, supporting their leg.
- Your opposite hand is palpating over the hip joint and stabilizing the pelvis.
- In this position, rotate the patient's leg down towards the plinth, pivoting the movement through the hip joint.
- Hip joint medial rotation is approximately 50°.

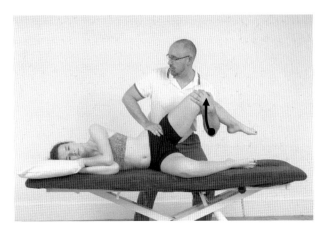

T9.4 Side-lying lateral rotation of the hip joint

- With the patient lying on their side, stand behind the patient.
- Place your corresponding hand under the patient's knee, supporting their leg.
- Your opposite hand is palpating over the hip joint and stabilizing the pelvis.
- In this position, rotate the patient's leg up towards you while pivoting the movement through the hip joint.
- Hip joint lateral rotation is approximately 40°.

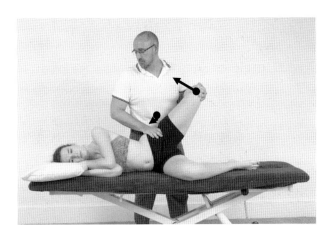

T9.5 Side-lying abduction of the hip joint

- With the patient lying on their side, stand behind patient.
- Place your corresponding hand under the patient's knee, supporting the leg.
- Your opposite hand is palpating over the hip joint and supporting the pelvis.
- With your arm, lift the patient's leg up in an arching motion.
- Hip joint abduction is approximately 50°.

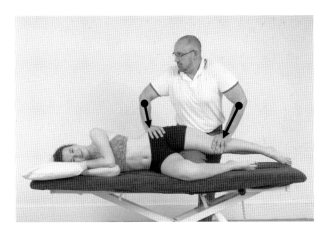

T9.6 Side-lying distraction of the hip joint

- With the patient lying on their side, stand behind patient, placing your closest leg on the plinth.
- Place the patient's leg on to your leg. With your corresponding hand, fix above the knee joint.
- Place your palpating hand over the hip joint.
- Using your leg as a fulcrum, place a downward movement from your corresponding hand to allow distraction to occur at the hip joint.

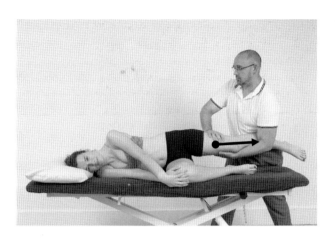

T9.7 Side-lying traction of the hip joint

- With the patient lying on their side, stand behind the patient.
- Ask the patient to hold on to their bottom leg.
- Place your corresponding hand and palpating hand above the knee, securing the knee joint, and place the patient's lower leg between your body and elbow, stabilizing the patient's leg.
- In this position, lean back to cause a traction through the hip joint.

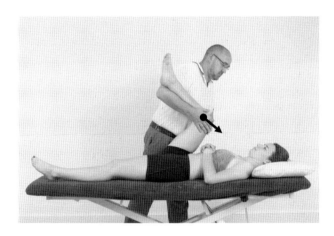

T9.8 Supine flexion of the hip joint

- With the patient supine, stand to the side of the patient.
- Place your corresponding hand below the knee and your palpating hand on top of the knee, securing the knee complex.
- Hold the knee just above 90°.
- Have the leg furthest away from the plinth in front of the back leg.
- With a forward movement of your arm and body, bring the patient's leg forward and up in an arching motion.
- Hip joint flexion is approximately 115–125°.

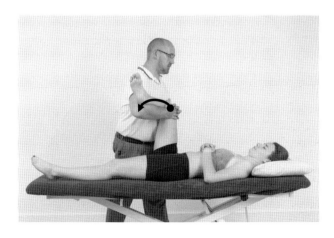

T9.9 Supine external (lateral) rotation of the hip joint

- With the patient supine, stand to the side of the patient.
- Flex the knee and place your corresponding hand below and to the inner side of the knee.
- Place your palpating hand around the front of the knee, securing the knee joint.
- In this position, rotate the patient's knee in an outward motion, pivoting the movement through the hip joint.
- Hip joint external (lateral) rotation is approximately 30–45°.

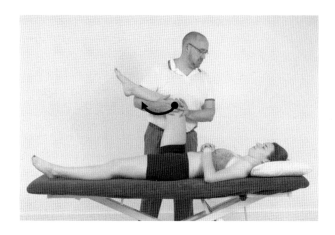

T9.10 Supine medial rotation of the hip joint

- With the patient supine, stand to the side of the patient.
- Flex the knee and place your corresponding hand below and to the inner side of the knee.
- Place your palpating hand around the front of the knee, securing the knee joint.
- In this position, rotate the patient's knee inwards, pivoting the movement through the hip joint.
- Hip joint medial rotation is approximately 40–60°.

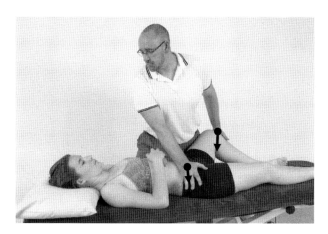

T9.11 Supine abduction of the hip joint

- With the patient supine, stand to the side of the patient.
- Place your palpating hand on the front of the anterior superior iliac spine (ASIS) furthest away from you.
- Palpate, with your fingers pointing down and away from the patient.
- Flex the closest leg and place your corresponding hand just below and in front of the patella.
- Draw the leg out towards you while supporting the patient's knee on to your upper thigh.
- Hip abduction is approximately 50°.

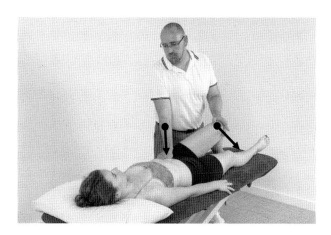

T9.12 Supine adduction of the hip joint

- With the patient supine, stand to the side of the patient.
- Place your palpating hand on the front of the ASIS closest to you, with your fingers pointing away from the patient and stabilizing the pelvis.
- Flex the closest leg and place your corresponding hand in front of the knee.
- Draw the leg in towards the patient, pivoting through the hip joint.
- Hip joint adduction is approximately 30°.

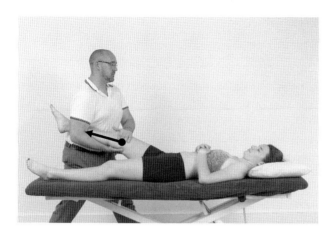

T9.13 Supine traction of the hip joint

- With the patient supine, stand to one side, facing them.
- Place your corresponding hand above the knee joint, supporting the lower leg between your body and arm.
- Place the palpating hand above the patient's knee.
- With a backward movement of your body, draw the patient's leg in a backward motion, tractioning the hip joint.

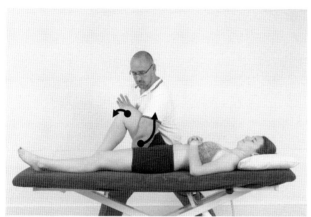

T9.14 Supine distraction of the hip joint (method 1)

- With the patient supine, stand to the side of them, with your body facing towards their feet.
- Flex the knee and place your corresponding hand on to the inner side of the patient's upper thigh.
- Note: you can place a pillow across the patient's inner thigh to act as a barrier or for comfort.
- Place the palm of your hand to the side of the patient's knee.
- In this position, rotate your body in an inward motion towards the plinth as well as gently pushing on to the side of the knee.
- Note: this motion should come from your waist and with a stable base of one foot behind the other.

T9.15 Supine distraction of the hip joint (method 2)

- With the patient supine, stand to the side of the patient.
- Flex the knee and place both hands around the inner side of the patient's upper thigh by holding on to your elbows.
- Note: you can place a pillow across the patient's inner thigh to act as a barrier or for comfort.
- In this position, add an element of compression and a 'J'-like motion by bringing your elbows in to your abdomen and lifting.
- From knees bent, straighten up while compressing around the thigh at all times.

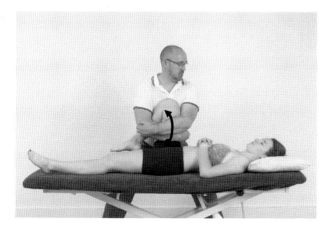

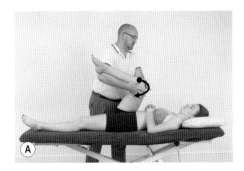

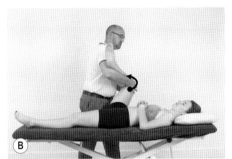

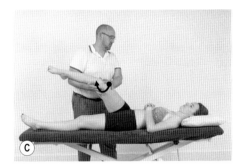

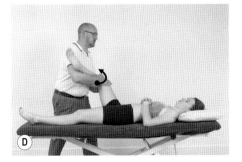

T9.16 Supine circumduction of hip joint

- With the patient supine, stand to the side of the patient.
- Flex the knee at 90° and allow the patient's leg to rest on your forearm.
- Place one hand on each side of the patient's knee joint.
- In this position, rotate the patient's leg as well as your body in all ranges of movement in a circular motion, pivoting through the hip joint.
- The amplitude of this movement depends on the tissues you want to influence.

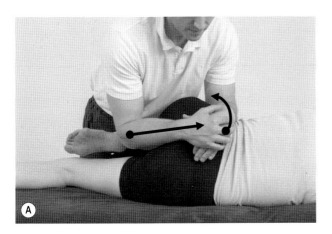

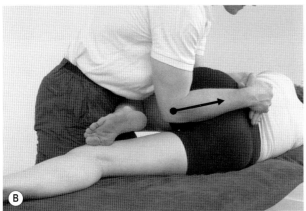

T9.17 Anterior rotation of the innominate – side-lying

- Stand to the side of the patient, with the patient lying on their side facing you.
- Flex the top leg and support the knee on your upper thigh – always retain body contact with the patient's supporting leg.
- Place your palpating hand around the side and back of the innominate, palpating the posterior superior iliac spine (PSIS).
- The forearm of the corresponding hand is on the ischial tuberosity.
- Compress and keep close body contact with the patient's leg.
- Movement is generated by shifting your weight from front foot to back foot and pulling through the superior portion of the innominate and pushing up through the ischial tuberosity.

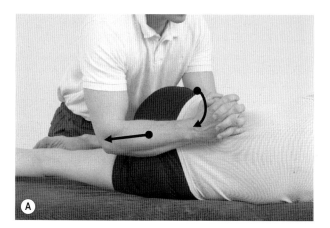

(A)

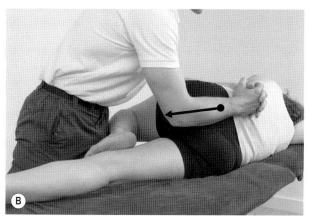

(B)

T9.18 Posterior rotation of the innominate – side-lying

- While the patient is side-lying, flex their top leg and support it.
- Place one forearm over the posterior portion of the ischial tuberosity.
- Place the forearm of your opposite hand over the iliac crest and interlock your fingers.
- Compress and keep close body contact with the patient's leg.
- Movement is generated by shifting your weight from the back foot to the front foot.
- With a posterior movement of your arms, move the patient's ileum backwards in an arching movement.

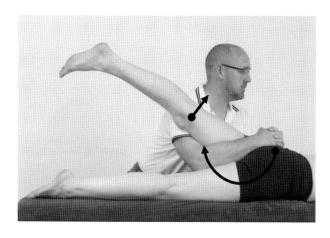

T9.19 Prone anterior rotation of the innominate bone / Sacroiliac joint articulation 1

- With the patient prone, stand to the side of the patient.
- Flex the leg closest to you.
- Now place your forearm under the patient's thigh and above the knee.
- Interlace your fingers together, cupping around the back of the innominate and PSIS.
- Keep close body contact with the patient's leg.
- From flexed knees, stand up straight to allow for a forward movement of the pelvis.

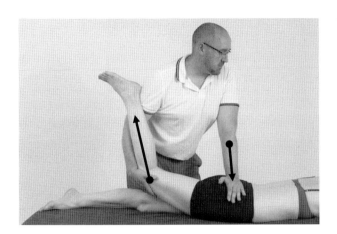

T9.20 Prone anterior rotation of the innominate bone / Sacroiliac joint articulation 2

- With the patient lying on their front, stand to the side of the patient.
- Flex and lift the leg furthest away from you with the corresponding hand by supporting the front of the knee. Have your forearm parallel to the patient's leg.
- Place your palpating hand on the PSIS, with your fingers pointing away from the patient.
- From flexed knees, stand up straight and lift your hand, supporting the knee in an upward motion to allow for a forward movement of the pelvis.

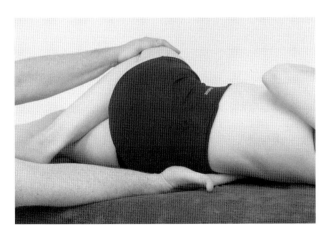

T9.21 Supine examination of the sacroiliac joint, hand position

- To palpate the sacroiliac joint, rotate the patient away from you and locate the PSIS.
- The area of the sacroiliac joint is slightly medial and inferior of the PSIS.

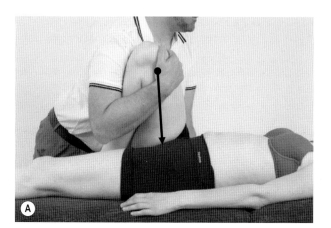

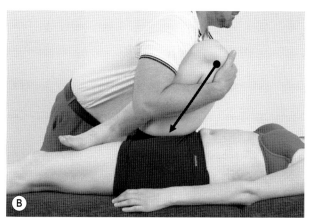

T9.22 Supine gapping of the sacroiliac joint

- With the patient supine, stand to the side of the patient.
- Flex the patient's leg and place your corresponding hand around the patient's thigh, supporting the leg.
- Place the palpating hand on the sacroiliac joint.
- With a downward pressure from your body, compress the adducted leg towards the plinth, thus gapping the sacroiliac joint.
- Vary the amount of hip adduction and flexion to apply a gapping force through the sacroiliac joint, as shown in photograph **b**.

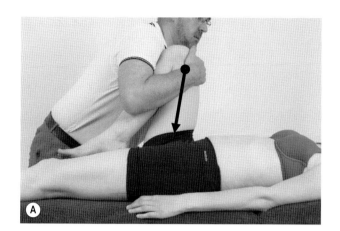

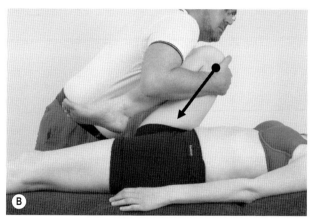

T9.23 Supine shearing of the sacroiliac joint

- With the patient supine, stand to the side of the patient.
- Flex the patient's leg and place your corresponding hand around the patient's thigh, supporting the leg.
- Place the palpating hand on the sacroiliac joint.
- With a downward pressure from your body, compress the abducted leg towards the plinth, thus gapping the sacroiliac joint.
- Vary the amount of hip abduction and flexion to apply a gapping force through the sacroiliac joint, as shown in photograph **b**.

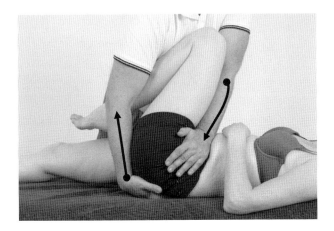

T9.24 Supine posterior rotation articulation of the sacroiliac joint

- With the patient supine, stand to the side of the patient.
- Flex the opposite leg.
- Place your hand under the patient's ischial tuberosity, supporting the leg against your body.
- Place your opposite hand on the patient's ASIS.
- Lean forward with your body, allowing for a posterior rotation of the patient's innominate.

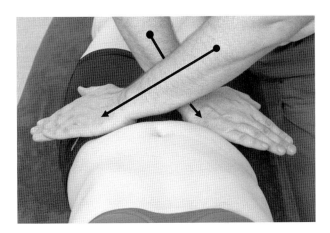

T9.25 Supine sacral iliac springing

- The patient should lie supine.
- With crossed forearms, compress on the ASIS with the heel of your hand.
- Apply an oblique inferior pressure onto the ASIS.
- This movement will generate a short lever sacroiliac shearing/spring of the joint that you will feel with proprioception.

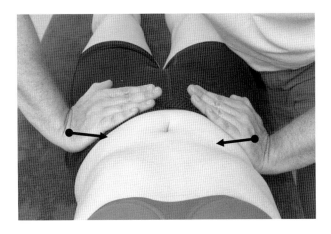

T9.26 Supine sacral iliac springing/gapping

- The patient should lie supine.
- Locate the anterior portion of the iliac crests.
- With the heel of your hand, compress towards the patient's midline.
- This short lever technique will cause a 'flaring' of the innominates posteriorly, thus creating a gapping of the sacroiliac joint.

REFERENCES

Baxter RE (2003). Pocket Guide to Musculoskeletal Assessment. Philadelphia: WB Saunders.

Becker I, Woodley SJ, Stringer MD (2010). The adult human pubic symphysis: a systematic review. Journal of Anatomy 217(5):475-487.

Boyd KT, Peirce NS, Batt ME (1997). Common hip injuries in sport. Sports Medicine 24(4):273-288.

Braly BA, Beall DP, Martin HD (2006). Clinical examination of the athletic hip. Clinics in Sports Medicine 25(2):199-210.

Brantingham JW, Globe G, Pollard H et al (2009). Manipulative therapy for lower extremity conditions: expansion of literature review. Journal of Manipulative and Physiological Therapeutics 32(1):53-71.

Byrd JT (1996). Labral lesions: an elusive source of hip pain case reports and literature review. Arthroscopy: The Journal of Arthroscopic and Related Surgery 12(5):603-612.

Choi H, McCartney M, Best TM (2008). Treatment of osteitis pubis and osteomyelitis of the pubic symphysis in athletes: a systematic review. British Journal of Sports Medicine, bjsports50989.

Cibulka MT, Delitto A (1993). A comparison of two different methods to treat hip pain in runners. Journal of Orthopaedic and Sports Physical Therapy 17(4):172-176.

Cibulka MT, Rose SJ, Delitto A et al (1986). Hamstring muscle strain treated by mobilizing the sacroiliac joint. Physical Therapy 66(8):1220-1223.

Cibulka MT, White DM, Woehrle J et al (2009). Hip pain and mobility deficits – hip osteoarthritis: Clinical practice guidelines linked to the international classification of functioning, disability, and health from the Orthopaedic Section of the American Physical Therapy Association. Journal of Orthopaedic and Sports Physical Therapy 39(4):A1-A25.

Coelho LFDS (2008). The muscular flexibility training and the range of movement improvement: a critical literature review. Motricidade 4(3):61-72.

Cohen SP, Chen Y, Neufeld NJ (2013). Sacroiliac joint pain: a comprehensive review of epidemiology, diagnosis and treatment. Expert Review of Neurotherapeutics 13(1):99-116.

Daniels L, Worthingham C (1972). Muscle Testing: Techniques of Manual Examination, 3rd ed. Philadelphia: WB Saunders.

Delarue Y, de Branche B, Anract P et al (2007). Supervised or unsupervised exercise for the treatment of hip and knee osteoarthritis. Clinical practice recommendations. Annales de Réadaptation et de Médecine Physique: Revue Scientifique de la Société Française de Rééducation Fonctionnelle de Réadaptation et de Médecine Physique 50(9):759-68.

Dreyfuss P, Dreyer SJ, Cole A et al (2004). Sacroiliac joint pain. Journal of the American Academy of Orthopaedic Surgeons 12(4):255-265.

Ekstrand J, Gillquist J (1983). The avoidability of soccer injuries. International Journal of Sports Medicine 4(2):124-128.

Ekstrand J, Hilding J (1999). The incidence and differential diagnosis of acute groin injuries in male soccer players. Scandinavian Journal of Medicine and Science in Sports 9:98-103.

Emery CA, Meeuwisse WH (2001). Risk factors for groin injuries in hockey. Medicine and Science in Sports and Exercise 33(9):1423-1433.

Fabry G (2010). Clinical practice: the hip from birth to adolescence. European Journal of Pediatrics 169(2):143-8.

Foley BS, Buschbacher RM (2006). Sacroiliac joint pain: anatomy, biomechanics, diagnosis, and treatment. American Journal of Physical Medicine and Rehabilitation 85(12):997-1006.

Gabbe BJ, Bailey M, Cook JL et al (2009). The association between hip and groin injuries in the elite junior football years and injuries sustained during elite senior competition. British Journal of Sports Medicine, bjsports 62554.

Gray H (1958). Gray's Anatomy: Descriptive and Applied. Longmans, Green & Co.

Harris NH, Murray RO (1974). Lesions of the symphysis in athletes. British Medical Journal 4(5938):211-214.

Hegedus EJ, Stern B, Reiman MP et al (2013). A suggested model for physical examination and conservative treatment of athletic pubalgia. Physical Therapy in Sport 14(1):3-16.

Henschke N, Maher CG, Refshauge KM (2007). Screening for malignancy in low back pain patients: a systematic review. European Spine Journal 16(10):1673-1679.

Herding D, Kessler RM (1990). Management of Common Musculoskeletal Disorders. Physical Therapy Principles and Methods, 4. Philadelphia: Lippincott Williams & Wilkins.

Hoeksma HL, Dekker J, Ronday HK et al (2004). Comparison of manual therapy and exercise therapy in osteoarthritis of the hip: a randomized clinical trial. Arthritis Care and Research 51(5):722-729.

Hölmich P, Amager AC (2014). Groin Injuries in Athletes – Development of Clinical Entities, Treatment, and Prevention. Doctoral thesis.

Hoppenfeld S (1976). Physical Examination of the Spine and Extremities. New York: Appleton-Century-Crofts.

Hunter DJ, Lo GH (2008). The management of osteoarthritis: an overview and call to appropriate conservative treatment. Rheumatic Disease Clinics of North America 34(3):689-712.

Idjadi J, Meislin R (2004). Symptomatic snapping hip: targeted treatment for maximum pain relief. The Physician and Sportsmedicine 32(1):25-31.

Illingworth CM (1978). 128 limping children with no fracture, sprain, or obvious cause. Seven were found to have Perthes' disease, 76 seemed to have transient synovitis of the hip, and in 45 the cause seemed to be in the ankle or knee. Clinical Pediatrics 17(2):139-142.

Jain S, Eedarapalli P, Jamjute P et al (2006). Symphysis pubis dysfunction: a practical approach to management. The Obstetrician and Gynaecologist 8:153-158.

Kampen WU, Tillmann B (1998). Age-related changes in the articular cartilage of human sacroiliac joint. Anatomy and Embryology 198(6):505-513.

Kendall HO, Kendall FP, Wadsworth GE (1973). Muscles, testing and function. American Journal of Physical Medicine and Rehabilitation 52(1).

Kibsgård T J, Røise O, Stuge B et al (2012). Precision and accuracy measurement of radiostereometric analysis applied to movement of the sacroiliac joint. Clinical Orthopaedics and Related Research® 470(11):3187-3194.

Kirkaldy-Willis WH, Cassidy JD (1985). Spinal manipulation in the treatment of low-back pain. Canadian Family Physician 31:535.

Kovacevic D, Mariscalco M, Goodwin RC (2011). Injuries about the hip in the adolescent athlete. Sports Medicine and Arthroscopy Review 19(1):64-74.

Larkin B (2010). Epidemiology of hip and pelvis injury. In: PH Seidenberg, JD Bowen eds. The Hip and Pelvis in Sports Medicine and Primary Care. New York: Springer; 1-7.

Larson CM, Pierce BR, Giveans MR (2011). Treatment of athletes with symptomatic intra-articular hip pathology and athletic pubalgia/sports hernia: a case series. Arthroscopy: The Journal of Arthroscopic and Related Surgery 27(6):768-775.

Lavernia CJ, Sierra RJ, Grieco FR (1999). Osteonecrosis of the femoral head. Journal of the American Academy of Orthopaedic Surgeons 7(4):250-261.

Li Z, Alonso JE, Kim JE et al (2006). Three-dimensional finite element models of the human pubic symphysis with viscohyperelastic soft tissues. Annals of Biomedical Engineering 34(9):1452-1462.

McCann S, Wise E (2014). Anatomy Coloring Book. Wokingham: Kaplan Publishing.

McFadden DP, Seidenberg PH (2010). Physical examination of the hip and pelvis. In: PH Seidenberg, JD Bowen eds. The Hip and Pelvis in Sports Medicine and Primary Care. New York: Springer; 9-36.

Maclennan AH, Maclennan SC (1997). Symptom-giving pelvic girdle relaxation of pregnancy, postnatal pelvic joint syndrome and developmental dysplasia of the hip. Acta Obstetricia et Gynecologica Scandinavica 76(8):760-764.

McRae R (2010). Clinical Orthopaedic Examination, 6th ed. Edinburgh: Elsevier Health Sciences; 62-67.

Mader SS (2004). Understanding Human Anatomy and Physiology, 5th ed. New York: McGraw-Hill Science.

Makofsky H, Panicker S, Abbruzzese J et al (2007). Immediate effect of grade IV inferior hip joint mobilization on hip abductor torque: a pilot study. Journal of Manual and Manipulative Therapy 15(2):103-110.

Mens JM, Pool-Goudzwaard A, Stam HJ (2009). Mobility of the pelvic joints in pregnancy-related lumbopelvic pain: a systematic review. Obstetrical and Gynecological Survey 64(3):200-208.

Meyers WC, Foley DP, Garrett WE et al (2000). Management of severe lower abdominal or inguinal pain in high-performance athletes. The American Journal of Sports Medicine 28(1):2-8.

Meyers WC, Yoo E, Devon ON et al (2012). Understanding 'sports hernia' (athletic pubalgia): the anatomic and pathophysiologic basis for abdominal and groin pain in athletes. Operative Techniques in Sports Medicine 20(1):33-45.

Mohr T (1989). Musculoskeletal analysis: the hip. In: RM Scully, MR Barnes eds. Physical Therapy. Philadelphia: JB Lippincott Co; 369-380.

Moore K, Dalley A (1999). Lower limb. In: Clinically Oriented Anatomy, 4th ed. Baltimore: Lippincott Williams & Wilkins.

NICE National Collaborating Centre for Chronic Conditions (UK) (2008). Osteoarthritis: National Clinical Guideline for Care and Management in Adults. London: Royal College of Physicians.

NICE (2011). The management of hip fracture in adults. Available from: https://www.nice.org.uk/guidance/cg124/evidence/full-guideline-183081997 [Accessed 15 February 2016].

Omar IM, Zoga AC, Kavanagh EC et al (2008). Athletic pubalgia and 'sports hernia': Optimal MR imaging technique and findings 1. Radiographics 28(5):1415-1438.

OpenStax College (2013). Anatomy and physiology. Available from: http://cnx.org/content/col11496/latest [Accessed 4 February 2016].

Prather H, Harris-Hayes M, Hunt D et al (2010). Hip range of motion and provocative physical examination tests reliability and agreement in asymptomatic volunteers. PM & R: The Journal of Injury, Function, and Rehabilitation 2(10):888-895.

Reiman MP, Thorborg K (2014). Invited clinical commentary. Clinical examination and physical assessment of hip joint-related pain in athletes. International Journal of Sports Physical Therapy 9(6):737-755.

Roach KE, Miles TP (1991). Normal hip and knee active range of motion: the relationship to age. Physical Therapy 71(9):656-665.

Samuel CS, Butkus ALDONNA, Coghlan JP et al (1996). The effect of relaxin on collagen metabolism in the nonpregnant rat pubic symphysis: the influence of estrogen and progesterone in regulating relaxin activity. Endocrinology 137(9):3884-3890.

Schmid A, Brunner F, Wright A et al (2008). Paradigm shift in manual therapy? Evidence for a central nervous system component in the response to passive cervical joint mobilisation. Manual Therapy 13(5):387-396.

Schünke M, Ross LM, Schulte E et al (2006). Thieme Atlas of Anatomy: General Anatomy and Musculoskeletal System. Thieme.

Schwellnus M (2008). Flexibility and joint range of motion. In: WR Frontera ed. Rehabilitation of Sports Injuries: Scientific Basis. Blackwell Science; 232-257.

Seidenberg PH (2010). Adult hip and pelvis disorders. In: PH Seidenberg, JD Bowen eds. The Hip and Pelvis in Sports Medicine and Primary Care. New York: Springer; 115-147.

Seidenberg PH, Childress MA (2005). Evaluating hip pain in athletes. Journal of Musculoskeletal Medicine 22(5):246-254.

Sing R, Cordes R, Siberski D (1995). Osteitis pubis in the active patient. Physician and Sportsmedicine 23(12):66-73.

Spahn G, Schiele R, Langlotz A et al (2005). Hip pain in adolescents: Results of a cross-sectional study in German pupils and a review of the literature. Acta Paediatrica 94(5):568-573.

Standring S (2008). Gray's Anatomy: The Anatomical Basis of Clinical Practice, 40th ed. New York: Churchill Livingstone-Elsevier.

Steinberg ME (1997). Avascular necrosis: diagnosis, staging, and management. Journal of Musculoskeletal Medicine 14:13-25.

Sturesson B, Uden A, Vleeming A (2000a). A radiostereometric analysis of movements of the sacroiliac joints during the standing hip flexion test. Spine 25:364-368.

Sturesson B, Uden A, Vleeming A (2000b). A radiostereometric analysis of the movements of the sacroiliac joints in the reciprocal straddle position. Spine 25:214-217.

Tate P (2009). Anatomy of Bones and Joints. Seeley's Principles of Anatomy and Physiology. New York: McGraw-Hill; 149-196.

Thompson JP (2002). Netter's Concise Atlas of Orthopaedic Anatomy. Teterboro, NJ: Icon Learning Systems.

Tüchsen F, Hannerz H, Burr H et al (2003). Risk factors predicting hip pain in a 5-year prospective cohort study. Scandinavian Journal of Work, Environment and Health 29(1):35-39.

Tullberg T, Blomberg S, Branth B et al. (1998). Manipulation does not alter the position of the sacroiliac joint. A roentgen stereophotogrammetric analysis. Spine 23:1124-1128.

Van den Bruel A, Haj-Hassan T, Thompson M et al (2010). Diagnostic value of clinical features at presentation to identify serious infection in children in developed countries: a systematic review. The Lancet 375(9717):834-845.

Vleeming A, Schuenke MD, Sturesson B et al (2013). Authors' response to the letter to the Editors by Professor MT Cibulka: a critical interpretation of sacroiliac joint movement studies. Journal of Anatomy 222(3):391-395.

Watkins J, Peabody P (1996). Sports injuries in children and adolescents treated at a sports injury clinic. The Journal of Sports Medicine and Physical Fitness 36(1):43-48.

Yoder E (1990). Physical therapy management of non-surgical hip problems in adults. In: L Echternach ed. Physical Therapy of the Hip. New York, NY: Churchill Livingstone.

Zhang W, Moskowitz RW, Nuki G et al (2008). OARSI recommendations for the management of hip and knee osteoarthritis, Part II: OARSI evidence-based, expert consensus guidelines. Osteoarthritis and Cartilage 16(2):137-162.

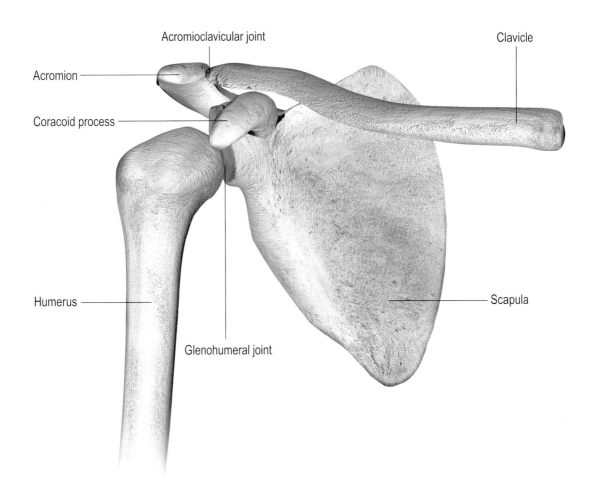

Acromioclavicular joint

Clavicle

Acromion

Coracoid process

Humerus

Glenohumeral joint

Scapula

Figure 10.1
The shoulder

Introduction

Shoulder pain is the most common musculoskeletal peripheral joint pain and the third most common site of pain reported after cervical and lumbar spine (Chen 2012). In the year 2000 the cost of treating shoulder dysfunction in the United States was estimated at $7 billion (Meislin et al 2005). In the US 200,000 rotator cuff operations are performed annually (Hettrich et al 2014).

Shoulder dysfunction is most commonly found in the elderly, in people with occupations that involve repetitive movements, in sportsmen and women practicing certain sports, such as racquet sports, swimming or sports that involve throwing, and in people with some medical conditions, such as diabetes.

Occupations that have been shown to have a high occurrence of shoulder complaints include manual handlers (Silverstein et al 1998, Roquelaure 2006), dentists (Lalumandier et al 2001, Dajpratham et al 2010, Harutunian et al 2011), people who work at computers (Brandt et al 2004, Bongers et al 2006), and musicians who play instruments with their arm/arms in a raised position (Nyman et al 2007, Leaver et al 2011).

The most regular injury in swimming is to the shoulder (Kluemper et al 2006, Ludewig & Reynolds 2009) with some studies stating that up to 76% of reported injuries in swimmers are shoulder-related (Weldon & Richardson 2001). Other sports include tennis (Pluim et al 2006), baseball (Wyland et al 2012) and, as would be predicted, contact sports such as rugby (Headey et al 2007, Usman et al 2011, Horsley & Herrington 2014) and (American) football (Dick et al 2007). Although volleyball has a lower injury rate than these sports, players also have a high rate of shoulder over-use injuries (Reeser et al 2006).

One common cause of persistent shoulder pain is adhesive capsulitis, more commonly known as frozen shoulder. It can affect 2–5% of the population (Prestgaard 2015), most often individuals of 50–70 years of age. Interestingly, it still has no precise definition (Zuckerman & Rokito 2011). Its etiology can be linked to several conditions such as diabetes mellitus, heart disease and thyroid dysfunction. It can also be linked to prolonged lack of use, stroke and, in rare occurrences, Parkinson's disease. There is growing evidence that end-range articulation of the shoulder complex can be very effective in treating adhesive capsulitis (Vermeulen et al 2000, Kisner & Colby 2012). Yang et al (2007) also found that end-range articulation of the shoulder was more effective than mid-range articulation of the joint.

Some interesting work by Mintken and colleagues (2010) suggests that treatment to the cervical and thoracic spine can help in the treatment of persistent shoulder pain, although the authors acknowledge that further research is needed. Brantingham et al (2011) found that there is 'fair evidence' that manual treatment of the shoulder complex is beneficial, especially when combined with exercise rehabilitation.

Anatomy

The shoulder joint is the most complex biomechanical structure in the human body. It is formed by the union of three bones that connect the superior extremity to the axial skeleton. These are the humerus (upper arm bone), the scapula (shoulder blade) and the clavicle (collarbone), positioned in a special harmony that allows very considerable movement of the shoulder in different stages of motion (Halder et al 2000). Movement of the shoulder joint, which is the most flexible and mobile joint in the body, results from a complex dynamic relationship of bony articulations, tendonous restraints, ligament constraints and dynamic muscle forces (Terry & Chopp 2000).

From the structural point of view, ligaments of the shoulder, including the transverse humeral, coracohumeral and three glenohumeral ligaments, work primarily to maintain the joint's range of motion, and the concave glenoid fossa of the scapula forms the socket for the joint and permits extensive rotational movement. Overall, the articular capsule arrangement is loose, affording considerable separation between the joint bones, which allows the extensive range of motion (Williams et al 1989).

The shoulder joint's hyperactive mobility affords the upper extremity a myriad range of motions, including abduction, adduction, internal and external rotation, extension, flexion and up to 180° rotation in three different planes. In addition, the shoulder permits scapular extension, elevation, depression and retraction (Quillen et al 2004).

This extensive range of motion enables the arm of the athlete, for example, to perform a very wide range of sports activities. But the wide range of motion comes at a cost, as it leads the shoulder to an increased risk of injury (Sofu et al 2014), such as torn rotator cuff muscles, frozen shoulder, tendinitis, bursitis, fractures, strains, sprains, dislocations and separations. Furthermore, the shoulder joint lacks strong ligaments; it therefore relies heavily on muscles for stability, with its primary stabilizers including glenohumeral articulation, glenohumeral ligaments, labrum, deltoid muscle and rotator cuff (Bigliani et al 1996).

Two aspects of the range of movement of the shoulder can be measured: movement of the shoulder complex and movement of its individual parts. Table 10.1 shows the range of movement for the shoulder complex and later in the chapter we will look at the individual joints' range of movement.

Bony anatomy

Humerus

The humerus is the longest bone in the upper limb, running from the shoulder to the elbow. It articulates with the scapula and connects the two lower arm bones: the ulna and the radius. Its upper portion is cylindrical in shape and consists of a rounded head, a constricted neck, proximal humeral shaft and two eminences, the greater and lesser tubercles (also known as tuberosities). The body of the humerus is more prismatic in the lower part. The lower portion

Movement type	Range of motion (°)
Abduction	180
Adduction	45
Extension	60
Flexion	180
Lateral (external) rotation	90
Medial (internal) rotation	70–90

Table 10.1
Range of motion of the shoulder complex
Data from Norkin & White (2009)

includes two processes (capitulum and trochlea), two epicondyles (lateral and medial) and three fossae (coronoid, olecranon and radial) (Ashalatha & Deepa 2012).

The humeral head is inclined to the proximal shaft at an angle between 130° and 150° at the anatomical neck, and the retroversion is between 26° and 31° from the medial and lateral epicondylar plane (Kronberg et al 1990). The greater tubercle has three separate facets, which attach the supraspinatus, infraspinatus and teres minor tendons. The lesser tubercle is the point of insertion of the subscapularis, ending the rotator cuff (Terry & Chopp 2000).

Scapula

The scapula is a large triangular-shaped bone, which is placed on the posterolateral aspect of the thorax, partly covering ribs 2 to 7. It connects the humerus with the clavicle and forms the back of the shoulder girdle. It serves primarily as a site of muscle attachment and provides a stable environment for upper extremity movement. Four muscles of the rotator cuff – the subscapularis, supraspinatus, infraspinatus and teres minor – that act on the shoulder originate from the scapula. These muscles attach to the scapula surface and are accountable for the internal and external rotation of the shoulder joint, along with humeral abduction (Marieb & Hoehn 2007).

Clavicle

The clavicle is a long S-shaped bone that connects the trunk to the shoulder girdle and forms the anterior portion. It is the only bone in the human body that is placed horizontally. The clavicle is subcutaneous in its full extent and has a dual curve along its long axis. It has two articulations: the sternoclavicular joint and the acromioclavicular joint (Ljunggren 1979).

The clavicle serves as a barrier that protects underlying neurovascular structures, a site for the attachments of muscle, a strut between the scapula and the sternum, and a stabilizer of the shoulder complex (Rockwood Jr et al 2009). Furthermore, it helps to prevent the shoulder girdle's inferior migration via the strong coracoclavicular ligaments (Terry & Chopp 2000).

Joint articulations

Glenohumeral joint

The glenohumeral (GH) joint is the major joint of the shoulder. It is a multi-axial ball-and-socket synovial joint, which is formed between the humeral head and the lateral scapula (the glenoid fossa). The articular surfaces are oval, although reciprocally curved, and are not portions of true spheres. Because the GH has a large humeral head and small glenoid cavity, it enables extensive mobility (Villaseñor-Ovies et al 2012).

The GH is loosely packed, and the surfaces are mismatching and asymmetrical. In any position of the joint, only 25–30% of the humeral head can be in articulation with the glenoid fossa (Bigliani et al 1996). However, in spite of this lack of articulating surface coverage, the normal shoulder specifically restrains the head of the humerus between 1 mm and 2 mm of the glenoid fossa center throughout most of the arc of motion (Terry & Chopp 2000). Full congruence and the close-packed situation are attained when the humerus rotates laterally, and is abducted (Peat 1986). Properties of the articulating surfaces are summarized in Table 10.2.

The GH joint's static stabilizers include the joint capsule, the labrum glenoidal, the articulating surfaces, the glenohumeral ligaments and the coracohumeral ligament. Although these play an important role in stabilization,

Articular surface	Average dimension (mm)	Radius of curvature (mm)
Humeral head	Vertical: 48	2-5
	Transverse: 45	22
Glenoid fossa	Vertical: 35	Anteroposterior view: 32.2 ± 7.6
	Transverse: 25	Axillary–lateral view: 40.6 ± 14.0

Table 10.2

Properties of the articulating surfaces

Data from Sarrafian (1983), McPherson et al (1997), Peterson & Bronzino (2007)

the GH joint heavily relies on the rotator cuff muscles for stability (Cooper et al 1992). The range of motion for the GH joint is summarized in Table 10.3.

Acromioclavicular joint

The acromioclavicular (AC) joint is a synovial joint between the lateral end of the clavicle and the medial edge of the acromion. It is covered by a fibrous capsule and is strengthened by the coracoacromial ligaments: the trapezoid and conoid ligaments. The average size of an AC joint in the adult is about 9 mm–19 mm (Terry & Chopp 2000). Static stabilizers of the joint include

Movement type	Range of motion (°)
Abduction	90–120
Adduction	45
Extension	20
Flexion	90–110
Lateral (external) rotation	90
Medial (internal) rotation	70–90

Table 10.3

Range of motion of the glenohumeral joint

Data from Norkin & White (2009)

Movement type	Range of motion (°)
Abduction/adduction	30
Anteroposterior movement	20–40
Combined internal and external rotation	30–40

Table 10.4
Range of motion of the acromioclavicular joint
Data from McClure (2001), Ludewig & Reynolds (2009)

Movement type	Range of motion (°)
Upward elevation	30–35
Anteroposterior movement	35
Rotation around the clavicle's long axis	45–50

Table 10.5
Range of motion of the sternoclavicular joint
Data from Rockwood Jr et al (1991)

the ligaments, intra-articular disc and capsule. The AC joint is essentially important for shoulder stability, because it not only helps in transmitting forces between the clavicle and the acromion but also contributes to total arm movement (McCluskey & Todd 1994).

The AC joint also has little motion (see Table 10.4). However, the motion does not occur individually; rather it is coupled with the motion of the sternoclavicular joint, which includes depression, elevation, retraction, protraction and rotation of the clavicle around its axis. Movements of this joint can be notable when the arm is abducted about 90°: about 6° of internal rotation around a vertical axis and about 15° of elevation along the anteroposterior axis (Teece et al 2008). Within the joint is an articular disc which can vary in size among individuals, and can change in size through life. Due to use of the shoulder complex, the AC can become more mobile and the articular space can expand and develop a meniscoid (Cailliet 1991), thus leading to possible entrapment symptoms.

Acromioclavicular joint injuries usually result from an inferiorly directed force to the upper extremity of the shoulder, such as a fall directly on to the shoulder or fall on to an outstretched hand. Common separation injuries characterize degrees of injury level, first to the acromioclavicular joint and then to the coracoclavicular ligaments (Rockwood Jr et al 1991).

Sternoclavicular joint

The sternoclavicular (SC) joint is a synovial double-plane joint that represents the true articulation between the axial skeleton and the superior extremity. It is a saddle-type joint formed by the connection of the sternum's upper portion and the clavicle's medial end. It has a thick capsule and it consists of two sections, partitioned by a complete disc or meniscus, which is made from fibrocartilage. Although there is no similarity in structure, the SC joint's function mostly resembles a ball-and-socket articulation (Van Tongel et al 2012).

The SC joint's static stabilizers include its joint capsule and supporting ligaments: costoclavicular, interclavicular and (anterior and posterior) sternoclavicular ligaments. However, due to the great incongruence in size between the smaller articular surface of the sternum and the large bulbous end of the clavicle, stability of the joint is mostly attributed to the surrounding ligamentous structures (Terry & Chopp 2000).

The SC joint allows the clavicle to move freely in nearly all planes, enabling elevation, depression, protraction as well as retraction (see Table 10.5). The axis for movements lies close to the clavicular attachment of the costoclavicular ligament (Frankel & Nordin 1980). This freedom of movement provides the shoulder with the ability to thrust forward.

Epidemiology

Shoulder pain

Shoulder pain comprises a diverse range of pathologies. It occurs as a result of problems in various regions of the body, including the GH joint, AC joint, SC joint, rotator cuff, neck and other soft tissues surrounding

Injury	Description	Reference
Clavicle fracture	A common acute shoulder injury frequently caused by a fall on the lateral shoulder Accounts for 2.6–5% of all fractures (about 1 in every 20 fractures) and 44% of all shoulder girdle injuries in adults Accounts for 10–16% of all fractures in childhood Affects 30–60 cases per 100,000 population globally Occurs 2.5 times more commonly in men than in women	Zlowodzki et al (2005), Jeray (2007), Khan et al (2009)
Proximal humerus fracture	A quite rare fracture and has a poor prognosis Responsible for 1–3% of all fractures, and roughly 20% of all fractures of the bone Annual incidence in people 16 years or older is 14.5 per 100,000 but gradually increases from the fifth decade Occurs more frequently in elderly people Usually results from a fall on to an outstretched arm	Balfour et al (1982), Ward et al (1998), Ekholm et al (2006)
Glenohumeral dislocation	Occurs when the articulation between the head of the humerus and the glenoid fossa is moved out of contact Approximately 96% of all shoulder dislocations are anterior, with the rest being posterior The annual incidence rate is 17 per 100,000 population Usually occurs in young and middle-aged people	Krøner et al (1989), Dala-Ali et al (2014)
Acromioclavicular sprain	A common injury in athletes and active persons Usually results when a direct blow or force is applied to the acromion with the humerus adducted Accounts for roughly 12% of all shoulder dislocations More commonly affects males than females, with a ratio of around 5:1 Men between their second and fourth decades of life have the highest frequency of incidence	Bucholz et al (2002), Quillen et al (2004), Lynch et al (2013)

Table 10.6
Common shoulder injuries

the shoulder. Risk factors include higher body mass index (BMI), decreased flexibility, imbalances in the rotator cuff muscle, disproportions in scapular stabilizing muscles, duration of injury, old age, use of a manual wheelchair and poor seated posture (Dyson-Hudson & Kirshblum 2003).

Shoulder pain affects about one-quarter of the population in the UK, based on risk factors and age. Murphy and Carr (2010) stated that every year in the UK about 1% of adults of 45 years or older suffer a new episode of shoulder pain. The authors estimated that the prevalence might be between 4% and 26%. Van der Windt et al (1995) state that for every 1000 patients seen in primary care, 15 are there for shoulder pain. But Chakravarty and Webley (1993) discovered in their research that only 47% of elderly patients who had shoulder pain reported their symptoms to their GP.

Ongoing pain in the shoulder can be the result of several conditions, including adhesive capsulitis, tendonitis, bursitis, and degenerative conditions such as osteoarthritis. Rotator cuff syndromes, adhesive capsulitis and osteoarthritis of the glenohumeral joint are often the cause of chronic shoulder pain representing 10%, 6%, and 2–5%, of all shoulder complaints respectively (Meislin et al 2005).

Shoulder injuries

Shoulder injury is the third most common musculoskeletal issue seen in general practice, and it is a potential source of disability and morbidity in the overall population (Chen 2012). Linsell et al (2006) suggested that the yearly prevalence and incidence of patients consulting for a shoulder problem in UK was 2.36% and 1.47% respectively. Risk factors include participation in athletic events, young or old age, and male gender. The reappearance of shoulder injury is also a major problem. A study to evaluate the recurrence of shoulder instability reported that, after a standard non-operative treatment, about 87% of young patients presented recurring injuries during a 5-year follow-up (Robinson et al 2006).

Common shoulder injuries are summarized in Table 10.6.

Shoulder examination

Medical history

During a shoulder joint examination, taking a detailed medical history of the patient is as essential as the physical examination itself. The healthcare provider should assess whether the injury or underlying condition hampers regular physical activities, sports and hobbies. The patient should be asked about pain, stiffness, instability, catching, locking, swelling or any other issues related to the shoulder. In most cases, the narrative provided by the patient will give information critical to narrowing the differential diagnosis and facilitate the shoulder examination.

Red flags

The clinician should make an immediate note of any signs of red flag conditions (see Table 10.7).

Physical examination

Physical examinations of shoulder problems should be done in a systematic manner. Burbank et al (2008)

Condition	Signs and symptoms
Acute rotator cuff tear	Trauma
	Acute disabling pain in the shoulder, sensory deficits
	Significant muscle weakness
	Positive drop arm test
Neurological lesion	Unexplained wasting
	Significant neurological deficit (e.g. sensory or motor)
	Persistent headaches
Radiculopathy	Severe radiating pain
	Pins and needles sensation in shoulder
Dropped head syndrome	Severe neck extensor muscle weakness
	Profound, sparing of flexors
	Chin-on-chest deformity
	Neck stiffness
	Weakness of shoulder girdle
Unreduced dislocation	Major trauma
	Epileptic fit
	Electric shock
	Loss of rotation and normal shape
Tumor	History of cancer (e.g. breast carcinoma, lung carcinoma)
	Suspected malignancy
	Unexplained deformity, mass or swelling
Infection, septic arthritis	Red skin
	Systemically unwell such as loss of appetite or unusual fatigue (malaise)
	Constitutional symptoms such as recent fever, chills or unexplained weight loss
	Recent bacterial infection
	Severe and/or persisting shoulder complaints

Table 10.7

Red flags for serious pathology in the shoulder region

Data from Mitchell et al (2005), Mutsaers & van Dolder (2008) suggest that the preferred approach to a complete physical examination should include inspection, palpation, range of motion and strength tests, and special tests. The examination should also include the neck and the elbow, so that the practitioners can dismiss the chance of a shoulder pain arising from a pathological condition in any of these parts.

Inspection

The physical examination process should start with a careful visual inspection of the patient. The inspection should include all the involved body parts, particularly the entire shoulder. The patient should be suitably undressed to allow complete inspection of the anterior, lateral and posterior shoulder. Cutaneous rashes, such as herpes zoster, presence of deformity and atrophy of muscles around the shoulder often indicate shoulder symptoms; therefore, a thorough inspection is very important (Burbank et al 2008).

Palpation

When examining the shoulder, several important bony and soft-tissue structures need to be palpated to identify areas of pathology. Palpation should comprise examination of the AC and SC joints, the anterior GH joint, the cervical spine, the clavicle, the subacromial bursae, the coracoid process and the scapula. In addition, the practitioner should palpate both shoulders, since some structures, such as biceps tendon, can cause a painful sensation, even in a healthy shoulder (Woodward & Best 2000).

Range of motion

Movement of the shoulder should be evaluated in internal and external rotation, abduction and flexion. Both active and passive movements should be assessed; however, these ranges of motion should be examined separately. Active range of motion tests the power of different muscles, so start with that first. Assess the unaffected side first to determine the patient's normal range. If the patient has a limitation in active movements, assess the passive range of motion. Passive movements test joint function and associated periarticular joint tissues (Buchanan et al 1997).

Special tests

See Table 10.8.

There have been several studies on the reliability of clinical shoulder tests (Park et al 2005, Hegedus et al 2008, Hughes et al 2008, Silva et al 2008, Nomden et al 2009, Cadogan et al 2011). Although the tests are sensitive to reproducing pain, all of the studies question the specificity of the tests as a single entity and the usefulness of them to differentially diagnose. This is why all tests must be supported with an accurate case history and other testing and examinations.

Test	Procedure	Positive sign	Interpretation
Hawkins' impingement test	The examiner should forward flex the patient's arm and elbow to 90°. A force is then applied to the arm to internally rotate the shoulder at the glenohumeral joint.	Pain on internal rotation	Subacromial impingement or rotator cuff tendonitis
Drop-arm rotator cuff test	The practitioner should passively abduct the patient's arm to 160°. The patient is then instructed to slowly lower the arm to the waist.	Inability to control the maneuver as far as the side	Supraspinatus or rotator cuff tear
Empty-can test	The examiner should abduct the patient's arms to 90°. The arms are then forward flexed to 30°. The thumbs of the patient should be turned downward. The examiner applies pressure while the patient actively resists a downward force.	Pain or weakness compared with the contralateral side	Supraspinatus tendon or muscle tear

(Continued)

Test	Procedure	Positive sign	Interpretation
Lift-off subscapularis test	The examiner should instruct the patient to rotate the arm internally behind the back. The examiner should be resisting the patient's attempt to force the arm away from the back.	Inability to lift the back of the hand off the lower back	Rotator cuff disorder involving subscapularis
Cross-body adduction test	The examiner adducts the patient's shoulder and arm horizontally across the body.	Pain at the AC joint	AC joint pathology
Yergason test	The examiner should instruct the patient to flex the elbow to 90°, with the thumbs upward. The examiner should grasp the patient's wrist and resist the patient's attempts to actively supinate the arm and flex the elbow.	Pain during this maneuver	Biceps tendonitis
Apprehension test	The patient should be in a supine or seated position. The examiner should apply slight anterior pressure on the humerus while externally rotating the patient's arm.	Sensation of apprehension or resistance	Glenohumeral instability
Relocation test	The patient should be in a supine position. The examiner should apply posterior pressure on the proximal humerus while externally rotating the patient's arm.	A decrease in pain or apprehension	Glenohumeral instability

Table 10.8

Special tests for shoulder examination

Data from Magee (2014), Burbank et al (2008), Woodward & Best (2000)

Shoulder muscles

Name	Origin	Insertion	Action	Nerve supply
Levator scapulae	Transverse processes of C1–C4	Superior part of medial border of scapula	Elevates the scapula and assists in pulling the scapula medially and upward	Dorsal scapular nerve (C5)
Trapezius	Medial third of superior nuchal line, external occipital protuberance, ligamentum nuchae, spinous processes and supraspinous ligaments of C1–T12	Lateral third of clavicle, acromion and crest of spine of scapula, medial portion of spine of scapula	Elevates, retracts and depresses the scapula. Rotation of the scapula during arm elevation	Accessory nerve (C3–C4)
Latissimus dorsi	Spinous processes of thoracic T6–T12, thoracolumbar fascia, iliac crest and inferior 3 or 4 ribs	Floor of bicipital groove of humerus	Extends, adducts and medially rotates the arm. Draws the shoulder downward and backward. Keeps the inferior angle of the scapula against the ribcage, accessory muscle of respiration	Thoracodorsal nerve (C6–C8)
Rhomboid major	Spinous processes of T2–T5 vertebrae	Medial border of scapula, inferior to the insertion of rhomboid minor muscle	Retracts the scapula and rotates it to depress the glenoid cavity. Also fixes the scapula to the thoracic wall	Dorsal scapular nerve (C4–C5)
Rhomboid minor	Ligamentum nuchea, spinous processes of C7–T1 vertebrae	Medial border of scapula, superior to the insertion of rhomboid major muscle	Retracts the scapula and rotates it to depress the glenoid cavity. Also fixes the scapula to the thoracic wall	Dorsal scapular nerve (C4–C5)
Serratus anterior	Upper 8 or 9 ribs and fascia of first intercostal space	Costal aspect of medial margin of scapula	Protracts and rotates the scapula	Long thoracic nerve (C5–C7)

(Continued)

Name	Origin	Insertion	Action	Nerve supply
Pectoralis major	Anterior surface of the medial half of the clavicle Sternocostal head: anterior surface of the sternum, the superior six costal cartilages	Lateral lip of bicipital groove of humerus	Clavicular head: flexes the humerus Sternocostal head: extends the humerus As a whole, adducts and medially rotates the humerus. Also draws the scapula anteriorly and inferiorly	Lateral pectoral nerve and medial pectoral nerve Clavicular head: (C5–C6) Sternocostal head: (C7–T1)
Pectoralis minor	Third to fifth ribs	Medial border and superior surface of coracoid process of scapula	Stabilizes the scapula by drawing it inferiorly and anteriorly against the thoracic wall	Medial pectoral nerves (C8, T1)
Subclavius	First rib	Subclavian groove of clavicle	Depresses the clavicle	Subclavian (C5–C6)
Supraspinatus	Supraspinous fossa of scapula	Superior facet of greater tubercle of humerus	Abduction of the arm and stabilizes the humerus	Suprascapular nerve (C5)
Infraspinatus	Infraspinous fossa of scapula	Middle facet of greater tubercle of humerus	Lateral rotation of the arm, adduction of the arm and stabilizes the humerus	Suprascapular nerve (C5–C6)
Subscapularis	Subscapular fossa	Lesser tubercle of humerus	Rotates medially the humerus; stabilizes the shoulder	Upper and lower subscapular nerve (C5–C6)
Teres minor	Lateral border of scapula	Inferior facet of greater tubercle of humerus	Laterally rotates and adducts the arm	Axillary nerve (C5)
Teres major	Posterior aspect of inferior angle of scapula	Medial lip of intertubercular sulcus of humerus	Internal rotation of the humerus	Lower subscapular nerve (C5–C6)
Deltoid	Clavicle, acromion, spine of scapula	Deltoid tuberosity of humerus	Shoulder abduction, flexion and extension	Lower subscapular nerve (C5–C6)
Coracobrachialis	Coracoid process of scapula	Medial humerus	Flexes at the shoulder joint	Musculocutaneous nerve (C5–C6)

(Continued)

Name	Origin	Insertion	Action	Nerve supply
Biceps brachii	Short head: coracoid process of scapula Long head: supraglenoid tubercle	Radial tuberosity	Flexes the elbow and supinates the forearm	Musculocutaneous nerve (C5–C6)
Brachialis	Anterior surface of humerus, particularly distal half of this bone	Coronoid process and tuberosity of ulna	Flexion at the elbow joint	Musculocutaneous nerve (C5–C6)
Triceps brachii	Long head: infraglenoid tubercle of scapula Lateral head: posterior humerus, superior to radial groove Medial head: posterior humerus, inferior to radial groove	Olecranon of ulna	Extends the forearm, long head helps in adduction from abduction	Radial nerve (C7–C8)

Table 10.9
Shoulder muscles

Techniques: shoulder

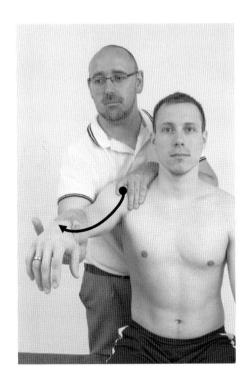

T10.1 Flexion of the shoulder (seated)

- Stand behind the patient to one side.
- Place your hand under the patient's forearm, supporting the wrist. Your elbow should then be parallel with theirs.
- Your opposite hand is palpating over the shoulder, palm over the acromioclavicular (AC) joint, with the fingers palpating the anterior portion of the shoulder while your forearm is stabilizing the patient.
- With a forward movement of your arm, lift the patient's arm forward and up in an arcing motion.
- Shoulder complex flexion is approximately 180°; glenohumeral flexion is approximately 90–110°.

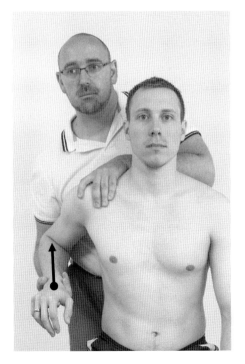

T10.2 Extension of the shoulder (seated)

- Stand behind the patient to one side.
- Place your hand under the patient's forearm, supporting the wrist. Your elbow should then be parallel with theirs.
- Your opposite hand is palpating over the shoulder, palm over the AC joint, with the fingers palpating the anterior portion of the shoulder while your forearm is stabilizing the patient.
- With your arm, lift the patient's arm out to their side in an arcing motion. You may wish to take a small side step to help support the arm.
- Shoulder complex abduction is approximately 180°; glenohumeral abduction is approximately 90–120°.

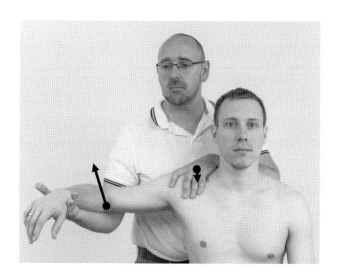

T10.3 Abduction of the shoulder (seated)

- Stand behind the patient to one side.
- Place your hand under the patient's forearm, supporting the wrist. Your elbow should then be parallel with theirs.
- Your opposite hand is palpating over the shoulder, palm over the AC joint, with the fingers palpating the anterior portion of the shoulder while your forearm is stabilizing the patient.
- With a backward movement of your arm, move the patient's arm backwards towards and past your body.
- Shoulder complex extension is approximately 60°; glenohumeral extension is approximately 20°.

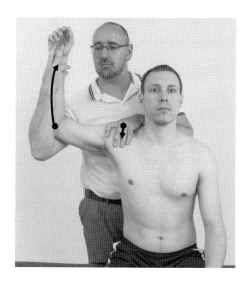

T10.4 Lateral (external) rotation (seated)

- Stand behind the patient to one side.
- Place your hand under the patient's forearm, supporting the wrist. Your elbow should then be parallel with theirs. (In this picture you can see how the wrist and hand are supported by the practitioner.)
- Your opposite hand is palpating over the shoulder, palm over the AC joint, with the fingers palpating the anterior portion of the shoulder while the forearm is stabilizing the patient.
- In the abducted position, let the patient's forearm drop towards the floor while pivoting the movement through the upper arm.
- Shoulder complex and glenohumeral internal (medial) rotation is approximately 70–90°.

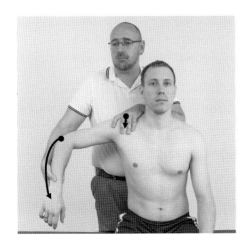

T10.5 Internal (medial) rotation (seated)

- Stand behind the patient to one side.
- Place your hand under the patient's forearm, supporting the wrist. Your elbow should then be parallel with theirs. (In this picture you can see how the wrist and hand are supported by the practitioner.)
- Your opposite hand is palpating over the shoulder, palm over the AC joint, with the fingers palpating the anterior portion of the shoulder while the forearm is stabilizing the patient.
- In the abducted position, rotate the patient's forearm up towards you while pivoting the movement through the upper arm.
- Shoulder complex and glenohumeral lateral (external) rotation is approximately 90°.

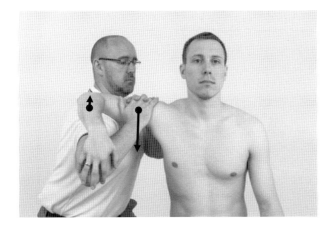

T10.6 Inferior traction of the glenohumeral capsule (seated)

- Stand to the side of the patient.
- Use your corresponding arm to abduct the shoulder to 90°, and rest their elbow on your shoulder.
- Ask the patient to hold on to your elbow.
- Place both hands (with fingers interlocked) on the superior aspect of the humerus (keeping your wrists straight).
- By straightening your legs slightly, the elbow will abduct further and drive the humerus in an inferior direction to the capsule.

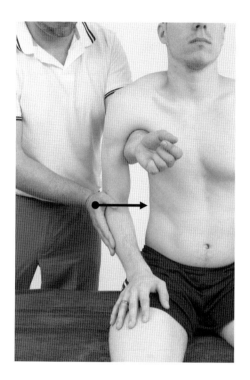

T10.7 Distraction of the glenohumeral joint (seated)

- Stand behind the patient to one side.
- Rest the patient's hand on their thigh.
- Place your opposite forearm superiorly into the axilla. (For effectiveness, always make sure your fulcrum is as close to the joint you are affecting as possible.)
- Place your corresponding hand on the lateral elbow of the patient, to ease the elbow into adduction (towards the patient's ribs).
- Proprioceptively, feel the humerus distracting from the joint.

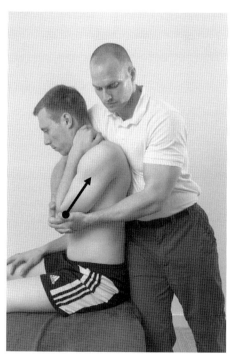

T10.8 Posterior shearing of the glenohumeral and acromioclavicular joints (seated) 1

- Stand behind the patient, at a slight angle.
- Ask the patient to bend their elbow and place one hand around their neck.
- Place both of your hands on the patient's elbow, interlocking your fingers.
- Fix the patient's thoracic spine against your body.
- Using your arms, move the humerus in an anterior and posterior direction, keeping body contact with the patient, thus blocking the scapula, to articulate the shoulder joint.
- Try different angles when articulating the joint.

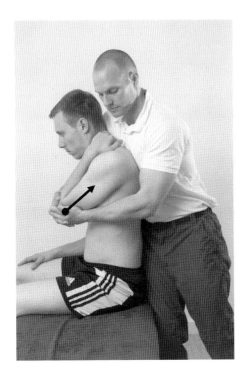

T10.9 Posterior shearing of the glenohumeral and acromioclavicular joint (seated) 2

- Stand behind the patient, at a slight angle.
- Ask the patient to bend their elbow and place one hand around their neck.
- Place both of your hands on the patient's elbow, interlocking your fingers.
- Fix the patient's thoracic spine against your body.
- Using your arms, move the humerus in an anterior and posterior direction, keeping body contact with the patient, thus blocking the scapula, to articulate the shoulder joint.
- Try different angles when articulating the joint.

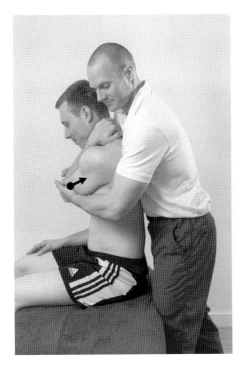

T10.10 Posterior shearing of the glenohumeral and acromioclavicular joint (seated) 3

- Stand behind the patient.
- Ask the patient to bend their elbow and place one hand around their neck.
- Keep your hips parallel to the patient.
- Place both of your hands on the patient's elbow, interlocking your fingers.
- Fix the patient's thoracic spine against your body.
- Using your arms, move the humerus in an anterior and posterior direction, keeping body contact with the patient, thus blocking the scapula, to articulate the acromioclavicular joint.

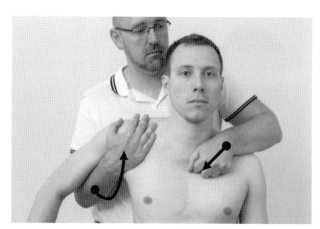

T10.11 Sterno-clavicular articulation (seated)

- Stand behind the patient, slightly to one side.
- Place your corresponding arm under the axilla, and hold the anterior portion of the shoulder.
- Place your opposite hand on the superior portion of the sternum to fix it in place.
- Use your body and the shoulder complex of the patient to move the shoulder in all directions, creating an articulation at the sternoclavicular joint.

T10.12 Sternoclavicular articulation (supine)

- Lay the patient supine.
- Stand to the side of your patient.
- Place one hand on the distal end of the patient's clavicle.
- Place your other hand on their sternum.
- In a 'seesaw' movement, shift your weight between your two hands, to articulate the sternoclavicular joint.

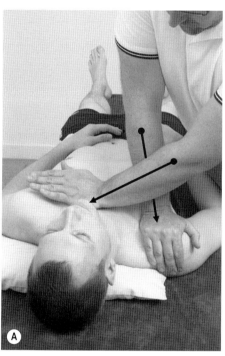

A

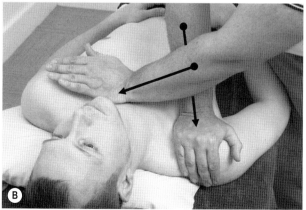

B

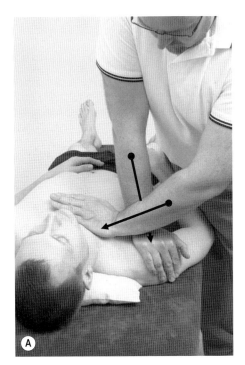

T10.13 Acromioclavicular articulation (supine)

- Lay the patient supine.
- Stand to the side of your patient.
- Place one hand on the distal end of the patient's shoulder over the acromion.
- Place your other hand on the proximal end of the clavicle.
- In a 'seesaw' movement, shift your weight between your two hands, to articulate the acromioclavicular joint.

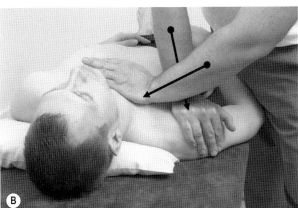

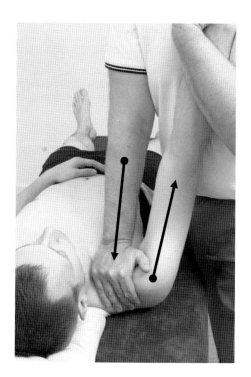

T10.14 Acromioclavicular articulation (supine)

- Lay the patient supine.
- Stand to the side of your patient.
- Hold the patient's arm against your body, supporting their wrist.
- Place your lower hand on the distal aspect on the clavicle, and fix it in a depressed position.
- Use the long lever of the arm to move the acromioclavicular joint in a superior and inferior direction, in a slow motion.

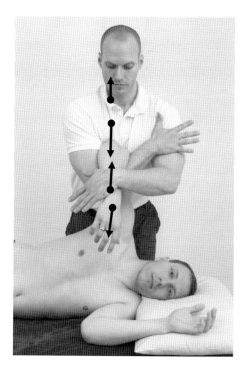

T10.15 Glenohumeral articulation (side-lying)

- Position your patient side lying, towards the back of the plinth.
- Stand behind the patient.
- Hook your corresponding arm under the elbow of the patient's upper arm, and allow the wrist to fall in front.
- Place your opposite arm on the distal aspect of the patient's forearm.
- Lift the humerus in a superior direction to create traction in the joint and, using gentle movements, articulate the humerus in the shoulder capsule.

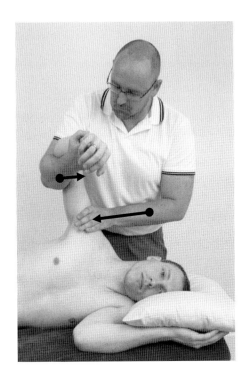

T10.16 Inferior distraction (side-lying)

- Stand behind the patient.
- Use your corresponding arm to abduct the shoulder to 90°.
- Keep the elbow at right angles to the shoulder, and support the patient's wrist with your hand. Fix their elbow against your body.
- Place your opposite hand on the superior aspect of the humerus (keeping your wrist straight), and drive the humerus in an inferior direction to the capsule.

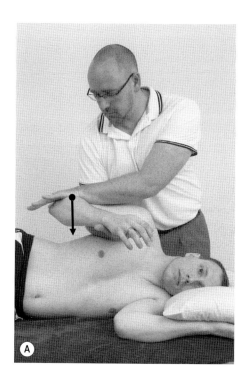

T10.17 Glenohumeral distraction (side-lying)

- Stand behind the patient with them in a side lying position.
- Place your arm high into the axilla of the patient's upper arm to create a fulcrum. Support their wrist with your hand. (For effectiveness, always make sure your fulcrum is as close to the joint you are affecting as possible.)
- Place your other hand on the lateral elbow of the patient, to ease the elbow inferiorly (towards the patient's ribs).
- Proprioceptively, feel the humerus distracting from the joint.

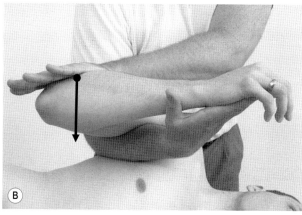

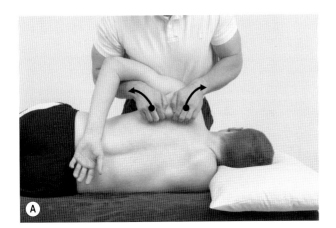

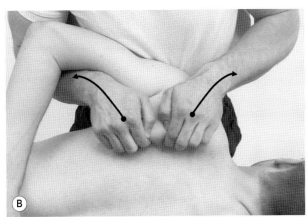

T10.18 Scapulothoracic articulation (side-lying)

- Stand in front of your patient, with your hips parallel to the plinth.
- Place your lower hand under the patient's elbow, and allow their hand to fall behind their lower back to expose the scapula.
- Fix your fingers under the medial border of the scapula.
- Lift your costal margin over the patient's shoulder, and maintain contact with your body.
- Using your body, move the scapula in all directions, moving it as one with your body.
- Use slow, rhythmic movements to articulate the scapula against the thorax.

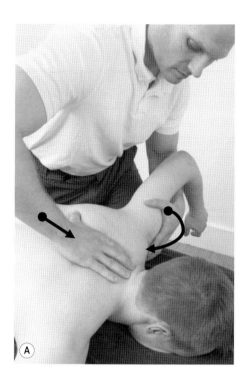

T10.19 Glenohumeral articulation (prone)

- Lay the patient in a prone position.
- Ask the patient to allow their arms to drape off the sides of the plinth.
- Stand to the side of the patient.
- Place your closest hand around the medial border of the patient's scapula.
- Place your far arm on the anterior portion of the patient's humerus, with their elbow hooked over your forearm.
- Use your body to move the humerus around in the joint, in a slow motion.

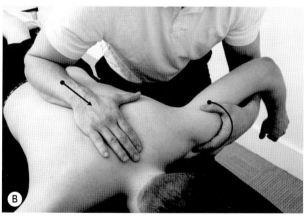

REFERENCES

Ashalatha PR, Deepa G (2012). Textbook of Anatomy and Physiology for Nurses. London: JP Medical Ltd.

Balfour GW, Mooney V, Ashby ME (1982). Diaphyseal fractures of the humerus treated with a ready-made fracture. Journal of Bone and Joint Surgery American 64:11-13.

Bigliani LU, Kelkar R, Flatow EL et al (1996). Glenohumeral stability: biomechanical properties of passive and active stabilizers. Clinical Orthopaedics and Related Research 330:13-30.

Bongers PM, Ijmker S, Van den Heuvel S et al (2006). Epidemiology of work-related neck and upper limb problems: psychosocial and personal risk factors (part I) and effective interventions from a bio behavioural perspective (part II). Journal of Occupational Rehabilitation 16(3):272-295.

Brandt LP, Andersen JH, Lassen CF et al (2004). Neck and shoulder symptoms and disorders among Danish computer workers. Scandinavian Journal of Work, Environment and Health 30(5):399-409.

Brantingham JW, Cassa TK, Bonnefin D et al (2011). Manipulative therapy for shoulder pain and disorders: expansion of a systematic review. Journal of Manipulative and Physiological Therapeutics 34(5)314-346.

Buchanan WW, DeCeulaer K, Balint GP (1997). Clinical Examination of the Musculoskeletal System: Assessing Rheumatic Conditions, 2nd ed. Philadelphia: Lippincott Williams & Wilkins.

Bucholz RW, Heckman JD, Tornetta P et al (2002). Rockwood and Green's Fractures in Adults. Philadelphia: Lippincott Williams & Wilkins.

Burbank KM, Stevenson JH, Czarnecki GR et al (2008). Chronic shoulder pain: part I. Evaluation and diagnosis. American Family Physician 77(4):453-460.

Cadogan A, Laslett M, Hing W et al (2011). Interexaminer reliability of orthopaedic special tests used in the assessment of shoulder pain. Manual Therapy 16(2):131-135.

Cailliet R (1991). Shoulder Pain, 3rd ed. Philadelphia: FADavies..

Chakravarty K, Webley M (1993). Shoulder joint movement and its relationship to disability in the elderly. Journal of Rheumatology 20(8):1359-1361.

Chen J (2012). Effectiveness of Passive Joint Mobilisation for Shoulder Dysfunction: A Review of the Literature. INTECH Open Access Publisher.

Cooper DE, Arnoczky SP, O'Brien SJ et al (1992). Anatomy, histology, and vascularity of the glenoid labrum. An anatomical study. Journal of Bone and Joint Surgery, American Volume 74(1):46-52.

Dajpratham P, Ploypetch T, Kiattavorncharoen S et al (2010). Prevalence and associated factors of musculoskeletal pain among the dental personnel in a dental school. Journal of the Medical Association of Thailand 93(6):714-721.

Dala-Ali B, Penna M, McConnell J et al (2014). Management of acute anterior shoulder dislocation. British Journal of Sports Medicine 48(16):1209-1215.

Dick R, Ferrara MS, Agel J et al (2007). Descriptive epidemiology of collegiate men's football injuries: National Collegiate Athletic Association Injury Surveillance System, 1988–1989 through 2003–2004. Journal of Athletic Training 42(2):221-233.

Dyson-Hudson TA, Kirshblum SC (2003). Shoulder pain in chronic spinal cord injury, Part I: Epidemiology, etiology, and pathomechanics. Journal of Spinal Cord Medicine 27(1):4-17.

Ekholm R, Adami J, Tidermark J et al (2006). Fractures of the shaft of the humerus an epidemiological study of 401 fractures. Journal of Bone and Joint Surgery, British Volume 88(11):1469-1473.

Frankel VH, Nordin M (1980). Basic Biomechanics of the Skeletal System. Philadelphia: Lea & Febiger.

Halder AM, Itoi E, An KN (2000). Anatomy and biomechanics of the shoulder. Orthopedic Clinics of North America 31(2):159-176.

Harutunian K, Gargallo Albiol J, Figueiredo R et al (2011). Ergonomics and musculoskeletal pain among postgraduate students and faculty members of the School of Dentistry of the University of Barcelona (Spain). A cross-sectional study. Medicina Oral, Patología Oral y Cirugia Bucal 16(3):425-429.

Headey J, Brooks JH, Kemp SP (2007). The epidemiology of shoulder injuries in English professional rugby union. American Journal of Sports Medicine 35(9):1537-1543.

Hegedus EJ, Goode A, Campbell S et al (2008). Physical examination tests of the shoulder: a systematic review with meta-analysis of individual tests. British Journal of Sports Medicine 42(2):80-92.

Hettrich CM, Gasinu S, Beamer BS et al (2014). The effect of mechanical load on tendon-to-bone healing in a rat model. The American Journal of Sports Medicine 42(5):1233-1241.

Horsley I, Herrington L (2014). Optimal management of glenohumeral joint injuries in athletes playing rugby. Trauma and Treatment 3:193.

Hughes PC, Taylor NF, Green RA (2008). Most clinical tests cannot accurately diagnose rotator cuff pathology: a systematic review. Australian Journal of Physiotherapy 54:159-170.

Jeray KJ (2007). Acute midshaft clavicular fracture. Journal of the American Academy of Orthopaedic Surgeons 15(4):239-248.

Khan LK, Bradnock TJ, Scott C et al (2009). Fractures of the clavicle. Journal of Bone and Joint Surgery, American Volume 91(2):447-460.

Kisner C, Colby LA (2012). Therapeutic exercise: foundations and techniques. Philadelphia: FA Davis.

Kluemper M, Uhl T, Hazelrigg H (2006). Effect of stretching and strengthening shoulder muscles on forward shoulder posture in competitive swimmers. Journal of Sport Rehabilitation 15(1):58-70.

Kronberg M, Broström LÅ, Söderlund V (1990). Retroversion of the humeral head in the normal shoulder and its relationship to the normal range of motion. Clinical Orthopaedics and Related Research 253:113-117.

Krøner K, Lind T, Jensen J (1989). The epidemiology of shoulder dislocations. Archives of Orthopaedic and Trauma Surgery 108(5):288-290.

Lalumandier JA, McPhee SD, Parrott CB et al (2001). Musculoskeletal pain: prevalence, prevalence, prevention, and differences among dental office personnel. General Dentistry 49:160-166.

Leaver R, Harris EC, Palmer KT (2011). Musculoskeletal pain in elite professional musicians from British symphony orchestras. Occupational Medicine 61(8):549-555.

Linsell L, Dawson J, Zondervan K et al (2006). Prevalence and incidence of adults consulting for shoulder conditions in UK primary care; patterns of diagnosis and referral. Rheumatology 45(2):215-221.

Ljunggren AE (1979). Clavicular function. Acta Orthopaedica 50(3): 261-268.

Ludewig PM, Reynolds JF (2009). The association of scapular kinematics and glenohumeral joint pathologies. Journal of Orthopaedic and Sports Physical Therapy 39(2):90-104.

Lynch TS, Saltzman MD, Ghodasra JH et al (2013). Acromioclavicular joint injuries in the National Football League: epidemiology and management. American Journal of Sports Medicine 41(12):2904-2908.

McClure P (2001). Direct 3-dimensional measurement of scapular kinematics during dynamic movements in vivo. Journal of Shoulder and Elbow Surgery 10:269.

McCluskey GM 3rd, Todd J (1994). Acromioclavicular joint injuries. Journal of the Southern Orthopaedic Association 4(3):206-213.

McPherson EJ, Friedman RJ, An YH et al (1997). Anthropometric study of normal glenohumeral relationships. Journal of Shoulder and Elbow Surgery 6(2):105-112.

Magee DJ (2014). Orthopedic Physical Assessment, 6th ed. St Louis, Mo: Elsevier Health Sciences.

Marieb EN, Hoehn K (2007). Human Anatomy and Physiology. New York: Pearson Education.

Meislin RJ, Sperling JW, Stitik TP (2005). Persistent shoulder pain: epidemiology, pathophysiology, and diagnosis. American Journal of Orthopedics (Belle Mead, NJ) 34(12 Suppl):5-9.

Mintken PE, Cleland JA, Carpenter KJ et al (2010). Some factors predict successful short-term outcomes in individuals with shoulder pain receiving cervicothoracic manipulation: a single-arm trial. Physical Therapy 9(1):26-42.

Mitchell C, Adebajo A, Hay E et al (2005). Shoulder pain: diagnosis and management in primary care. British medical Journal 331(7525): 1124-1128.

Murphy RJ, Carr AJ (2010). Shoulder pain. Clinical Evidence (Online) 1107.

Mutsaers B, van Dolder R (2008). 'Red flags' of the neck and shoulder area: a review of the literature. Available from: http://vanpend.nl/Publicatie20_DTO_PDF.pdf [Accessed 16 February 2016].

Nomden JG, Slagers AJ, Bergman GJ et al (2009). Interobserver reliability of physical examination of shoulder girdle. Manual Therapy 14:152-159.

Norkin CC, White DJ (2009). Measurement of Joint Motion: A Guide to Goniometry. Philadelphia: FA Davis.

Nyman T, Wiktorin C, Mulder M et al (2007). Work postures and neck shoulder pain among orchestra musicians. American Journal of Independent Medicine 50:370-376.

Park HB, Yokota A, Gill HS et al (2005). Diagnostic accuracy of clinical tests for the different degrees of sub-acromial impingement syndrome. Journal of Bone and Joint Surgery, American Volume 87:1446-1455.

Peat M (1986). Functional anatomy of the shoulder complex. Physical Therapy 66(12):1855-1865.

Peterson DR, Bronzino JD eds (2007). Biomechanics: Principles and Applications. Boca Raton, Fl: CRC Press.

Pluim BM, Staal JB, Windler GE et al (2006). Tennis injuries: occurrence, aetiology, and prevention. British Journal of Sports Medicine 40(5):415-423.

Prestgaard TA (2015). Frozen shoulder (adhesive capsulitis). http://www.uptodate.com/contents/frozen-shoulder-adhesive-capsulitis [Accessed 6 February 2016].

Quillen DM, Wuchner M, Hatch RL (2004). Acute shoulder injuries. American Family Physician 70(10):1947-1954.

Reeser JC, Verhagen EALM, Briner WW et al (2006). Strategies for the prevention of volleyball-related injuries. British Journal of Sports Medicine 40(7):594-600.

Robinson CM, Howes J, Murdoch H et al (2006). Functional outcome and risk of recurrent instability after primary traumatic anterior shoulder dislocation in young patients. Journal of Bone and Joint Surgery 88(11):2326-2336.

Rockwood CA Jr, Matsen FA III, Wirth MA et al (2009). The Shoulder. St Louis, Mo: Elsevier Health Sciences.

Rockwood CA Jr, Williams GR, Young DC (1991). Injuries to the acromioclavicular joint. In: CA Rockwood Jr, DP Green, RW Bucholz eds. Rockwood and Green's Fractures in Adults. Philadelphia: Lippincott Williams & Wilkins.

Roquelaure Y, Ha C, Leclerc A et al (2006). Epidemiologic surveillance of upper-extremity musculoskeletal disorders in the working population. Arthritis Care and Research 55(5):765-778.

Sarrafian SK (1983). Gross and functional anatomy of the shoulder. Clinical Orthopaedics and Related Research 173:11-19.

Silva L, Andreu JL, Munoz P et al (2008). Accuracy of physical examination in subacromial impingement syndrome. Rheumatology 47:679-683.

Silverstein B, Welp E, Nelson N et al (1998). Claims incidence of work-related isorders of the upper extremities: Washington State, 1987 through 1995. American Journal of Public Health 88:1827-1833.

Sofu H, Gürsu S, Koçkara N et al (2014). Recurrent anterior shoulder instability: Review of the literature and current concepts. World Journal of Clinical Cases 2(11):676-682.

Teece RM, Lunden JB, Lloyd AS et al (2008). Three-dimensional acromioclavicular joint motions during elevation of the arm. Journal of Orthopaedic and Sports Physical Therapy 38(4):181-190.

Terry GC, Chopp TM (2000). Functional anatomy of the shoulder. Journal of Athletic Training 35(3):248-255.

Usman J, McIntosh AS, Best JP (2011). The epidemiology of shoulder injuries in rugby union football. British Journal of Sports Medicine 45(4):379.

Van der Windt DA, Koes BW, de Jong BA et al (1995). Shoulder disorders in general practice: incidence, patient characteristics, and management. Annals of the Rheumatic Diseases 54(12):959-964.

Van Tongel A, MacDonald P, Leiter J et al (2012). A cadaveric study of the structural anatomy of the sternoclavicular joint. Clinical Anatomy 25(7):903-910.

Vermeulen HM, Obermann WR, Burger BJ et al (2000). End-range mobilization techniques in adhesive capsulitis of the shoulder joint: a multiple-subject case report. Physical Therapy 80(12):1204-1213.

Villaseñor-Ovies P, Vargas A, Chiapas-Gasca K et al (2012). Clinical anatomy of the elbow and shoulder. Reumatología Clínica 8:13-24.

Ward EF, Savoie FH, Hughes JL (1998). Fractures of the diaphyseal humerus. Skeletal Trauma 2:1177-1193.

Weldon EJ, Richardson AB (2001). Upper extremity overuse injuries in swimming. A discussion of swimmer's shoulder. Clinics in Sports Medicine 20:423-438.

Williams PL, Warwick R, Dyson M et al (1989). Gray's Anatomy, 37th ed. Edinburgh: Churchill Livingstone.

Woodward TW, Best TM (2000). The painful shoulder: Part I. Clinical evaluation. American Family Physician 61(10):3079-3089.

Wyland DJ, Pill SG, Shanley E et al (2012). Bony adaptation of the proximal humerus and glenoid correlate within the throwing shoulder of professional baseball pitchers. American Journal of Sports Medicine 40(8):1858-1862.

Yang JL, Chang CW, Chen SY et al (2007). Mobilization techniques in subjects with frozen shoulder syndrome: randomized multiple-treatment trial. Physical Therapy 87(10):1307-1315.

Zlowodzki M, Zelle BA, Cole PA et al (2005). Treatment of acute midshaft clavicle fractures: systematic review of 2144 fractures: on behalf of the Evidence-Based Orthopaedic Trauma Working Group. Journal of Orthopaedic Trauma 19(7):504-507.

Zuckerman JD, Rokito A (2011). Frozen shoulder: a consensus definition. Journal of Shoulder and Elbow Surgery 20(2):322-325.W

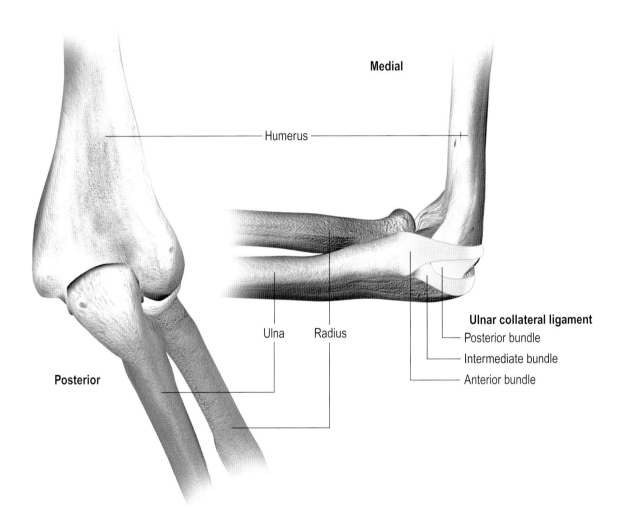

Medial

Humerus

Ulna   Radius

Posterior

Ulnar collateral ligament
Posterior bundle
Intermediate bundle
Anterior bundle

Figure 11.1
The elbow: posterior and medial views

Introduction

The elbow joint (or elbow complex) is a more complex joint than most people believe. It plays an extremely important part in dynamic movements of the upper extremity such as reaching, lifting and the orientation of the hand, and loss of mobility through the elbow can have a huge impact on quality of life and independency (Turpin et al 2012).

Common injuries in the elbow are associated with overstrain and repetitive movements, resulting in tendinopathies or epicondylitis. The etiology of this can be from occupational stresses as well as recreational or sporting, but lateral epicondylitis is commonly called 'tennis elbow' (or 'lawn tennis arm' – Morris 1882) and medial epicondylitis is commonly classified as 'golfer's elbow'. Lateral epicondylitis is one of the most common upper extremity complaints and it has an estimated occurrence of 0.7–4.0% in the population (Coombes et al 2009, Shiri & Viikari-Juntura 2011). It affects the dominant upper extremity predominantly (Shiri et al 2006, Smidt et al 2006). A study by Silverstein et al (1998) found that 11.7% of work-associated injury claims in Washington between 1987 and 1995 were related to either lateral or medial epicondylitis. These resulted in an average compensation of $6593 per case. Walker-Bone et al (2012) reported that 5% of the participants in their study had taken sickness absence due to epicondylitis, and they took an average of 29 days' absence in a year due to their symptoms.

Many researchers have investigated the occupational epidemiology of epicondylitis, which shows higher rates of occurrence in occupations involving manual tasks (Walker-Bone et al 2003, Shiri et al 2006, Fan et al 2009, van Rijn et al 2009). An interesting occupation that has a high incidence is the meat-handling trade; this is possibly due to the repetitive movements involved in sausage making, packing and the cutting of the meat (Kurppa et al 1991, Shiri & Viikari-Juntura 2011, Walker-Bone et al 2012). The US National Institute for Occupational Safety and Health (NIOSH) recognizes a strong link between occupations that involve a combination of factors such as force, repetition and vibration and the risk of developing epicondylitis, but limited evidence is found when looking at these factors individually (Bernard 1997). In the United Kingdom, the Health and Safety Executive (HSE) defines epicondylitis as pain and tenderness over the epicondylar (lateral or medial) region and pain with resisted flexion of the wrist for medial epicondylitis and resisted extension for lateral epicondylitis (Harrington et al 1998). Work by Schaefer and Speier (2012) found studies that recorded incidences of musculoskeletal disorders of the elbow in musicians between 56.8% and 77%, mainly in string musicians. Other studies into epicondylitis have found a possible predisposition in females compared to males, although this is still unclear (Shiri et al 2006), and possible links with obesity (Werner et al 2005). Studies have demonstrated that articulation of the elbow joint/complex can be beneficial in hypoalgesia and improving the symptoms associated with epicondylitis (Abbott et al 2001, Paungmali et al 2003, Vicenzino 2003, Vicenzino et al 2007).

Distal and partial ruptures of the biceps brachii also affect the elbow, as does tendinitis of the distal biceps, although these are less common than epicondylitis. They typically affect the dominant arm and are most common in men between 40 and 50 years of age. Factors that are associated with these include smoking (smokers are 7.5 times more likely to suffer than non-smokers), previous injury and use of anabolic steroids (Taylor & Hannafin 2012).

Anatomy

The elbow joint is a large, complex structure. Although it appears to be a much simpler joint than the shoulder, it is one of the most intricately constructed joints in the body. In fact, it is a complex hinge between three bones: the humerus in the upper arm, and the ulna and radius in the forearm. These bones are attached by various ligaments and tendons and are influenced by a number of muscles that cross the joint (Alcid et al 2004). The elbow is one of the most highly congruent and stable joints in the body. Anteriorly, it is constrained by the radial head and coronoid process; posteriorly, it is protected by the olecranon, the bony eminence at the very tip of the elbow (Bain 1999). A single fibrous capsule encloses the entire joint complex, which is strengthened by both the medial and lateral ligaments (Morrey et al 1981).

The elbow joint consists of three separate articulations: the humeroulnar joint, the humeroradial joint and the superior radioulnar joint. These three joints comprise a single compound joint and work in coordination to allow flexion and extension of the upper limb and, at the same time, supination and pronation of the forearm and wrist (Villaseñor-Ovies et al 2012) (see Table 11.1).

The average carrying angle of the elbow is 10–15° in males and is about 5° greater in females (An et al 2009). Sharma et al (2013) found in their study and other research that the carrying angle increases in both males and females during puberty and also that it is greater in the non-dominant extremity. There have been many theories as to the cause of variation in the carrying angle, including the shape and position of the inner (medial) lip or edge of the trochlea, the angle of the trochlear groove, curvature of the shaft of the ulna, the coronoid process or the olecra-

Movement type	Range of motion (°)
Flexion	150
Extension	Males: 0 Females: 10–15
Pronation and supination	80–90

Table 11.1
Range of motion of the elbow complex

non (Purkait & Chandra 2004, Kumar et al 2010), but none of these has been statistically proven to be the main determinant of the angle.

The elbow joint acts as the mechanical link in the upper limb between the shoulder and the hand. This interconnection provides the arm with much of its versatility and allows the hand to move toward and away from the body. The major functions of the elbow are placing the hand in space, serving as a hinge or support for the forearm, allowing sturdy grasping, and affording fine movements of the hand and wrist. Injury of the elbow joint can result in significant disability and upset activities of daily living and job-related tasks. A sound understanding of the anatomy and biomechanics of the elbow is therefore essential for physiotherapists, surgeons and researchers, among others (Fornalski et al 2003).

Bony anatomy

Humerus

The distal humerus contributes two humeral condyles – the capitellum laterally and the trochlea medially – to the articular surfaces of the elbow joint. The humeral condyle is a round prominence that is covered in articular cartilage, a tube-like structure that covers most of the distal end space of the humerus (An & Morrey 2000). On the lateral aspect of the humeral condyle are the medial and lateral epicondyles. The medial epicondyle protects the ulnar nerve and is more prominent than the lateral epicondyle. It gives attachment to the ulnar collateral ligament and flexor–pronator group. The less prominent lateral epicondyle is the region where the radial collateral ligament and extensor–supinator group are attached. Anteriorly, the radial fossa (superior to the capitulum) and the coronoid fossa (superior to the trochlea) accommodate the head of the radius and the coronoid process of the ulna, respectively, when in full flexion. Posteriorly, the olecranon fossa accommodates the olecranon process of the ulna in full extension (Celli 2008).

Ulna

The ulna is prismatic in shape and is the larger of the two long bones (ulna and radius) in the forearm. It articulates with both the humerus and the radius.

Articulation	From	To	Joint type	Motion
Humeroulnar joint	Trochlear notch of the ulna	Trochlea of humeral condyle	Synovial hinge joint	Flexion and extension
Humeroradial joint	Superior aspect of the radial head	Capitulum of the humeral condyle	Combined hinge and pivot joint	Flexion and extension as well as rotation of the radial head on the capitellum
Superior radioulnar joint	Radial head	Radial notch of the ulna	Pivot-type synovial joint	Pronation or supination movement

Table 11.2

Articulations of the elbow joint

Data from Kuxhaus (2008), Fornalski et al (2003)

The ulna proximally contributes the articulation of the elbow with an intrinsic stability, particularly in full extension. It provides the articular cartilage-covered trochlear notch to the hinge of the elbow joint and articulates with the trochlea of the humerus as a hinge joint. It articulates with the radius near the elbow as a pivot joint. The ulna includes the olecranon (the bony process where triceps muscle tendon attaches) and the coronoid process (a triangular eminence where the brachialis attaches) (Fornalski et al 2003).

Radius

The radius is a prism-shaped long bone, which runs parallel to the ulna and extends from the elbow's lateral part to the thumb side of the wrist. It includes the head of the radius or radial head, which articulates with both the capitellum of the humerus and the radial notch of the ulna. Distal to the radial head is a narrowing of the bone, known as the radial neck. Medial to the radius, and just distal to the radial neck, is an oval projection, referred to as the radial tuberosity, which receives the biceps tendon (An & Morrey 2000).

Joint articulations

The articulations of the elbow joint are summarized in Table 11.2.

Ligaments

The ligamentous complexes reinforce osseous stability and serve as stabilizers for the elbow joint. The triangular medial (or ulnar) collateral ligament is formed by the medial capsular thickenings. It extends from the medial humeral epicondyle to the olecranon and coronoid process of the ulna. The medial complex contributes valgus stability to the flexed elbow (Morrey et al 1991) and comprises three components: the anterior, posterior and transverse bundles. The anterior bundle gives the highest elbow stability, the posterior bundle inhibits pronation of the ulna in cooperation with the bony articulations, and the transverse bundle helps to extend the trochlear notch (Jackson & McKeag 1997).

The lateral (or radial) collateral ligament is formed by the lateral capsular thickenings. It originates from the lateral epicondyle of the humerus and distally blends with the annular ligament of the radius. The radial collateral ligament supports the annular ligament during varus stress (Chumbley et al 2000) and helps stabilize the lateral humeroulnar joint, precisely by inhibiting supination of the ulna (Bain 1999).

Epidemiology

Elbow injuries

The elbow is the most common site of injury in athletes of all ages and skill levels, especially in sports

Condition	Description	Reference
Lateral epicondylitis (tennis elbow)	A condition in which the lateral epicondyle of the humerus becomes sore and tender Involves an acute or chronic inflammation of the tendons Results from overuse of the wrist extensor musculature, such as extensor carpi radialis brevis Occurs in more than 50% of athletes that use overhead arm motions Annual incidence: 4–7 cases per 1000 patients Peak incidence: 40–50 years of age	Field & Savoie (1998), Smidt & van der Windt (2006), Johnson et al (2007)
Medial epicondylitis (golfer's elbow)	An inflammatory condition of the tendons Characterized by pain and repetitive stress at the flexorpronator tendinous origin with pathology Results from repetitive valgus stress, flexion and pronation placed on the soft tissues of the medial elbow Causes tendinosis of the medial epicondyle of the humerus Most commonly affects men aged 20–49 years Peak incidence: third to fourth decades of life	Chumbley et al (2000), Gabel & Morrey (2000), Johnson et al (2007)
Dislocation of the radial head (pulled elbow)	Often comes with significant trauma Occurs when the radial head is pulled out of the annular ligament Results in displacement of radial head from its normal articulation with the humerus and the ulna In children, the head of the radius is more frequently subluxed than dislocated Occurs most commonly in male adults who are subject to high-force injury Peak incidence occurs in young children (under the age of 5), more frequently in girls	Ovesen et al (1990), Tosun et al (2008)
Olecranon bursitis (student's elbow)	An inflammation of the olecranon bursa, which is located just above the extensor aspect of the proximal end of the ulna Characterized by pain, swelling and redness near the olecranon process Usually develops as a result of prolonged pressure, single injury to the elbow, mild but repeated minor injuries, infection, trauma or other condition that aggravates inflammation Peak incidence occurs at older age	Snider (1997), Brinker & Miller (1999)
Pronator teres syndrome	A proximal median neuropathy of the forearm Causes paresthesia in the distribution of the median nerve Incidence: very rare and limited	Hartz et al (1981), Lee et al (2014a)
Radial tunnel syndrome	Classic feature is pain over the radial proximal forearm with little or no motor weakness Pain is centered over the lateral epicondyle (sometimes making differential diagnosis with lateral epicondylitis difficult)	Charalambous & Stanley (2008), Huisstede et al (2008)

(Continued)

Condition	Description	Reference
Cubital tunnel syndrome	Second most common nerve entrapment (carpal tunnel syndrome is first) Is a consequence of compression of the ulnar nerve, resulting in pain or paresthesia in the fourth and fifth digit and pain on the medial side of the elbow Manual workers are most prone	Bartels et al (2005), van Rijn et al (2009)

Table 11.3
Common pathological conditions of the elbow

involving overhead arm motions, such as throwing and racquet sports. Playing such sports involves considerable compression forces on the lateral radiocapitellar joint and tension forces on the medial side of the elbow, leading to a range of pathological conditions (Whiteside et al 1999).

Elbow injuries may occur at any of the functional structures in the region. However, the frequency of elbow pain and the type of injury vary greatly, depending on the type of athletic pursuit and, in some sports, on the athlete's position. Injuries to the elbow, wrist and forearm are responsible for roughly 25% of all injuries related to sports (Amadio 1990).

The majority of sporting elbow injuries are classified as either traumatic or overuse (Dugas & Cain Jr 2005). Azar et al (2000) found that ulnar collateral ligament (UCL) reconstruction had increased 50% from 1995 to the time of their study. Elbow injuries are particularly common in sports involving throwing, such as baseball (Fleisig et al 2011, Tyler et al 2014) and javelin (Dines et al 2012, Leigh et al 2013). In their review of elbow injuries, Frostick et al (1999) reported that approximately 30% of all baseball pitchers have a carrying-angle deformity and 50% have flexion contractures. Tullos and King (1973) found that two-thirds of pitchers who participated in their study had radiographic evidence of joint damage in the upper limb. They also suggested that about 50% of throwers participating in sports have either elbow or shoulder injuries which force them to cut short their careers. In a group of baseball pitchers undertaking treatment for chronic medial instability of the elbow, Conway et al (1992) found that 68% had a fixed flexion deformity. Additional studies have found that a sportsperson involved in a throwing sport has an increased chance of elbow pain/injury if they have an underlying shoulder injury (Shanley 2011, Fleisig & Andrews 2012). As a manual therapist, it is extremely important to assess and treat the shoulder complex when a patient presents with any elbow injury.

It is not only throwing sports that cause elbow injuries, however. Bethapudi et al (2013) found that over 50% of the elbow injuries sustained during the London 2012 Olympics were from judo and weightlifting. Other sports that are prone to elbow injury include wrestling (Molnár et al 2014), arm wrestling (Lee et al 2014b) and martial arts (Kreiswirth et al 2014).

Common elbow disorders

Elbow injuries may lead to a number of disorders, including lateral and medial epicondylitis, nerve compression syndromes and olecranon bursitis. These disorders of the elbow can occur following elbow dislocation, elbow instability, fractured bones, pulled muscles, ruptured tendons and sprained ligaments (see Table 11.3).

Elbow examination

Medical history

During the elbow joint examination, taking a detailed medical history of the patient is as essential as the physical examination itself. Chumbley et al (2000) suggest that the healthcare provider should seek information from the patient about recreational and occupational activities involving a repetitive load to the elbow, which could induce a chronic inflammation, cycle of microtrauma, necrosis, tissue degeneration and tendon rupture. The patient should be asked about pain, swelling, instability, locking or any other issues related to the elbow. In most cases, the narrative provided by the patient will provide information critical for narrowing the differential diagnosis and facilitating the elbow examination.

Red flags

The examiner must be aware of and note the presence of any of the red flag conditions listed in Table 11.4.

Physical examination

Physical examinations of the elbow joint should be carried out in a systematic manner. A complete evaluation of the elbow should include inspection, palpation, range of motion, neurological tests, examination of connected areas, and a variety of special tests.

Inspection

The physical examination process should start with a careful visual inspection of the patient. The inspection

Table 11.4
Red flags for serious pathology in the elbow
Data from Harvey (2001), Jawed et al (2001), Hunter et al (2002), Reiman (2016)

Condition	Signs and symptoms
Compartment syndrome	History of trauma or surgery
	Persistent forearm pain and tightness
	Pain intensified with stretch applied to affected muscles
	Increased tension in the involved compartment
	Tingling, burning or numbness
	Paresthesia, paresis and sensory deficits
	Symptoms unchanged by position or movement
Radial head fracture	History of fall on an outstretched arm
	Radial head tenderness
	High guard position of the upper extremity
	Elbow joint effusion
	Restricted or painful supination and pronation AROM
Avascular necrosis	Pain and stiffness in the upper arm
	Gradual onset of pain
	History of excessive alcohol use
	Prolonged use of oral steroids
	Previous history of undergoing chemotherapy and radiation (less common)
Malignancy	Asymmetric or irregular shape lesion
	Unexplained deformity, mass or swelling
	Chronic pain in bones
	Unexplained weight loss
	Extreme tiredness (fatigue)
	Repeated infection
	Persistent low-grade fever, either constant or intermittent
Infection	Fever, chills, malaise and weakness
	Recent bacterial infection such as urinary tract or skin infection
	Recent cut, scrape or puncture wound
	Loss of appetite

should include all the involved body parts, particularly the entire elbow. The examiner should look for abnormal contours of the elbow. The carrying angle of the elbow on both sides should be measured (normal range in adults: 11° of valgus in men and 13° of valgus in women) (Beals 1976). Muscle wasting and both generalized and localized swelling of the joint should be looked for. If any bruising, laceration, ecchymosis or visible malalignment is present, it should be noted immediately. The examiner should also look for signs of joint effusion. Evaluation of the possible existence of joint effusion is usually performed with the elbow flexed between 30° and 40° (Dugas & Cain Jr 2005).

Palpation

The examiner should carry out the palpation of the anatomic landmarks in a systematic fashion. The examination should begin with joint palpation via the full range of motion to look for joint crepitus and effusion. Several important bony structures, including the epicondyles, olecranon, radial head and ulna shaft, should be palpated to identify areas of pathology. If the epicondyles are tender on palpation, tennis elbow or golfer's elbow may be present. Tenderness with olecranon palpation indicates olecranon bursitis. Pain and symptoms radiating into the fourth and fifth digits found with ulnar nerve palpation are indicative of cubital tunnel syndrome (Buchanan et al 1996, Cooper 2007).

Range of motion

For assessment of range of motion, the examiner should place the patient in a sitting position. Active, active-resisted and passive range of motion should be tested. If a patient with loss of extension is found with a bony end feel, it may indicate heterotopic ossification, osteophyte formation, fracture malunion or loose bodies. Conversely, a soft end feel may suggest a tendinous or capsular contracture (Dugas & Cain Jr 2005). Movement in pronation or supination should also be measured. If a patient presents with restricted pronation or supination of the elbow, it may indicate distal radioulnar joint disease (McRae 2010).

Special tests

Table 11.5 details special tests that may be carried out for the elbow examination.

Test	Procedure	Positive sign	Interpretation
Tennis elbow test	**Method 1:** The examiner pronates the patient's forearm and flexes the wrist with ulnar deviation. Finally, the examiner instructs the patient to extend the elbow.	Pain over the lateral humeral epicondyle	Lateral epicondylitis
	Method 2: The examiner stabilizes the involved elbow with one hand and instructs the patient to make a fist, pronate the forearm, and radially deviate and extend the wrist against the examiner's resisting force at the fist.	Sharp, sudden or severe pain over the lateral humeral epicondyle	Lateral epicondylitis
Golfer's elbow test	The examiner palpates the patient's medial epicondyle of the humerus, then passively supinates the forearm and extends the elbow and wrist fully with radial deviation.	Pain along the medial epicondyle of the humerus	Medial epicondylitis
Varus stress test	The patient is sitting with elbow flexed to 15–20°. The examiner stabilizes the arm, with one hand placed at the elbow and the other hand placed above the wrist. Finally, the examiner applies a varus force to the elbow.	Lateral (radial) pain and/or increased laxity when compared with uninvolved	Lateral collateral ligament injury
Valgus stress test	The patient is sitting with elbow flexed to 15–20°. The examiner stabilizes the arm, with one hand placed at the elbow and the other hand placed above the wrist. Finally, the examiner applies a valgus force to the elbow.	Medial (ulnar) pain and/or increased laxity when compared with uninvolved	Medial collateral ligament injury
Elbow flex test	The examiner flexes the patient's elbow with the forearm supinated and wrist extended and holds it for 60 seconds.	Pain and symptoms radiating into the fourth and fifth digits	Cubital tunnel syndrome

Table 11.5

Special tests for the elbow joint examination

Data from Baxter (2003), Cooper (2007), McRae (2010)

Elbow muscles

Name	Origin	Insertion	Action	Nerve supply
Biceps brachii	Short head: coracoid process of scapula Long head: supraglenoid tubercle of scapula	Radial tuberosity, bicipital aponeurosis into the deep fascia of forearm	Flexes the elbow and supinates the forearm	Musculocutaneous nerve (C5–C6)
Brachialis	Anterior surface of humerus	Coronoid process and tuberosity of ulna	Flexion of the elbow joint	Musculocutaneous nerve (C5–C6)
Triceps brachii	Long head: infraglenoid tubercle of scapula Lateral head: upper posterior humerus, superior to radial groove Medial head: lower posterior humerus, inferior to radial groove	Posterior surface of olecranon	Extends the elbow joint, adducts when the arm is abducted	Radial nerve (C7–C8)
Anconeus	Posterior surface of lateral epicondyle of humerus	Lateral surface of olecranon process and superior/posterior surface of ulna	Extends the forearm	Radial nerve (C7–C8)
Pronator teres	Humeral head: medial epicondyle and medial supracondylar ridge of humerus (common flexor tendon) Ulnar head: medial portion of coronoid process of ulna	Pronator tuberosity on lateral surface of radius	Pronation and flexion of the elbow	Median nerve (C6–C7)
Flexor carpi radialis	Medial epicondyle of humerus (common flexor tendon)	Bases of second and third metacarpal bones	Flexion and abduction of the wrist	Median nerve (C6–C7)
Palmaris longus	Medial epicondyle of humerus (common flexor tendon)	Flexor retinaculum and palmar aponeurosis	Flexes the wrist	Median nerve (C6–C7)

(Continued)

Name	Origin	Insertion	Action	Nerve supply
Flexor carpi ulnaris	Humeral head: medial epicondyle of humerus (common flexor tendon) Ulnar head: medial border of olecranon of ulna	Pisiform, hook of hamate and base of fifth metacarpal	Flexion and adduction of the wrist	Ulnar nerve (C8–T1)
Flexor digitorum superficialis	Humeroulnar head: medial epicondyle of humerus (common flexor tendon), medial border of coronoid process of ulna Radial head: shaft of radius, anterior surface	Anterior surface of middle phalanges of four fingers	Flexion of the fingers	Median nerve (C7–T1)
Flexor digitorum profundus	Upper three-quarters of anterior and medial surface of ulna, medial surface of coronoid process and interosseous membrane	Base of distal phalanges of fingers	Flexes the fingers	Medial portion: ulnar nerve (C8–T1) Lateral portion: median nerve (C8–T1)
Flexor pollicis longus	Anterior surface of radius, interosseous membrane, medial epicondyle of humerus and occasionally coronoid process of ulna	Base of the distal phalanx of thumb	Flexion of the thumb	Median nerve (C8–T1)
Extensor digitorum	Lateral epicondyle of humerus (common extensor tendon)	Lateral and dorsal surfaces of phalanges of all fingers	Extension of the wrist and fingers	Radial nerve (C7–C8)
Extensor digiti minimi	Lateral epicondyle of humerus (common extensor tendon)	Dorsal surface of base of phalanx of little finger	Extension of the little finger	Radial nerve (C7–C8)
Extensor carpi ulnaris	Common extensor tendon (lateral epicondyle), ulna	Dorsal surface of base of phalanx of little finger	Extends and adducts the wrist	Radial nerve (C7–C8)
Brachioradialis	Upper two-thirds of lateral supracondylar ridge of humerus	Radial styloid process	Flexion of the forearm	Radial nerve (C5–C6)

(Continued)

Name	Origin	Insertion	Action	Nerve supply
Extensor carpi radialis longus	Lower third of lateral supracondylar ridge of humerus	Base of metacarpal of index finger	Extension and abduction of the wrist	Radial nerve (C6–C7)
Extensor carpi radialis brevis	Lateral epicondyle of humerus (common extensor tendon)	Base of metacarpal of middle finger	Extension and abduction of the wrist	Radial nerve (C7–C8)
Supinator	Lateral epicondyle of humerus, supinator crest of ulna, radial collateral ligament, annular ligament	Posterior and lateral surfaces of proximal third of radius	Supinates the forearm	Radial nerve (C5–C6)

Table 11.6
Elbow muscles

Techniques: elbow

All elbow joint techniques shown are with the patient supine.

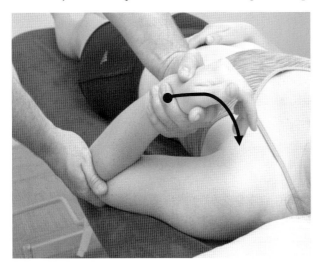

T11.1 Flexion

- Stand facing the patient on the side you wish to assess.
- Hold the forearm by placing the corresponding hand around the patient's wrist, thus supporting the area.
- Your opposite hand is under the patient's elbow, palpating the olecranon.
- Induce flexion by moving the patient's hand towards their glenohumeral joint.
- Elbow flexion is approximately 145°.

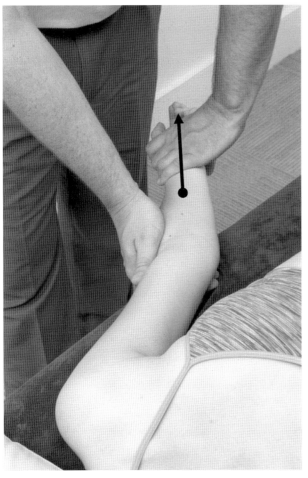

T11.2 Extension

- Stand facing the patient on the side you wish to assess.
- Hold the arm by supporting around the wrist.
- Your opposite hand is under the patient's elbow, palpating the olecranon.
- Induce extension by moving the patient's hand towards the floor, with the palm facing upwards.
- Elbow extension is approximately 0–15°.

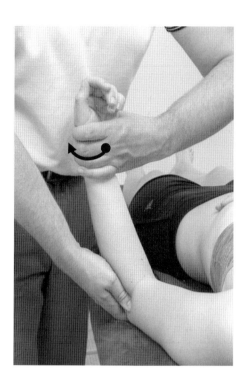

T11.3 Supination

- Stand facing the patient on the side you wish to assess.
- Hold the arm by supporting around the wrist.
- Place the palpating hand under the patient's elbow, with the fingers palpating the radial head.
- Using your body, rotate the forearm in a lateral (external) direction.
- Elbow supination is approximately 90°.

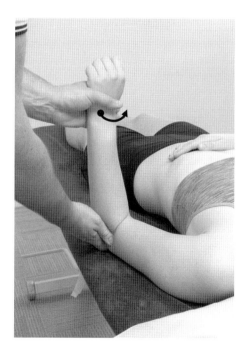

T11.4 Pronation

- Stand facing directly across the patient on the side you wish to assess.
- Hold the arm by supporting around the wrist.
- Place the palpating hand under the patient's elbow, with the fingers palpating the radial head.
- Using your body, rotate the forearm in a medial (internal) direction.
- Elbow pronation is approximately 85°.

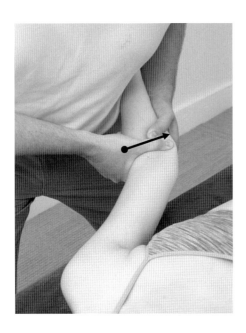

T11.5 Medial gapping

- Stand facing directly across the patient on the side you wish to assess.
- Stabilize the patient's arm by placing their forearm between your corresponding arm and your body.
- Hold the medial aspect of the upper forearm.
- Place your other hand over the lateral aspect of the forearm, level with the elbow joint.
- Using your body, rotate towards the patient to induce medial (internal) gapping of the humeral–ulnar joint.

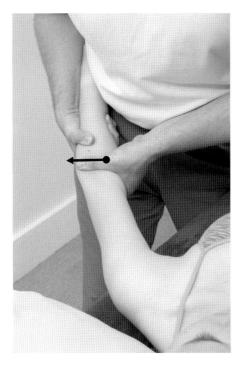

T11.6 Lateral gapping

- Stand facing directly across the patient on the side you wish to assess.
- Stabilize the patient's arm by placing their forearm between your corresponding arm and your body.
- Hold the lateral aspect of the patient's upper forearm.
- Place your other hand over the medial aspect of the forearm, level with the elbow joint.
- Using your body, rotate away from the patient to induce lateral (external) gapping of the humeral–ulnar joint.
- To gap the humeral–radial joint, follow the above instructions but externally rotate the patient's arm first.

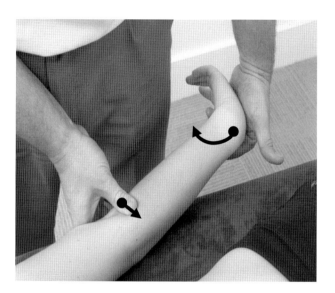

T11.7 Radial head articulation

- Stand facing directly across the patient on the side you wish to assess.
- Support around the patient's wrist over the radial side of their lower forearm.
- Place the thumb of the palpating hand behind the radial head.
- Keeping the patient's elbow on the plinth, with a positive pressure on the radial head, articulate the joint by inducing pronation and slight extension at the elbow and palmar flexion at the wrist.

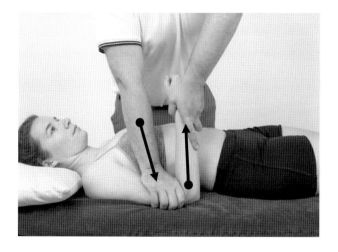

T11.8 Radial head traction

- Stand facing directly across the patient on the opposite side you wish to assess.
- Hold the patient's forearm by the wrist with your corresponding hand.
- Place your opposite hand fully extended on the distal aspect of the humerus, inducing a force down towards the plinth.
- While maintaining this downwards force, traction the radial head by bringing the patient's wrist in a superior direction.

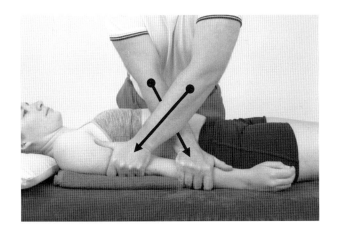

T11.9 Radial head articulation

- Stand facing directly across from the patient on the opposite side you wish to assess.
- While adopting a cross-handed position, place one hand on the distal aspect of the patient's humerus.
- Place your opposite hand on the proximal aspect of their forearm.
- Impulse is driven towards the plinth in the direction of the forearms (see photograph).
- A small fulcrum of a towel or pillow can be used (as shown).

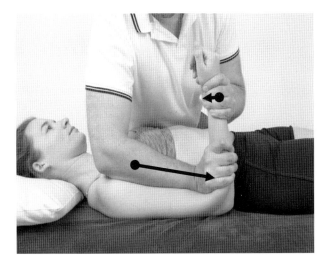

T11.10 Humeral–ulnar traction

- Stand facing directly across from the patient on the opposite side you wish to assess.
- Hold the elbow at 90°, supporting the patient's forearm by holding around their wrist.
- Place the other hand on the superior part of the patient's forearm.
- Apply a force parallel to the humerus, thus inducing humeral–ulnar traction.

REFERENCES

Abbott JH, Patla CE, Jensen RH (2001). The initial effects of an elbow mobilization with movement technique on grip strength in subjects with lateral epicondylalgia. Manual Therapy 6(3):163-169.

Alcid JG, Ahmad CS, Lee TQ (2004). Elbow anatomy and structural biomechanics. Clinics in Sports Medicine 23(4):503-517.

Amadio PC (1990). Epidemiology of hand and wrist injuries in sports. Hand Clinics 6(3):379-381.

An KN, Morrey BF (2000). Biomechanics of the elbow. In: BF Morrey ed. The Elbow and its Disorders. Philadelphia: WB Saunders; 43-60.

An KN, Zobitz ME, Morrey BF (2009). Biomechanics of the elbow. In: BF Morrey, J Sanchez-Sotelo eds. The Elbow and its Disorders. St Louis, Mo: Elsevier Health Sciences.

Azar FM, Andrews JR, Wilk KE et al (2000). Operative treatment of ulnar collateral ligament injuries of the elbow in athletes. American Journal of Sports Medicine 28:16-23.

Bain GI (1999). A review of complex trauma to the elbow. Australian and New Zealand Journal of Surgery 69(8):578-581.

Bartels RH, Termeer EH, van der Wilt GJ et al (2005). Simple decompression or anterior subcutaneous transposition for ulnar neuropathy at the elbow: a cost-minimization analysis – Part 2. Neurosurgery 56(3):531-536.

Baxter RE (2003). Pocket Guide to Musculoskeletal Assessment. Philadelphia: WB Saunders.

Beals RK (1976). The Normal Carrying Angle of the Elbow: A Radiographic Study of 422 Patients. Clinical Orthopaedics and Related Research 119:194-196.

Bernard BP (1997). Musculoskeletal Disorders (MSDs) and Workplace Factors. Cincinnati: US Department of Health and Human Services.

Bethapudi S, Robinson P, Engebretsen L et al (2013). Elbow injuries at the London 2012 Summer Olympic Games: demographics and pictorial imaging review. American Journal of Roentgenology 201(3):535-549.

Brinker MR, Miller MD (1999). Fundamentals of Orthopaedics. Philadelphia: WB Saunders.

Buchanan WW, DeCeulaer K, Balint GP (1996). Regional examination of the limb and spine. In: Clinical Examination of the Musculoskeletal System: Assessing Rheumatic Conditions. Philadelphia: Lippincott Williams & Wilkins.

Celli A (2008). Anatomy and biomechanics of the elbow. In: Treatment of Elbow Lesions. Milan: Springer; 1-11.

Charalambous CP, Stanley JK (2008). Posterolateral rotatory instability of the elbow. Journal of Bone and Joint Surgery, British Volume 90(3):272-279.

Chumbley EM, O'Connor FG, Nirschl RP (2000). Evaluation of overuse elbow injuries. American Family Physician 61(3):691-700.

Conway JE, Jobe FW, Glousman RE et al (1992). Medial instability of the elbow in throwing athletes. Treatment by repair or reconstruction of the ulnar collateral ligament. The Journal of Bone and Joint Surgery 74(1):67-83.

Coombes BK, Bisset L, Vicenzino B (2009). A new integrative model of lateral epicondylalgia. British Journal of Sports Medicine 43(4):252-258.

Cooper G (2007). Pocket Guide to Musculoskeletal Diagnosis. New York: Springer Science+Business Media.

Dines JS, Jones KJ, Kahlenberg C et al (2012). Elbow ulnar collateral ligament reconstruction in javelin throwers at a minimum 2-year follow-up. The American Journal of Sports Medicine 40(1):148-151.

Dugas JR, Cain EL Jr (2005). Elbow injuries in sports. Orthopaedic Sports Medicine 1(4):1-12.

Fan ZJ, Silverstein BA, Bao S et al (2009). Quantitative exposure–response relations between physical workload and prevalence of lateral epicondylitis in a working population. American Journal of Industrial Medicine 52(6):479-490.

Field LD, Savoie FH (1998). Common elbow injuries in sport. Sports Medicine 26(3):193-205.

Fleisig GS, Andrews JR, Cutter GR et al (2011). Risk of serious injury for young baseball pitchers: a 10-year prospective study. The American Journal of Sports Medicine 39(2):253-257.

Fleisig GS, Andrews JR (2012). Prevention of elbow injuries in youth baseball pitchers. Sports Health: A Multidisciplinary Approach 1941738112454828.

Fornalski, S, Gupt, R, Lee TQ (2003). Anatomy and biomechanics of the elbow joint. Techniques in Hand and Upper Extremity Surgery 7(4):168-178.

Frostick SP, Mohammad M, Ritchie DA (1999). Sport injuries of the elbow. British Journal of Sports Medicine 33(5):301-311.

Gabel GT, Morrey BF (2000). Medial epicondylitis. In: BF Morrey ed. The Elbow and its Disorders. Philadelphia: WB Saunders; 537-542.

Harrington JM, Carter JT, Birrell L et al (1998). Surveillance case definitions for work related upper limb pain syndromes. Occupational and Environmental Medicine 55(4):264-271.

Hartz CR, Linscheid RL, Gramse RR et al (1981). The pronator teres syndrome: compressive neuropathy of the median nerve. Journal of Bone and Joint Surgery, American Volume 63(6): 885-890.

Harvey C (2001). Compartment syndrome: When it is least expected. Orthopaedic Nursing 20(3):15-25.

Huisstede B, Miedema HS, van Opstal T et al (2008). Interventions for treating the radial tunnel syndrome: a systematic review of observational studies. The Journal of Hand Surgery 33(1):72-78.

Hunter JM, Mackin EJ, Callahan AD (2002). Rehabilitation of the Hand and Upper Extremity, 5th ed. Maryland Heights: Mosby.

Jackson MD, McKeag DB (1997). Anatomy and biomechanics of the elbow and forearm. In: Essentials of Sports Medicine. St Louis: Mosby; 294-306.

Jawed S, Jawad ASM, Padhiar N et al (2001). Chronic exertional compartment syndrome of the forearms secondary to weight training. Rheumatology 40(3):344-345.

Johnson GW, Cadwallader K, Scheffel SB et al (2007). Treatment of lateral epicondylitis. American Family Physician 76(6):843-848.

Kreiswirth EM, Myer GD, Rauh MJ (2014). Incidence of injury among male Brazilian jiu-jitsu fighters at the World Jiu-Jitsu No-Gi Championship 2009. Journal of Athletic Training 49(1):89.

Kumar B, Pai S, Ray B et al (2010). Radiographic study of carrying angle and morphometry of skeletal elements of human elbow. Romanian Journal of Morphology and Embryology 51(3):521-526.

Kurppa K, Viikari-Juntura E, Kuosma E et al (1991). Incidence of tenosynovitis or peritendinitis and epicondylitis in a meat-processing factory. Scandinavian Journal of Work, Environment and Health 17(1):32-37.

Kuxhaus L (2008). Development of a feedback-controlled elbow simulator: design validation and clinical application. ProQuest. Doctoral thesis.

Lee HJ, Kim I, Hong JT et al (2014a). Early surgical treatment of pronator teres syndrome. Journal of Korean Neurosurgical Society 55(5):296-299.

Lee YS, Chou YH, Chiou HJ et al (2014b). Use of sonography in assessing elbow medial collateral ligament injury after arm wrestling. Journal of the Chinese Medical Association 77(3):163-165.

Leigh S, Dapena J, Gross M et al (2013). Associations between javelin throwing technique and upper extremity kinetics. In: ISBS-Conference Proceedings Archive (Vol 1, No 1).

McRae R (2010). Clinical Orthopaedic Examination, 6th ed. Edinburgh: Elsevier Health Sciences.

Molnár SL, Hidas P, Kocsis G et al (2014). Operative elbow injuries among Hungarian elite wrestlers. International Journal of Therapy and Training 19(6).

Morrey BF, Askew LJ, Chao EY (1981). A biomechanical study of normal functional elbow motion. The Journal of Bone and Joint Surgery 63(6):872-877.

Morrey BF, Tanaka S, An KN (1991). Valgus stability of the elbow: a definition of primary and secondary constraints. Clinical Orthopaedics and Related Research 265:187-195.

Morris H (1882). The rider's sprain. Lancet 120:133-134.

Ovesen O, Brok KE, Arreskøv J et al (1990). Monteggia lesions in children and adults: an analysis of etiology and long-term results of treatment. Orthopedics 13(5):529-534.

Paungmali A, O'Leary S, Souvlis T et al (2003). Hypoalgesic and sympathoexcitatory effects of mobilization with movement for lateral epicondylalgia. Physical Therapy 83(4):374-383.

Purkait R, Chandra H (2004). An anthropometric investigation into the probable cause of formation of carrying angle: A sex indicator. Journal of Indian Academy of Forensic Medicine 26(1):0971-0973.

Reiman MP (2016). Orthopedic Clinical Examination. Champaign, Illinois: Human Kinetics.

Schaefer PT, Speier J (2012). Common medical problems of instrumental athletes. Current Sports Medicine Reports 11(6):316-322.

Shanley E, Rauh MJ, Michener LA et al (2011). Shoulder range of motion measures as risk factors for shoulder and elbow injuries in high school softball and baseball players. The American Journal of Sports Medicine 39(9):1997-2006.

Sharma K, Mansur DI, Khanal K et al (2013). Variation of carrying angle with age, sex, height and special reference to side. Kathmandu University Medical Journal 44(4):315-318.

Shiri R, Viikari-Juntura E, Varonen H et al (2006). Prevalence and determinants of lateral and medial epicondylitis: a population study. American Journal of Epidemiology 164(11):1065-1074.

Shiri R, Viikari-Juntura E (2011). Lateral and medial epicondylitis: role of occupational factors. Best practice & research. Clinical Rheumatology 25:43.

Silverstein B, Welp E, Nelson N et al (1998). Claims incidence of work-related disorders of the upper extremities: Washington State, 1987 through 1995. American Journal of Public Health 88(12):1827-1833.

Smidt N, Lewis M, Windt DAVD et al (2006). Lateral epicondylitis in general practice: course and prognostic indicators of outcome. The Journal of Rheumatology 33(10):2053-2059.

Smidt N, van der Windt DA (2006). Tennis elbow in primary care: corticosteroid injections provide only short term pain relief. British Medical Journal 333(7575):927-928.

Snider RK (1997). Olecranon bursitis. In: RK Sinder ed. Essentials of Musculoskeletal Care. Rosemont, IL: American Academy of Orthopaedic Surgeons; 114-119.

Taylor SA, Hannafin JA (2012). Evaluation and management of elbow tendinopathy. Sports Health: A Multidisciplinary Approach 4(5):384-393.

Tosun B, Selek O, Buluc L et al (2008). Chronic post-traumatic radial head dislocation associated with dissociation of distal radio-ulnar joint: a case report. Archives of Orthopaedic and Trauma Surgery 128(7):669-671.

Tullos HS, King JW (1973). Throwing mechanism in sports. The Orthopedic Clinics of North America 4(3):709.

Turpin JM, Cridelich C, Teboul B et al (2012). Actigraphy for assessment of elbow articular amplitude for articular assessment in gerontology. Gerontechnology 11(2):262.

Tyler TF, Mullaney MJ, Mirabella MR et al (2014). Risk factors for shoulder and elbow injuries in high school baseball pitchers: the role of preseason strength and range of motion. The American Journal of Sports Medicine 42(8):1993-1999.

van Rijn RM, Huisstede BM, Koes BW et al (2009). Associations between work-related factors and specific disorders at the elbow: a systematic literature review. Rheumatology 48(5):528-536.

Vicenzino B (2003). Lateral epicondylalgia: a musculoskeletal physiotherapy perspective. Manual Therapy 8(2):66-79.

Vicenzino B, Paungmali A, Teys P (2007). Mulligan's mobilization-with-movement, positional faults and pain relief: current concepts from a critical review of literature. Manual Therapy 12(2):98-108.

Villaseñor-Ovies P, Vargas A, Chiapas-Gasca K et al (2012). Clinical anatomy of the elbow and shoulder. Reumatología Clínica 8:13-24.

Walker-Bone KE, Palmer KT, Reading I et al (2003). Soft-tissue rheumatic disorders of the neck and upper limb: prevalence and risk factors. In: Seminars in Arthritis and Rheumatism (Vol 33, No 3). Philadelphia: WB Saunders; 185-203.

Walker-Bone K, Palmer KT, Reading I et al (2012). Occupation and epicondylitis: a population-based study. Rheumatology 51(2):305-310.

Werner R, Franzblau A, Gel N et al (2005). A longitudinal study of industrial and clerical workers: predictors of upper extremity tendonitis. Journal of Occupational Rehabilitation 15:37-46.

Whiteside JA, Andrews JR, Fleisig GS (1999). Elbow injuries in young baseball players. The Physician and Sportsmedicine 27(6):87-102.

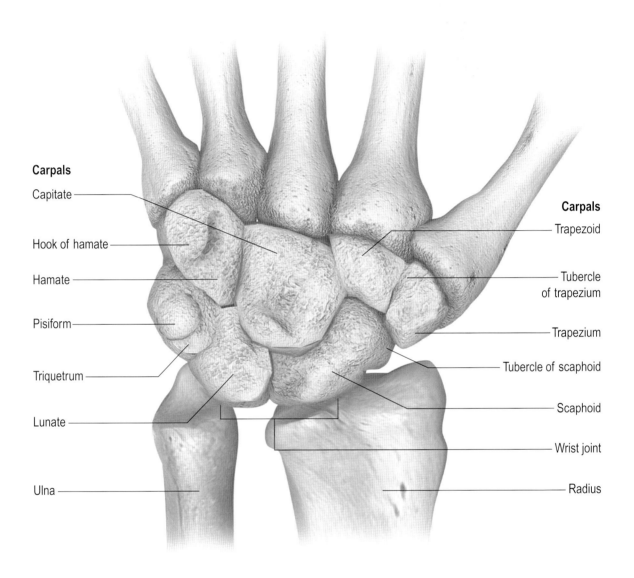

Carpals

Capitate

Hook of hamate

Hamate

Pisiform

Triquetrum

Lunate

Ulna

Carpals

Trapezoid

Tubercle
of trapezium

Trapezium

Tubercle of scaphoid

Scaphoid

Wrist joint

Radius

Figure 12.1
The carpal bones of the wrist

Introduction

The wrist and hand are extremely important for normal everyday functional living. Their extensive range of motion enables us to perform a variety of complex tasks, including notably object handling and communicating, and providing oppositional grip.

Anatomically, the hand and wrist comprise a complex system of static and dynamic structures – bones, muscles, tendons, ligaments and skin. These components have complex relationships with each other to allow and maintain variable mobility (Rhee et al 2006). The 'wrist joint' is not a single joint but a complex of radiocarpal, intercarpal, mid-carpal and carpal–metacarpal joints.

A common condition, and the most common peripheral nerve entrapment in the wrist, is carpal tunnel syndrome (Alfonso et al 2010). This is a compression and/or entrapment of the median nerve as it traverses through the carpal tunnel that causes impairment of motor and/or sensory nerve conduction, resulting in symptoms such as numbness, pain and paresthesia. It has a higher incidence in the elderly population, is more common in females than males (Newport 2000), and it can be associated with medical conditions such as diabetes, rheumatoid arthritis, hypothyroidism, renal disease and pregnancy (Katims et al 1989, Maghsoudipour et al 2008, Barcenilla et al 2012, O'Connor et al 2012). There is also evidence for an association with obesity and smoking (Becker 2002, Geoghegan et al 2004). Although there remains a lack of detailed understanding of its interconnection with occupation, some studies have hypothesized that 50% of all carpal tunnel syndrome presentations are connected to occupation (Dale et al 2013). Abbas et al (1998) and Palmer et al (2007) found that occupations that involve prolonged repetitive dorsiflexion/palmar flexion of the wrist and the operation of handheld vibration tools had high incidences, for example.

The total available evidence suggests that carpal tunnel syndrome can be associated with factors such as occupation, lifestyle and medical history, but that a person is more likely to develop it when multiple factors are present.

There have been a number of studies into the effectiveness of manual therapies in the treatment of carpal tunnel syndrome (e.g. Heebner & Roddey 2008, McKeon & Yancosek 2008, Carlson et al 2010). These have looked at articulation of the wrist and carpal bones, splinting and neural gliding, but the research to date is inconclusive: some have found that in mild presentations manual therapy has had beneficial results (Burke et al 2007, Meems et al 2014), while others have stated that there is no statistical evidence for this (Huisstede et al 2010, Page et al 2012). Although a recent paper by Meems and colleagues (2014) stated that traction of the wrist may be an alternative, if not yet fully evaluated, treatment option for carpal tunnel syndrome, the main medical approach is either corticosteroid injections or surgery to the palmar retinaculum to release the median nerve. The 'gold standard' approach is obviously, when possible, to address the mechanical cause of the carpal tunnel syndrome, whether work ergonomics, occupational causes or hobby, and then the use of night splints coupled with a structured manual therapy approach to the hand, wrist and upper extremity. If this does not succeed, surgery is possibly the best course of treatment.

Villafañe et al (2013) examined the effectiveness of manual therapy and exercise for osteoarthritis in the carpometacarpal joint and discovered that a combination of articulation, neural articulation and exercise was more effective than a sham intervention, although they acknowledged that further research is required.

A study by Rabin et al (2015) found that three out of four participants with De Quervain syndrome reported better reduction in symptoms with manual articulation, muscle training and electrical stimulation compared to corticosteroid injections. A case study by Walker-Bone and colleagues (2004) of a patient with radial wrist pain, which had been diagnosed 2 years before as De Quervain's syndrome, found that manual therapy of the hand and wrist decreased the patient's reported pain over a period of 4 weeks.

Van Tulder et al (2007) found that manual therapy, combined with exercise therapy and self-help advice, can be beneficial for repetitive strain injuries such as tenosynovitis and wrist impingement conditions, although the studies they reviewed were not large enough to be statistically significant.

Anatomy

Bony and joint anatomy

The hand is made up of 27 bones, which are divided into two groups: the carpus, containing 8 carpal bones that form the wrist and base of the hand, and the digits, comprising 5 metacarpals and 14 non-sesamoid bones of the phalanges. The wrist acts as a bridge between the forearm and the hand. In addition to the carpal bones, it comprises the proximal areas of the metacarpal bones and the distal ends of the ulna and radius. All of these bones take part in complex articulations, which enable a variety of movement of the hand and wrist (Taylor & Schwarz 1955).

Carpals

The carpal bones are pebble-like structures aligned in two rows – proximal and distal – of four each. The proximal row is located very close to the distal radius and represents an intercalated segment. It includes the scaphoid (boat-shaped), lunate (moon-shaped), triquetrum (three-cornered) and pisiform (pea-shaped). These bones are held together as a group by ligaments. The scaphoid, lunate and triquetrum contribute to the radiocarpal joint. The pisiform does not participate in the kinematics of the proximal row, because it is a sesamoid bone and has only one side that can articulate (Virginia 1999). Also contributing to the integrity of the joint is an articular disc that attaches to the distal radius and ulna and articulates with the triquetral and lunate bones. This articular disc with the distal radius forms a concave ellipsoidal articular surface that is mirrored by the convex shape of the proximal row.

The distal row is closely approximated to the metacarpus region of the hand and articulates with the roots of the five metacarpal bones. It includes the hamate (hook-shaped), capitate (head-shaped), trapezium (table-shaped figure with no two parallel sides), and trapezoid (table-shaped structure with two parallel sides). The carpal bones of the distal row are united to each other as a unit via intercarpal ligaments. These bones also form the carpometacarpal (CMC) joint by tightly binding to the metacarpal bones (McCann & Wise 2011).

Metacarpals

The metacarpals are long, narrow bones with knobby ends. They form the palm of the hand, located between the bones of the carpus and the bones of the phalanges. There are five metacarpal bones in the hand, and they are numbered I–V, beginning at the thumb (Virginia 1999).

Each metacarpal bone is characterized as having a proximal base, a shaft, a neck and a distal head. The distal head of each metacarpal articulates with the proximal phalanges of each digit, and forms a metacarpophalangeal joint. Each metacarpal end articulates proximally with one of the distal carpal bones, and these articulations are named carpometacarpal joints (Taylor & Schwarz 1955).

Phalanges

Phalanges are bones of the fingers and the thumb. There are a total of 14 phalanges in each hand. The thumb contains two phalanges: a proximal phalanx (plural: phalanges) and a distal phalanx. Each of the other digits comprises a proximal, a middle and a distal phalanx bone. These bones articulate with each other through the distal interphalangeal (DIP) and proximal interphalangeal (PIP) joints. The base of the proximal phalanges articulates with the metacarpal bones via the metacarpophalangeal (MCP) joints (Rhee et al 2006; McCann & Wise 2011).

Ligaments

There are a variety of ligaments in the wrist and hand region that primarily serve as the stabilizers of the joints.

The wrist joints are held together by an array of ligaments such as the palmar and dorsal radiocarpal ligaments, and the ulnar and radial

Motion unit	Movement type	Range of motion (°)	Reference
Functional range of motion in ADL	Flexion	45	Brigstocke et al (2013)
	Extension	50	
	Radial deviation	15	
	Ulnar deviation	40	
Average range of motion in ADL	Flexion	50	Nelson et al (1994)
	Extension	51	
	Radial deviation	12	
	Ulnar deviation	40	

Table 12.1
Functional and average range of motion of the wrist

collateral ligaments. These unite the radius and ulna with the carpal bones. The intercarpal articulations between the carpals are strengthened as a unit by a group of ligaments. These include the radiate carpal, pisohamate and intercarpal ligaments (Platzer 2004).

The carpometacarpal joints connect the distal row of carpals with the proximal bases of the metacarpals. These joints are supported by some strong ligaments, including the carpometacarpal and pisometacarpal ligaments. Like the intercarpal articulations, the intermetacarpal articulations between the metacarpals are also strengthened by a group of ligaments, such as the dorsal, palmar, and interosseous metacarpal ligaments (Platzer 2004).

The ligaments of the metacarpophalangeal joints unite the metacarpal bones with the proximal phalanges. The radial and ulnar collateral ligaments are the primary stabilizers of the metacarpophalangeal joints (Berger & Weiss 2003). However, specialized ligaments are also found at these joints, such as the deep transverse metacarpal ligament and the natatory ligament.

Like the metacarpophalangeal joints, the ligaments of the proximal interphalangeal, distal interphalangeal and the interphalangeal joints are all very similar in configuration (Petre & Deune 2013).

Range of motion

The wrist is capable of three types of movement: flexion and extension, pronation and supination, and radial or ulnar deviation. Palmer et al (1985) suggested that the functional range of the wrist is 5° of flexion, 30° of extension, 10° of radial deviation and 15° of ulnar deviation. In another study, Nelson et al (1994) reported that the average range of motion of the wrist in activities of daily living (ADL) is 50° of flexion, 51° of extension, 12° of radial deviation and 40° of ulnar deviation. Based on the goniometer measurement of wrist movement in 40 subjects, Ryu et al (1991) found an average maximum range of motion of 138° of flexion–extension (78° of flexion to 60° of extension) and 58° of radial–ulnar deviation (21° of radial deviation to 38° of ulnar deviation). See Tables 12.1 for an overview of wrist movement and Table 12.2 for information about the hand.

However, this extensive range of movement comes at a cost and leads to many hand and wrist disorders, most commonly traumatic injuries. On top of that, surgical processes may further complicate these injuries. For any physical therapist or general physician treating hand or wrist problems, detailed knowledge and understanding of hand/wrist anatomy is therefore essential to diagnose conditions accurately and deliver the best quality of care.

Epidemiology
Wrist and hand disorders

Wrist and hand disorders are the most common occupation-related musculoskeletal (MSK) diseases in the UK. The rate of incidence and prevalence of these disorders are also more predominant than any other MSK conditions. In a 3-year Musculoskeletal Occupational Surveillance Scheme (MOSS), Cherry et al (2001) found that upper limb disorders accounted for 66% of an estimated total of 8070 cases, with hand or wrist conditions comprising 44% of the total.

Motion unit	Joint name	Movement type	Range of motion (°)	
			Average	Total arc
Normal range of motion (thumb)	Metacarpophalangeal joint	Flexion	0–56 (in 85% population)	0–124
	Interphalangeal joint	Flexion	(-) 5–73	
Normal range of motion (finger)	Metacarpophalangeal joint	Flexion	0–100	0–290
	Distal interphalangeal joint	Flexion	0–85	
	Proximal interphalangeal joint	Flexion	0–105	
Functional range of motion (thumb)	Metacarpophalangeal joint	Flexion	21	40
	Interphalangeal joint	Flexion	18	
Functional range of motion (finger)	Metacarpophalangeal joint	Flexion	61	164
	Distal interphalangeal joint	Flexion	39	
	Proximal interphalangeal joint	Flexion	60	

Table 12.2

Normal and functional range of motion of the hand joints

Data adapted from Hume et al (1990)

Hand and wrist disorders tend to be predominant among adults in the general population and are more prevalent in women than in men. Walker-Bone et al (2004), in a two-stage cross-sectional study of 9696 healthy adults, reported that the prevalence rates of several hand and wrist conditions were higher in female adults than in male (see Table 12.3). Table 12.4 lists some common pathological conditions of the wrist and hand.

Table 12.3

Estimated prevalence of hand/wrist diagnoses in the general population

Data from Walker-Bone et al (2004)

Diagnosis	Prevalence in general population (%)	
	Men (n = 2696)	Women (n = 3342)
De Quervain syndrome	0.5	1.3
Tenosynovitis of the wrist	1.1	2.2
Carpal tunnel syndrome	0.9	1.2
Specific wrist/hand disorders	2.6	3.6
Nonspecific wrist/hand pain	8.7	11.5
Osteoarthritis, DIP joint	1.1	2.8
Osteoarthritis, thumb base	2.5	4.6

Condition	Description	Reference
De Quervain syndrome	A tenosynovitis of the sheath that involves abductor pollicis longus and the extensor pollicis brevis Occurs most commonly in the middle-aged Affects women 8–10 times more often than men Symptoms include difficulty gripping, pain and tenderness on certain movements of the wrist, and pain along the base of the thumb	McRae (2010)
Dupuytren's disease	Involves nodular thickening and a contracture of the palmar fascia Most commonly affects the ring finger, followed by the middle and little fingers Occurs predominantly in men over the age of 40 Typically affects people with northern European ancestry; rare in people from China, India and Africa May be associated with diabetes, epilepsy, gout or alcoholic cirrhosis	Burge (1999), Mir (2003)
Carpal tunnel syndrome	A condition in which the median nerve is compressed as it traverses the tunnel under the thick transverse carpal ligament Usually occurs in middle-aged (30–60 years age group), obese women Almost four times more prevalent in older women than in men May be associated with myxedema, acromegaly, pregnancy, obesity, rheumatoid arthritis, primary amyloidosis, tophaceous gout and repetitive work with the hand Symptoms include numbness, tingling, pain and weakness in the palm of the hand and the fingers	Silverstein et al (1987), Atroshi et al (1999)
Ulnar tunnel syndrome	A condition in which the ulnar nerve is compressed as it passes via the ulnar carpal canal Causes include ganglionic compression, repetitive trauma, ulnar artery disease, inflammatory arthritis and old carpal or metacarpal fractures Symptoms include small muscle wasting and weakness in the hand	Grundberg (1984), McRae (2010)
Rheumatoid arthritis	Commonest of the arthritides Progressively affects the tendons, joints, muscles, arteries and nerves of the hand and wrist Produces most severe deformities Has crippling effects on hand function Affects women three times more often than men Peak incidence: between 4th and 6th decades	Mir (2003)
Extensor tenosynovitis	An inflammation of the tendons at the back of the wrist Usually occurs in 20–40 years age group Often caused by a period of overactivity	McRae (2010)
Wrist bone fracture (scaphoid)	A common bone fracture in the carpus region May involve direct axial compression or hyperextension of the wrist Occurs more often in men than in women Most common in young men (age group: 15–29 years) following a fall, athletic injury, or traumatic injury on an outstretched hand Symptoms include pain in wrist motion, swelling around the wrist, and tenderness in the wrist and at the thumb base	Fisk (1970), Leslie & Dickson (1981)

(Continued)

Condition	Description	Reference
Mallet finger	An injury of the extensor digitorum tendon of the fingers	Wang & Johnson (2001), Anderson (2011)
	Results from interruption of the terminal extensor mechanism at the DIP joint	
	Usually occurs when an object strikes the finger hard and creates a forceful flexion of an extended DIP joint	
	Symptoms include tenderness just behind the nail, pain and swelling at the end of the injured finger, and inability to straighten the tip of that finger	
Tumors in the hand	Involve the soft tissues	McRae (2010)
	Common tumors include ganglions, mucous cysts, implantation dermoid cysts, chondroma osteoid osteoma and solitary glomus	

Table 12.4
Some common pathological conditions of the wrist and hand

Wrist and hand injuries

Fingers and wrists are two of the most injured parts of the body, accounting for 10% and 7% of all injuries, respectively (Health & Safety Authority 2011). A database query about all upper extremity injuries presented to US emergency departments in 2009 by Ootes et al (2012) found that fingers were the most injured region, accounting for 38.4% of all injuries. The authors also reported that the wrist accounted for 15.2% of all upper extremity injuries. The annual incidences of hand and wrist injuries are also shown to be higher than other injuries. According to the British Society for Surgery of the Hand (BSSH 2007), each year about 20% of patients (i.e. more than 1.36 million people) attend Accident and Emergency Departments for hand/wrist injuries in the UK.

Wrist and hand examination

Medical history

Taking a detailed medical history of the past and present problems of the patient is as essential as the physical examination itself. Apart from questioning about the patient's health in general, the healthcare provider should seek information about whether the patient performs repetitive activities that involve simultaneous wrist and finger extension or flexion. The patient should also be asked about pain, swelling, numbness, tingling or any other issues concerning the wrist, palm or fingers. In most cases, the narrative provided by the patient helps to narrow the differential diagnosis and facilitate the physical examination.

Red flags

Table 12.5 summarizes the signs and symptoms of serious conditions to look for in the wrist and hand region.

Physical examination

Physical examinations of the wrist and hand should be carried out in a systematic manner. A general evaluation of the wrist/hand should include inspection, palpation, range of motion and a variety of special tests.

Inspection

The physical examination process should start with a careful visual inspection of the patient's hand, wrist and forearm. The examiner should observe while the patient uses their hands. They should also inspect the nails, checking whether the color is normal or unusual (e.g. cyanotic or pale) and for infection, hemorrhages, abnormal flattening, and clubbing in the nails. Any type of swelling, nonalignment in joints, ecchymosis, joint asymmetry, functional deficits or bony deformities observed in the hands should be noted for further examination. In addition, signs of muscle wasting should be looked for by inspecting the thenar and hypothenar eminence (McRae 2010).

Condition	Signs and symptoms
Lunate fracture	Generalized wrist pain
	History of a dorsiflexion injury of the hand or a fall on to an outstretched hand
	Severe pain when gripping objects or moving the wrist
	Reduced grip strength
Scaphoid fracture	History of a fall on to an outstretched hand
	Pain with or without swelling or bruising at the base of the thumb
	Severe pain when grabbing or gripping objects
	Difficulty in moving and twisting the wrist or thumb
	Reduced movement around the wrist
Long flexor tendon rupture	An injury on the palm side of the hand
	Numbness in the fingertip
	Pain with bending the finger
	Inability to move or bend one or more joints of the finger, such as the DIP or PIP joint
	Forceful flexor contraction
Tumor	History of cancer
	Asymmetric or irregular-shaped lesion
	Suspected malignancy
	Unexplained deformity, mass or swelling
	Fair skin, history of sunburns
Infection	Fever, chills
	Recent bacterial infection
	Recent cut, scrape or puncture wound
	Unexplained weight loss
	Unexplained ulceration or open wounds

Table 12.5

Red flags for serious pathology in the wrist and hand region

Data from Hunter et al (2002), Weinzweig & Gonzalez (2002), Phillips et al (2004), Forman et al (2005)

Palpation

In the wrist and hand examination, several important bony and soft-tissue structures need to be palpated to identify areas of pathology. Palpation should include the anatomic snuffbox, radial and ulnar styloids, scaphoid tubercle, pisiform, hook of the hamate, extensor and flexor tendons, each finger and any enlarged joints (Cooper 2007). The lateral and medial aspects of each DIP and PIP joint should be palpated to assess abnormalities such as Heberden's and Bouchard's nodes. Palpation of the extensor tendon on the dorsum of the hand is important in patients with rheumatoid arthritis, because synovitis may result in rupture. Flexor tendons should be palpated to identify any contractures in the fingers (Lynch 2004).

Range of motion

The examiner should carefully assess the range of motion of the fingers and wrist. The strength of the thumb, fingers, wrist and forearms should also be tested. The range of both active and passive motion of the wrist as well as the MCP joint and IP joints of each digit should be measured and noted. The examiner may use a goniometer to assess the range of motion (McRae 2010). While examining the hand and wrist, the examiner should expose and evaluate the entire upper limb. The evaluation of the entire upper extremity is essential, because hand injuries are often associated with secondary stiffness and limited movement of other joints of the extremity and the part involved (Fisher 1984).

Special tests

See Table 12.6.

Test	Procedure	Positive sign	Interpretation
Tinel's sign test	The examiner lightly taps the volar aspect of the patient's wrist over the median nerve.	Tingling or paresthesia in the distribution of the nerve	Carpal tunnel syndrome
Phalen's test	The examiner instructs the patient to hold their wrists in a fully flexed position for 1–2 minutes.	Exacerbation of paresthesia in the median nerve distribution	Carpal tunnel syndrome
Wrinkle (shrivel) test	The patient's fingers are soaked in warm water for approximately 30 minutes. Examiner then removes the patient's fingers from the water and inspects whether skin on pulp of fingers is wrinkled or not.	No wrinkle of the fingers	Denervation of fingers
Murphy's sign test	The examiner asks the patient to make a fist and then observes the position of the third metacarpal.	Third metacarpal head is level with the second and fourth metacarpal heads	Dislocated lunate
Fromet's sign test	The patient is instructed to grasp a piece of paper between the thumb and index finger. The examiner then tries to pull it away.	Flexion of the patient's thumb IP joint due to weakness of adductor pollicis	Ulnar nerve paralysis
Flexor digitorum superficialis test	The examiner instructs the patient to flex the PIP joint of the involved finger while keeping the other fingers extended.	Inability to flex the PIP joint	Disrupted flexor digitorum superficialis
Flexor digitorum profundus test	The examiner instructs the patient to extend the DIP joint of the involved finger while keeping the other fingers extended.	Inability to flex the DIP joint	Disrupted flexor digitorum profundus
Allen's test	The examiner instructs the patient to make a tight fist and open it fully several times. The patient then squeezes their fist to 'pump' the blood out of the hand and fingers. The examiner compresses the radial and ulnar arteries. The patient relaxes their hand and the examiner releases one artery at a time, observing the color of the hand and fingers.	Failure of the radial or ulnar half of the hand to flush red immediately	Occlusion of radial or ulnar artery

Table 12.6

Special tests for the wrist and hand examination

Data adapted from Baxter (2003), Lynch (2004), Cooper (2007), McRae (2010)

Wrist and hand muscles

Name	Origin	Insertion	Action	Nerve supply
Flexor carpi radialis	Medial epicondyle of humerus (common flexor tendon)	Bases of second and third metacarpal bones	Flexion and abduction of the wrist	Median nerve (C6–C7)
Palmaris longus	Medial epicondyle of humerus (common flexor tendon)	Flexor retinaculum and palmar aponeurosis	Flexes the wrist	Median nerve (C6–C7)
Palmaris brevis	Flexor retinaculum, palmar aponeurosis	Skin of the palm	Wrinkles the skin of the palm	Ulnar nerve (C8–T1)
Flexor carpi ulnaris	Humeral head: medial epicondyle of the humerus (common flexor tendon) Ulnar head: medial border of olecranon of ulna	Pisiform, hook of hamate and base of fifth metacarpal	Flexion and adduction of the wrist	Ulnar nerve (C8–T1)
Flexor digitorum superficialis	Humeroulnar head: medial epicondyle of the humerus (common flexor tendon), medial border of coronoid process of ulna Radial head: shaft of radius, anterior surface	Anterior surface of the middle phalanges of the four fingers	Flexor of the fingers	Median nerve (C7–T1)
Flexor digitorum profundus	Upper three-quarters of anterior and medial surface of ulna, medial surface of coronoid process and interosseous membrane	Base of distal phalanges of fingers	Flexes the fingers	Medial portion: ulnar nerve (C8–T1) Lateral portion: median nerve (C8–T1)
Flexor pollicis longus	Anterior surface of the radius, interosseous membrane, medial epicondyle of the humerus and occasionally the coronoid process of the ulna	Base of the distal phalanx of thumb	Flexion of the thumb	Median nerve (C8–T1)
Extensor digitorum	Lateral epicondyle of the humerus (common extensor tendon)	Lateral and dorsal surface of phalanges of all fingers	Extension of the wrist and fingers	Radial nerve (C7–C8)
Extensor digiti minimi	Lateral epicondyle of the humerus (common extensor tendon)	Dorsal surface of base of phalanx of little finger	Extension of the little finger	Radial nerve (C7–C8)

(Continued)

Name	Origin	Insertion	Action	Nerve supply
Extensor carpi ulnaris	Common extensor tendon (lateral epicondyle), ulna	Dorsal surface of base of phalanx of little finger	Extends and adducts the wrist	Radial nerve (C7–C8)
Extensor carpi radialis longus	Lower third of lateral supracondylar ridge of the humerus	Base of metacarpal of index finger	Extensor and abduction of the wrist	Radial nerve (C6–C7)
Extensor carpi radialis brevis	Lateral epicondyle of humerus (common extensor tendon)	Base of metacarpal of middle finger	Extensor and abduction of the wrist	Radial nerve (C7–C8)
Abductor digiti minimi	Pisiform, tendon of flexor carpi ulnaris	Medial base of proximal phalanx of little finger	Abduction of the little finger	Ulnar nerve (C8–T1)
Flexor digiti minimi brevis	Hook of hamate	Medial base of proximal phalanx of little finger	Flexes the little finger	Ulnar nerve (C8–T1)
Opponens digiti minimi	Hook of hamate and flexor retinaculum	Medial border of metacarpal of little finger	Draws into opposition with the thumb, flexion	Ulnar nerve (C8–T1)
Lubricales (consist of four muscles)	Palmar tendons of flexor digitorum profundus	Tendon of extensor digitorum on lateral corresponding side	Flex the metacarpophalangeal joints, extend the interphalangeal joints	Lateral lumbricals: median nerve (C8–T1) Medial lumbricals: ulnar nerve (C8–T1)
Dorsal interossei	Via bicep formation to adjacent surfaces of metacarpals	Base of proximal phalanges	Abducts the fingers from the mid line (middle finger)	Ulnar nerve (C8–T1)
Palmar interossei	Thumb: medial base of metacarpal Index, ring and little finger: anterior surface of metacarpal	Thumb: medial base of proximal phalanx Index finger: medial base of proximal phalanx Ring and little finger: lateral base of proximal phalanx	Adducts the fingers from the mid line (middle finger), assists in palmar flexion	Ulnar nerve (C8–T1)
Opponens pollicis	Trapezium and flexor retinaculum	Lateral border of thumb metacarpal	Opposition of the thumb	Median nerve (C8–T1)

(Continued)

Name	Origin	Insertion	Action	Nerve supply
Flexor pollicis brevis	Trapezium, flexor retinaculum and thumb metacarpal	Base of proximal phalanx of thumb	Flexes the thumb, assists in abduction and rotation	Lateral part: median nerve (C8–T1) Medial part: ulnar nerve (C8–T1)
Abductor pollicis brevis	Scaphoid, trapezium and flexor retinaculum	Base of proximal phalanx of thumb	Abducts the thumb	Median nerve (C8–T1)
Adductor pollicis	Transverse head: anterior surface of metacarpal of middle finger Oblique head: anterior surface of metacarpal of thumb and index finger, trapezoid and capitate	Base of proximal phalanx of thumb and the ulnar sesamoid	Adducts the thumb	Ulnar nerve (C8–T1)

Table 12.7
Wrist and hand muscles

Techniques: wrist and hand

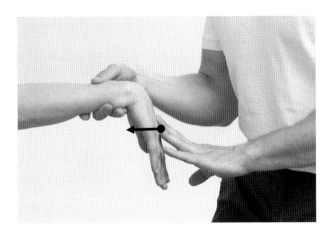

T12.1 Palmar flexion

- Stand in front of the patient, to the side of the hand you want to assess.
- With your opposite hand, grip over the distal forearm with the patient's hand in a pronated position.
- Place your corresponding finger pads over the upper dorsum of the patient's hand and introduce (palmar) flexion of the wrist until its end of range.
- Palmar flexion is approximately 45°.

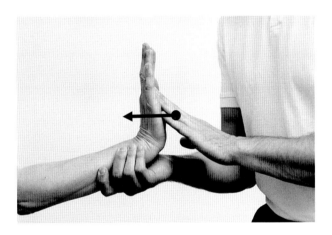

T12.2 Wrist extension

- Stand in front of the patient, to the side of the hand you want to assess.
- With your opposite hand, grip under the distal forearm.
- Place the corresponding finger pads over the upper palm of the patient's hand and introduce extension of the wrist.
- Dorsiflexion is approximately 50°.

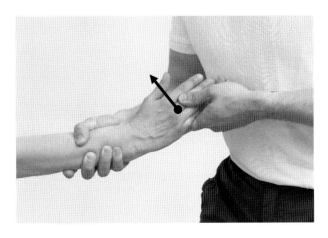

T12.3 Radial deviation

- With the patient supine, stand alongside the patient.
- Place the patient's wrist in a mid-supinated position, and place your hand around the distal forearm. Place your other hand around the medial wrist border.
- With your hand stabilizing the patient's forearm, compress towards the plinth.
- Your other hand introduces side bending (lateral/radial deviation) towards the radial bone.
- Radial deviation is approximately 15°.

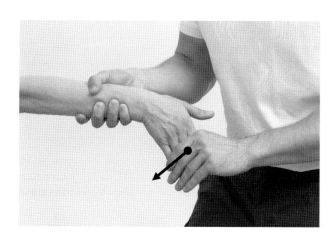

T12.4 Ulnar (medial) deviation

- With the patient supine, face the patient's head and grip their forearm with your inner hand. The patient's wrist should be in a mid-supinated position.
- With your opposite hand, grip the patient's outer phalanges.
- Whilst stabilizing the wrist, introduce ulnar (medial) deviation.
- Ulnar deviation is approximately 40°.

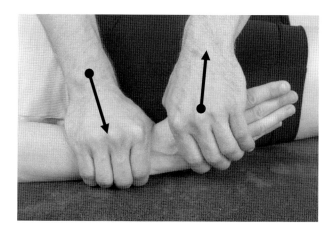

T12.5 Radial (lateral) articulation

- With the patient supine, face the patient's head and grip their forearm with your inner hand. The patient's wrist should be in a mid-supinated position.
- With your opposite hand, grip the patient's outer phalanges.
- Whilst stabilizing the wrist, introduce radial (lateral) deviation until an end of range is felt.

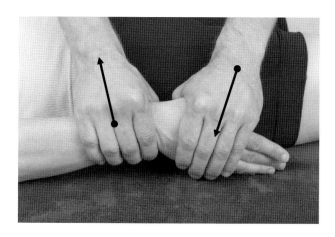

T12.6 Ulnar (medial) articulation

- With the patient supine, stand alongside the patient.
- Place the patient's wrist in a mid-supinated position, and place your hand around their distal forearm. Place your other hand around the medial wrist border.
- With the hand stabilizing the patient's forearm, lift up.
- Your other hand compresses and introduces side bending (medial/unlar deviation) towards the ulna bone.

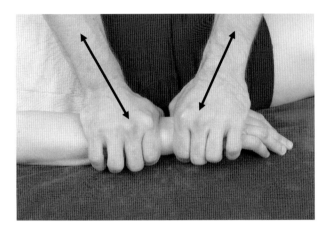

T12.7 Distal anterior–posterior carpal–metacarpal articulation

- With the patient supine, stand alongside the patient.
- Place the patient's wrist in a pronated position.
- With one hand, grip around the distal carpal row.
- With your other hand, grip over and around the base of the metacarpals.
- While fixing the distal carpal row by compressing towards the plinth, introduce a sheer movement by lifting up through the metacarpal bones.
- This movement can then be reversed by compressing through the distal hand and lifting up through the proximal hand.
- You can also do this movement through the radial proximal carpal row and intercarpal rows (see T12.8 Intercarpal anterior–posterior articulation).

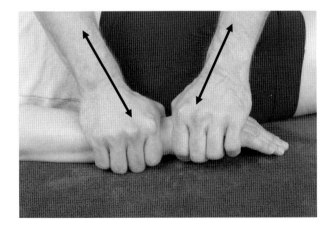

T12.8 Intercarpal anterior–posterior articulation

- With the patient supine, stand alongside the patient.
- Place the patient's wrist in a pronated position.
- With one hand, grip around the distal carpal row.
- With your other hand, grip over and around the proximal carpal row.
- While fixing the proximal carpal row by compressing towards the plinth, introduce a sheer movement by lifting up through the distal carpal row.
- This movement can then be reversed by compressing through the distal hand and lifting up through the proximal hand.

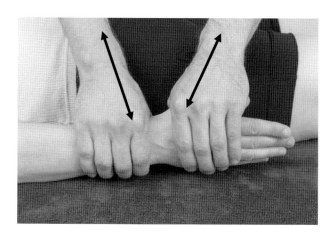

T12.9 Distal carpal metacarpal medial–lateral articulation

- With the patient supine, stand alongside the patient.
- Place the patient's wrist in a mid-pronated position.
- With one hand, grip around the distal carpal row.
- With your other hand, grip over and around the carpals.
- While fixing the base of the metacarpals by compressing towards the plinth, introduce a sheer movement by lifting up through the wrist.
- This movement can then be reversed by compressing through the distal hand and lifting up through the proximal hand.
- You can also do this movement through the radial proximal carpal row.

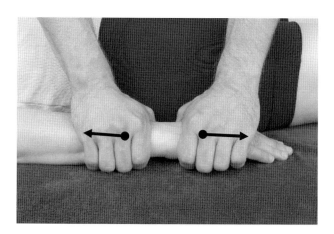

T12.10 Wrist traction

- Stand alongside the supine patient, level with and facing their wrist.
- Grip around the carpal rows, with the patient's wrist in a pronated position.
- With one hand, grip around the most distal portions of the radius and ulna. Slowly introduce traction by easing your hands apart.

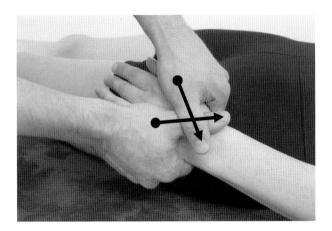

T12.11 Carpal articulation

- With the patient supine, stand alongside the patient.
- Overlap your thumbs over the choice of carpal bone while wrapping your other digits around the hand towards the palm.
- Compress your thumbs inwards to localize the carpal bones you want to treat and introduce a 'figure of 8' movement to articulate the joints. This will possibly include degrees of all ranges of motion.

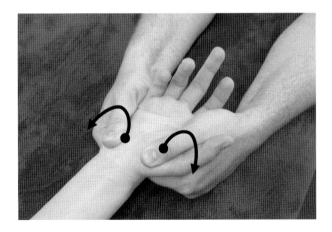

T12.12 Palmar retinaculum articulation

- With the patient supine, place their hand in a supinated and neutral position.
- While facing the patient's head, interlace the thumb of your outer hand between their first and second digits. Place the thumb of your inner hand along the outer palm of their hand.
- Introduce compression between your thumb and other digits on both hands while then supinating your hands to stretch the flexor retinaculum.

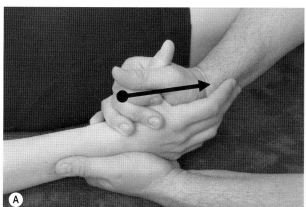

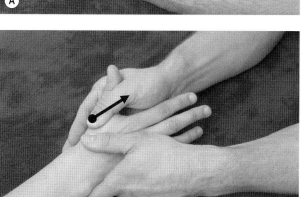

T12.13 Thumb articulation

- Stand alongside the supine patient.
- Using your outer hand, grip around the ulnar border of the patient's hand to stabilize the wrist and hand.
- With your inner hand, grip the base of the first phalangeal bone and introduce an anterior–posterior shear to the first metacarpophalangeal joint.
- Refer to photographs **a** and **b** for the different hand positions.

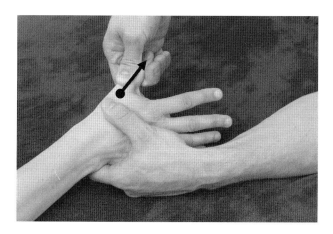

T12.14 Thumb traction

- Stand alongside the supine patient.
- Using your outer hand, grip your thumb around the dorsum of the hand and wrap your fingers into the palm, stabilizing the first metacarpal.
- With your inner hand, grip the base of the first phalangeal bone and introduce traction to the first metacarpophalangeal joint.

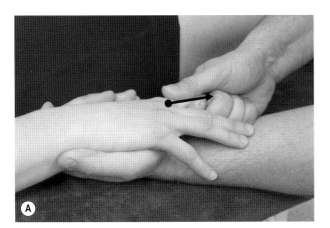

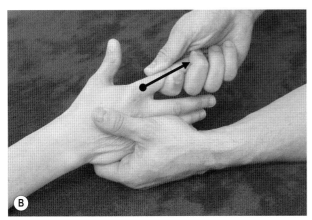

T12.15 Finger traction

- Stand alongside the supine patient, facing their head. Place the patient's wrist in a pronated position.
- Support the patient's palm by using your outer hand to stabilize the carpal rows and wrist.
- Using your inner hand, grip your thumb around the proximal phalanges and introduce traction to the metacarpophalangeal joints. This can be performed to all the digits.

REFERENCES

Abbas MA, Afifi AA, Zhang Z et al (1998). Meta-analysis of published studies of work-related carpal tunnel syndrome. International Journal of Occupational and Environmental Health 4:160-167.

Alfonso C, Jann S, Massa R et al (2010). Diagnosis, treatment and follow-up of the carpal tunnel syndrome: a review. Neurological Sciences 31(3):243-252.

Anderson D (2011). Mallet finger: management and patient compliance. Australian Family Physician 40(1/2):47.

Atroshi I, Gummesson C, Johnsson R et al (1999). Prevalence of carpal tunnel syndrome in a general population. Journal of the American Medical Association 282(2):153-158.

Barcenilla A, March LM, Chen JS et al (2012). Carpal tunnel syndrome and its relationship to occupation: a meta-analysis. Rheumatology 51(2):250-261.

Baxter RE (2003). Pocket Guide to Musculoskeletal Assessment. Philadelphia: WB Saunders.

Becker J, Nora DB, Gomes I et al (2002). An evaluation of gender, obesity, age and diabetes mellitus as risk factors for carpal tunnel syndrome. Clinical Neurophysiology 113(9):1429-1434.

Berger RA, Weiss APC eds (2003). Hand Surgery (Vol. 1). Philadelphia: Lippincott Williams & Wilkins.

Brigstocke G, Hearnden A, Holt CA et al (2013). The functional range of movement of the human wrist. Journal of Hand Surgery (European Volume) 38(5):554-556.

BSSH (2007). Hand Surgery in the UK: Manpower, resources, standards and training. London: British Society for Surgery of the Hand.

Burge P (1999). Genetics of Dupuytren's disease. Hand Clinics 15(1):63-71.

Burke J, Buchberger DJ, Carey-Loghmani MT et al (2007). A pilot study comparing two manual therapy interventions for carpal tunnel syndrome. Journal of Manipulative and Physiological Therapeutics 30(1):50-61.

Carlson H, Colbert A, Frydl J et al (2010). Current options for nonsurgical management of carpal tunnel syndrome. International Journal of Clinical Rheumatology 5(1):129-142.

Cherry NM, Meyer JD, Chen Y et al (2001). The reported incidence of work-related musculoskeletal disease in the UK: MOSS 1997–2000. Occupational Medicine 51(7):450-455.

Cooper G (2007). Pocket Guide to Musculoskeletal Diagnosis. New York: Springer Science+Business Media.

Dale AM, Harris-Adamson C, Rempel D et al (2013). Prevalence and incidence of carpal tunnel syndrome in US working populations: pooled analysis of six prospective studies. Scandinavian Journal of Work, Environment and Health 39(5):495.

Fisher TR (1984). The Hand. Examination and Diagnosis: American Society for Surgery of the Hand. Edinburgh: Churchill Livingstone.

Fisk GR (1970). Carpal instability and the fractured scaphoid. Annals of the Royal College of Surgeons of England 46(2):63-76.

Forman TA, Forman SK, Rose NE (2005). A clinical approach to diagnosing wrist pain. American Family Physician 72(9):1753-1758.

Geoghegan JM, Clark DI, Bainbridge LC et al (2004). Risk factors in carpal tunnel syndrome. The Journal of Hand Surgery (British and European Volume) 29(4):315-320.

Grundberg AB (1984). Ulnar tunnel syndrome. Journal of Hand Surgery (British and European Volume) 9(1):72-74.

Health & Safety Authority (2011). Summary of Workplace Injury, Illness and Fatality Statistics 2010–2011, pp. 1–40.

Heebner ML, Roddey TS (2008). The effects of neural mobilization in addition to standard care in persons with carpal tunnel syndrome from a community hospital. Journal of Hand Therapy 21(3):229-241.

Huisstede BM, Hoogvliet P, Randsdorp MS et al (2010). Carpal tunnel syndrome. Part I: Effectiveness of nonsurgical treatments – a systematic review. Archives of Physical Medicine and Rehabilitation 91(7):981-1004.

Hume MC, Gellman H, McKellop H et al (1990). Functional range of motion of the joints of the hand. The Journal of Hand Surgery 15(2): 240-243.

Hunter JM, Mackin EJ, Callahan AD (2002). Rehabilitation of the Hand and Upper Extremity, 5th ed. Maryland Heights, Mo: Mosby.

Katims JJ, Rouvelas P, Sadler B et al (1989). Current perception threshold: Reproducibility and comparison with nerve conduction in evaluation of carpal tunnel syndrome. Transactions of the American Society for Artificial Internal Organs 35:280-284.

Leslie IJ, Dickson RA (1981). The fractured carpal scaphoid. Natural history and factors influencing outcome. Journal of Bone and Joint Surgery (British Volume) 63(2):225-230.

Lynch JM (2004). Hand and wrist injuries: Part I. Nonemergent evaluation. American Family Physician 69(8)1941-1948.

McCann S, Wise E (2011). Kaplan Anatomy Coloring Book. Wokingham: Kaplan Publishing; 37-39.

McKeon JMM, Yancosek KE (2008). Neural gliding techniques for the treatment of carpal tunnel syndrome: a systematic review. Journal of Sport Rehabilitation 17(3):324-341.

McRae R (2010). Clinical Orthopaedic Examination, 6th ed. Edinburgh: Elsevier Health Sciences; 89-120.

Maghsoudipour M, Moghimi S, Dehghaan F et al (2008). Association of occupational and non-occupational risk factors with the prevalence of work related carpal tunnel syndrome. Journal of Occupational Rehabilitation 18(2):152-156.

Meems M, Den Oudsten B, Meems BJ et al (2014). Effectiveness of mechanical traction as a non-surgical treatment for carpal tunnel syndrome compared to care as usual: study protocol for a randomized controlled trial. Trials 15(1):180.

Mir MA (2003). Atlas of Clinical Diagnosis. Philadelphia: WB Saunders.

Nelson DL, Mitchell MA, Groszewski PG et al (1994). Wrist range of motion in activities of daily living. In: F. Schuind, KN An, WP Cooney III et al eds. Advances in the Biomechanics of the Hand and Wrist. New York: Springer; 329-334.

Newport ML (2000). Upper extremity disorders in women. Clinical Orthopaedics and Related Research 372:85-94.

O'Connor D, Page MJ, Marshall SC et al (2012). Ergonomic Positioning or Equipment for Treating Carpal Tunnel Syndrome. The Cochrane Library.

Ootes D, Lambers KT, Ring DC (2012). The epidemiology of upper extremity injuries presenting to the emergency department in the United States. Hand 7(1):18-22.

Page MJ, O'Connor D, Pitt V et al (2012). Exercise and Mobilisation Interventions for Carpal Tunnel Syndrome. The Cochrane Library.

Palmer AK, Werner FW, Murphy D et al (1985). Functional wrist motion: a biomechanical study. The Journal of Hand Surgery 10(1):39-46.

Palmer KT, Harris EC, Coggon D (2007). Carpal tunnel syndrome and its relation to occupation: a systematic literature review. Occupational Medicine 57:57-66.

Petre BM, Deune EG (2013). Anatomy of the Metacarpophalangeal and Interphalangeal Ligaments. Medscape.

Phillips TG, Reibach AM, Slomiany WP (2004). Diagnosis and management of scaphoid fractures. American Family Physician 70:879-892.

Platzer W (2004). Locomotor System. Color Atlas of Human Anatomy, Vol. 1. Stuttgart: Thieme.

Rabin A, Israeli T, Kozol Z (2015). Physiotherapy management of people diagnosed with de Quervain's disease: a case series. Physiotherapy Canada 67(3):263-267.

Rhee T, Neumann U, Lewis JP (2006). Human hand modeling from surface anatomy. In: Proceedings of the 2006 Symposium on Interactive 3D Graphics and Games. ACM; 27-34.

Ryu J, Cooney WP, Askew LJ et al (1991). Functional ranges of motion of the wrist joint. The Journal of Hand Surgery 16(3):409-419.

Silverstein BA, Fine LJ, Armstrong TJ (1987). Occupational factors and carpal tunnel syndrome. American Journal of Industrial Medicine 11(3):343-358.

Taylor CL, Schwarz RJ (1955). The anatomy and mechanics of the human hand. Artificial Limbs 2(2):22-35.

Van Tulder M, Malmivaara A, Koes B (2007). Repetitive strain injury. Lancet 369(9575):1815-1822.

Villafañe JH, Silva GB, Chiarotto A (2013). Effects of passive upper extremity joint mobilization on pain sensitivity and function in participants with secondary carpometacarpal osteoarthritis. Journal of Manipulative and Physiological Therapeutics 35(9):735-742.

Virginia C (1999). Bones and Muscles: An Illustrated Anatomy. New York: Wolf Fly Press; 84-86.

Walker-Bone K, Palmer KT, Reading I et al (2004). Prevalence and impact of musculoskeletal disorders of the upper limb in the general population. Arthritis Care and Research 51(4):642-651.

Wang QC, Johnson BA (2001). Fingertip injuries. American Family Physician 63(10):1961.

Weinzweig N, Gonzalez M (2002). Surgical infections of the hand and upper extremity: a county hospital experience. Annals of Plastic Surgery 49(6):621-627.

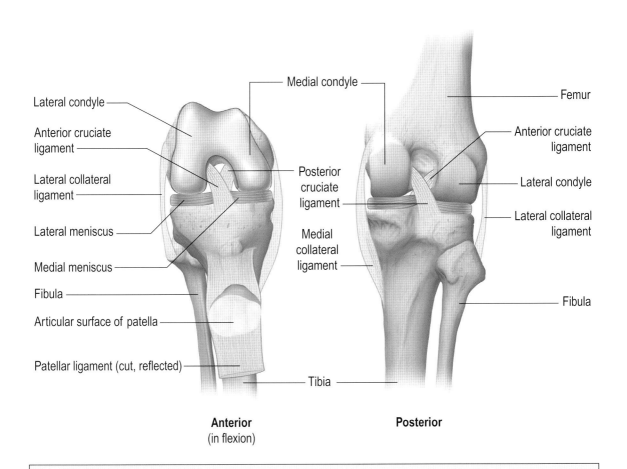

Lateral condyle

Anterior cruciate
ligament

Lateral collateral
ligament

Lateral meniscus

Medial meniscus

Fibula

Articular surface of patella

Patellar ligament (cut, reflected)

Medial condyle

Posterior
cruciate
ligament

Medial
collateral
ligament

Tibia

Anterior
(in flexion)

Femur

Anterior cruciate
ligament

Lateral condyle

Lateral collateral
ligament

Fibula

Posterior

Figure 13.1
The knee: posterior and anterior views

Introduction

The knee is the most common joint to develop osteo-arthritic changes globally, and it is reported in over 9 million people in the United States alone (Helmick et al 2008, Lawrence et al 2008). It is also the most reported joint for disability and symptoms (Corti & Rigon 2003, De Filippis et al 2004, Arden & Nevitt 2006). Osteoarthritic changes within the knee can be observed in approximately 70% of symptomatic individuals and approximately 40% of asymptomatic individuals aged 40 or over (Du et al 2005, Englund et al 2008).

Knee surgery, particularly arthroscopy, has been increasingly used over the past decade (Kim et al 2011, Bohensky et al 2012, Harris et al 2013, Thorlund et al 2014), although some would question the long-term benefits of this procedure (Katz et al 2013, Yim et al, 2013). There have always been protocols with regard to postoperative care for individuals following knee surgery, but there is growing evidence for both short- and long-term benefits from preoperative care (Ackerman & Bennell 2004, Wallis & Taylor 2011, Hoogeboom et al 2012), exercise-based or manual therapy. In the first stage of postoperative rehabilitation (2–3 weeks) following knee arthroscopy, it is recommended that articulation of the joint is performed to help aid the range of movement and fluid dynamics of the knee (UW Health 2011). Grella (2013) also suggests that early articulation of the joint is more beneficial than continuous passive motion of the knee following surgery.

Osteoarthritis: National Clinical Guideline for Care and Management in Adults (NICE 2008) recommends articulation as a core component of treatment of knee arthritis. Moss et al (2007) established that articulation of degenerative knees caused a neurological hypoalgesic effect in local and distal tissues. Sluka and colleagues (2006) discovered similar reductions in pain thresholds with the rhythmical articulation of chronically inflamed rat knee joints. It was also found that the decrease in pain threshold caused was bilateral, thus suggesting the involvement of a central neurological component. Pollard et al (2008) found that a short-term course of manual therapy to arthritic knees reduced reported pain symptoms.

Manual therapy combined with exercise can reduce the need for surgical intervention with arthroplasty and intra-articular injections (Deyle et al 2000). Fransen et al (2001) found that manual therapy of the knee caused not only a decrease in reported pain levels but also an increase in quality of life. In their trial, Crossley et al (2002) found that a course of 6 weeks of manual therapy and prescribed exercises decreased the perceived pain, disability and impairment of patients who suffered with patella–femoral pain. These findings are also reflected in studies by Taylor and Brantingham (2003), Stakes et al (2006) and Collins et al (2012).

Anatomy

The largest and most complex joint in the human body, the knee comprises bones, cartilage, ligaments and tendons. The knee joint connects the upper and lower leg bones, and is the anatomical region where four bones – the femur, tibia, fibula and patella – meet. Apart from the fibula, all these bones are functional in the knee joint (Kishner et al 2015).

The knee is a synovial (modified hinge) joint, consisting of three distinct and partially separated compartments. The main knee joints, known as the tibiofemoral joints, have a medial and a lateral compartment. These joints are formed between the medial and lateral condyles of the femur (thigh bone) and the medial and lateral condyles of the tibia (shin bone). Two wedge-shaped articular discs (the medial meniscus and lateral meniscus) provide padding and support between the femoral condyles and tibial condyles. The third knee joint, called the femoropatellar joint, is found between the kneecap (patella) and the distal femur. All of these joints are surrounded by a single articular capsule and the ligaments strap the inside and outside of these articulations (Tate 2009).

The knee is well constructed for transmitting the body weight in vertical and horizontal directions. It ensures weight-bearing support by allowing flexion and extension of the leg. It also allows a small amount of internal and external rotation when the knee is flexed, but not when it is extended. The stability and normal movements at the knee are essential in performing many daily activities, such as walking, running, kicking, sitting and standing (Mader 2004).

Bony anatomy

Femur

The femur is an important component of the appendicular skeleton and is the longest and strongest bone in the human body. The mean ratio of femur length to stature is 26.74%, with a very limited variation in both men and women and most ethnic groups (Feldesman et al 1990).

The femur is located in the thigh, extending from the hip to the knee. The proximal end of the femur has a smooth, spherical process called the femur head, which articulates with the acetabulum. The distal end of the femur has a double condyle that articulates with the proximal condyles of the tibia. The femurs support the weight of the body during many everyday activities, including walking, running, jumping and standing (OpenStax 2013).

Tibia

The tibia, also known as the shin bone, is the medial bone of the leg. It is located medial to the fibula and distal to the femur. It is the longest bone of the body after the femur and is larger and stronger than the fibula. It makes up the knee joint, articulating with the medial and lateral condyles of the femur; it forms the ankle joint, joining with the fibula and tarsus. The tibia articulates with the fibula by an interosseous membrane, forming a joint known as the syndesmosis joint (Standring 2008).

The tibia is the main bone of the lower leg that carries the weight of the body. The movement of the tibia is vital in executing numerous activities of the legs, such as running, walking and jumping.

Fibula

Also called the calf bone, the fibula is the slenderest of all the long bones. It runs parallel to the tibia and is found on the lateral side of the leg. It is connected to the tibia from above and below. It is smaller than the tibia and considerably thinner. The fibula has no articulation with the femur and patella (Mader 2004).

The fibula bears little or no weight of the body. It is largely surrounded by muscles and serves primarily for muscle attachment. It plays a major role in stabilizing the ankle and functions as a support for the tibia.

Patella

The patella, also known as the kneecap, is a large sesamoid bone. Although its shape may vary slightly from person to person, it is usually a flat triangular-shaped bone, with the apex facing downwards. The posterior region of the patella is connected with the femur; the base is attached to the tendon of the quadriceps extensor muscle, the large muscle group that covers the front and sides of the thigh. The patella has no articulation with the tibia. Functionally, it serves to protect the front of the knee joint (OpenStax 2013).

Ligaments

The knee joint has multiple ligaments that hold together the knee bones, protect the articular capsule and stabilize the joint. These ligaments are divided into two types: the extracapsular and

Movement type	Range of motion(°)
Flexion	120–150
Extension	5–10
Lateral (external) rotation (knee flexed 90°)	30–40
Medial (internal) rotation (knee flexed 90°)	10

Table 13.1
Normal range of motion of the knee
Data from Schünke et al (2006)

Age (years)	Movement type	Range of motion (°)		
		Males	Females	
2–8	Flexion	147.8 (146.6–149.0)	152.6 (151.2–154.0)	
	Extension	1.6 (0.9–2.3)	5.4 (3.9–6.9)	
9–19	Flexion	142.2 (140.4–144.0)	142.3 (140.8–143.8)	
	Extension	1.8 (0.9–2.7)	2.4 (1.5–3.3)	
20–44	Flexion	137.7 (136.5–138.9)	141.9 (140.9–142.9)	
	Extension	1.0 (0.6–1.4)	1.6 (1.1–2.1)	
45–69	Flexion	132.9 (131.6–134.2)	137.8 (136.5–139.1)	
	Extension	0.5 (0.1–0.9)	1.2 (0.7–1.7)	

Table 13.2
Reference values for normal knee range of motion
Data from Soucie et al (2011)

Movement type	Range of motion (°)		
	Visual estimation	Hand goniometry	Radiographic goniometry
Flexion	146	138	144
Extension	−3.5	−6.3	−4.2

Table 13.3
Comparison of three measurement methods of the knee for flexion and extension

the intracapsular ligaments. The extracapsular ligaments are found on the inner and outer sides of the knee joint. These ligaments include the fibular (lateral) collateral ligament, tibial (medial) collateral ligament, arcuate popliteal ligament, and oblique popliteal ligament. The intracapsular ligaments are located on the central part of the knee joint. They include the anterior cruciate ligament, posterior cruciate ligament and posterior meniscofemoral ligament (Kishner et al 2015).

Four of the knee ligaments – the lateral and medial collateral ligaments and the anterior and posterior cruciate ligaments – primarily serve to maintain the knee joint stability, restricting abnormal or excessive movements. The lateral and medial collateral ligaments prevent the femur from sliding side to side on the tibia. The anterior and posterior cruciate ligaments form an x-shape when they pass each other (hence their names) and prevent the femur from tipping backward and forward on the tibia (OpenStax 2013).

Range of motion

The knee joint allows flexion and extension, with slight internal and external rotation about the axis of the lower leg in the flexed position (see Table 13.1). Typical ranges of flexion and extension vary with age (see Table 13.2). The range of motion of the knee is typically measured using a hand goniometer but visual estimation and radiographic goniometry may also be used (see comparisons in Table 13.3).

Epidemiology

Knee pain

Knee pain is a very common condition and one that many people experience at some stage in their lives. It affects very large numbers of people indiscriminately across the world, and causes substantial social burden and persistent impairment of physical function.

Knee pain is common in all populations, including the very young and old, men and women, and athletes of

Condition	Description	Reference
Knee osteoarthritis	Represents a major cause of disability, functional limitation, morbidity, social isolation and reduced quality of life Extremely common in elderly people Prevalence rate: 14–34% (among people aged 45+ years) Symptoms include pain, impaired function, grating or grinding sensation, stiffness in the morning, and soft or hard swellings Risk factors include overweight, over 50 years of age, female sex, overwork, previous knee injury and family history of osteoarthritis	Dawson et al (2004), McRae (2010)
Patellar chondromalacia	The most common cause of runner's knee pain Characterized by softening or fibrillation of the patellar articular cartilage Occurs because of the repeated microtrauma or malalignment of the patella Commonest in females of 15–35 years age group Causes include a mechanical problem at the foot, tibia or hip, asynchronous muscle firing, connective tissue tightness and muscle tightness or weakness	Hartley (1995)
Osteochondritis dissecans	A common idiopathic condition that affects the articular cartilage and subchondral bone Occurs most commonly in men in the 2nd decade of life Male-to-female ratio: 2–3:1 Can affect both younger children and adults Causes 50% of loose bodies in the knee Affects the medial femoral condyle in 85% of cases	Jacobs (1992), Flynn et al (2004), McRae (2010)
Patellar tendonitis	An inflammation of the patellar tendon at the inferior patellar region or at the insertion of the quadriceps tendon at the base of the patella Occurs most commonly in teenage boys, particularly in athletes who actively participate in jumping sports Often associated with excessive foot pronation, patellar malalignment or patella alta Symptoms include anterior knee pain and localized swelling, thickening or nodules	Hartley (1995), Calmbach & Hutchens (2003b)
Iliotibial band syndrome	A common cause of lateral knee pain Occurs most frequently in people who are involved in repetitive knee flexion, such as cycling and running Often caused by friction between the iliotibial band and the lateral femoral epicondyle during flexion and extension of the knee Responsible for 12% of all running-related overuse injuries Risk factors include overpronation, genu varum, length discrepancy of the limb and myofascial restriction	Hartley (1995), Lavine (2010)

Table 13.4
Common disorders of the knee

numerous sports. In the UK general population aged 16+ years, the prevalence of knee pain (lasting for more than a week in the past month) was reported as 19% in 4515 respondents (Webb et al 2004). The same survey reported that the prevalence in participants over 45 years of age was slightly higher in females than in males and that, in people aged 75+ years, the prevalence in females was 36% while in males it was 27%. In pre-adolescent schoolchildren of 8–13 years of age, the prevalence of knee pain (occurring at least once a week) was 12% in 1756 participants (El-Metwally et al 2006).

The prevalence of knee pain increases with age in both men and women; thus, knee pain is a common complaint in the elderly. Over the past few decades, a number of studies have estimated the prevalence rate of knee pain in the elderly. In a narrative review, Peat et al (2001) suggested that rates in the UK were between 13% and 28%, with the variation being clarified by differences in study group design, survey methods, case definitions and the inclusion of questions. Furthermore, a recent community survey (with 6792 respondents) in the UK general population reported that 46.8% of people aged 50+ years had complained of knee pain in the last 12 months; of these, 33% consulted their GP (Jinks et al 2004). Although there are several theories regarding the etiology of osteoarthritis in the knee, it is known that there is a higher incidence in women than men (Lachance et al 2002). There is also a higher incidence of the development and progression of osteoarthritis in the knee associated with obesity and an increase in the need for total knee replacements (Messier et al 2000, Christensen et al 2005).

Synovial folds within the knee (called plicae or synovial plicae) can sometimes be symptomatic. These are caused by embryonic folds that separate the knee into compartments that normally disappear after birth, but occasionally they remain and will not be noticed until an arthroscopy is performed on the knee (Boles & Martin 2001, Kim et al 2006, Nakayama et al 2011). Occasionally, a plica may become aggravated, thickened and inflamed, normally associated with repetitive movement and strain (Duri et al 2002, Cothran et al 2003, Christoforakis et al 2006), and develop into 'plica syndrome' (Dupont 1997, Schindler 2004,

Demirag et al 2006). Plica is not generally listed as a common condition that affects the knee because it can be very difficult to clinically differentially diagnose it from other intra-articular conditions, such as damage to the articular cartilage or meniscus or osteochondritic changes to the knee (Fulkerson et al 2004, Christoforakis et al 2006, Kent & Khanduja 2010). In addition, although manual therapy can be effective in treating the symptoms of plica, in most circumstances the best treatment for knee plica is arthroscopy (Williams et al 2012, Schindler 2014, Vassiou et al 2015). Table 13.4 lists some common disorders of the knee.

Knee injuries

In athletes of various sports, the knee joint is the most common part of the body to be injured. According to a US epidemiological review, the incidence of knee injuries in patients presenting to the emergency departments was 2.29 per 1000 people (Gage et al 2012). Among all knee injuries, ligament injuries and meniscal tears are the most common, and they account for about 40% and 11% of all knee injuries, respectively (Nicholl et al 1991). Of the ligaments of the knee, the anterior cruciate and medial collateral ligaments are the most frequently injured, accounting for about 49% and 29% of all ligament injuries, respectively (Miyasaka et al 1991). The patellofemoral joint is also vulnerable and it can account for 25–40% of knee symptoms in active individuals (Boling et al 2010, Lankhorst et al 2012).

Knee examination

Medical history

A detailed medical history of the patient should be taken to help identify the red flags, characterize the severity of the pain, and facilitate the physical examination. The examiner should ask the patient presenting with knee pathology whether there is a history of trauma. If there is, the patient should be asked to discuss the history of the pain or injury (e.g. severity and type of pain, behavior since onset, history of swelling, duration of symptoms, and exacerbating and relieving factors).

If there is no history of trauma, other possible causes and risk factors should be taken into consideration, such as the patient's age, sex, weight and level of physical activity. Apart from questioning about pain, history of trauma or other issues related to the knee, the examiner should also find out whether the knee gives way or locks. If any of these symptoms is present in the patient, it indicates a possible meniscus injury.

Red flags

Table 13.5 summarizes red flag conditions of the knee.

Physical examination

The physical examination of the knee is considered crucial from several aspects: it helps confirm initial findings, fully explore the nature and extent of the problem, and make judgments. A general evaluation of the knee involves inspection, palpation, range of motion and a variety of special tests.

Inspection

A careful visual inspection of the patient's knee should be performed to compare the affected knee with the asymptomatic knee, and identify redness, swelling, bruising, deformity or skin changes. The examiner should start by observing movements of the knee during rising from a chair and standing, walking and in a sitting position. Any abnormalities observed, such as unusual ligamentary laxity, genu recurvatum, genu

Condition	Signs and symptoms
Knee fractures	History of recent trauma such as a knee injury or a fall from height
	Pain, bruising or swelling on the affected leg
	Numbness, tingling, or a pins-and-needles sensation
	Difficulty in bending the knee
	Inability to walk or bear weight on the involved leg
Compartment syndrome	History of trauma
	Severe, persistent pain and hardness to anterior compartment of shin
	Pain intensified with stretch applied to affected muscles
Extensor mechanism disruption	Ruptured quadriceps or patella tendon
	Altered position of the patella (superior translation)
Septic arthritis	Fever, chills
	Recent bacterial infection, surgery or injection
	Severe, constant pain
	Systemically unwell such as unusual fatigue (malaise) or loss of appetite
	Coexisting immunosuppressive disorder
	Red, swollen joint with no history of trauma
Cancer	Unremitting pain
	Previous history of cancer
	Atypical symptoms with no history of a trauma
	Systemic symptoms such as fever, chills, malaise and weakness
	Unexplained weight loss
	Suspected malignancy or unexplained deformity, mass or swelling

Table 13.5
Red flags for serious pathology in the knee region
Data from McGee & Boyko (1998), Gupta et al (2001), Ulmer (2002), Leeds Community Healthcare (2012)

varus, genu valgum and flexion deformity, should be noted immediately.

Palpation

While examining the knee, several important bony and soft-tissue structures should be palpated to determine areas of pathology. The examiner should palpate the patient's knee to check the warmth and effusion, assess muscle tone, determine the punctum maximum of pain, and qualify swelling. Point tenderness of anatomical structures should also be assessed, especially at the patella, epicondyles, joint lines, tibial tubercle, Gerdy's tubercle, quadriceps tendon, patellar tendon and proximal fibula.

Range of motion

Movements of the knee should be assessed to check the pain at movement, smoothness of motion, incidence of crepitus, and lateralization of the patella. The patient should be asked to flex and extend the knee as far as possible. The examiner may use a hand goniometer, visual estimation or radiographic goniometry to assess the range of motion. After measuring the range of motion of the knee, the examiner should compare the collected data with reliable standards (see Tables 13.1 and 13.2).

Special tests

A number of special tests can be included in the knee examination (Table 13.6).

Test	Procedure	Positive sign	Interpretation
Lachman's test	The patient lies supine and the injured knee is flexed 20–30°. The examiner stabilizes the distal femur with one hand and holds the proximal tibia with the other hand. The examiner then applies a gentle anterior force to pull up on the tibia anteriorly.	Excessive displacement of the tibia compared with the uninvolved knee	Compromised anterior cruciate ligament
Posterior drawer test	The patient lies supine with the hip flexed 45°, the knee flexed 90° and the tibia in neutral rotation. The examiner stabilizes the patient's foot and pushes posteriorly on the tibia.	Posterior displacement of the tibia with respect to the femur	Compromised posterior cruciate ligament
Valgus stress test	The patient lies in supine position. The examiner holds the lateral aspect of the knee joint with one hand and places the other hand on the medial aspect of the distal tibia. Next, the examiner gently applies valgus stress on the knee at both 0° (full extension) and 30° of flexion.	Laxity of the medial collateral ligament on valgus stress	Compromised posterior cruciate ligament in addition to medial collateral ligament
Varus stress test	The patient lies in supine position. The examiner holds the medial aspect of the knee with one hand and places the other hand on the lateral aspect of the distal fibula. Next, the examiner gently applies varus stress on the knee, first at 0° (full extension) and then at 30° of flexion.	Laxity of the lateral collateral ligament on varus stress	Torn lateral collateral ligament, also indicates torn posterior cruciate ligament

(Continued)

Test	Procedure	Positive sign	Interpretation
McMurray's test	The patient is in supine position. The examiner grasps the patient's heel with one hand and places the other hand on the knee, palpating the joint line (medial and lateral). To test the lateral meniscus, the examiner rotates the tibia internally and extends the knee from full flexion to 90°. A valgus stress is applied across the knee joint while the knee is being extended. To test the lateral meniscus, the examiner rotates the tibia externally and extends the knee from full flexion to 90°. A varus stress is applied across the knee joint while the examiner extends the knee.	Palpable click or pop and pain along joint line	Posterior meniscal tears
Apprehension test	The patient is in a sitting position with the knees fully extended. The examiner then applies medial and lateral force to the patella.	Patient reports a feeling of patella dislocation and shows apprehension	Patellar subluxation or hypermobility

Table 13.6

Special tests for knee examination

Data from Hartley (1995), Baxter (2003), Calmbach & Hutchens (2003a), Boonen et al (2015)

Knee muscles

Name	Origin	Insertion	Action	Nerve supply
Sartorius	Anterior superior iliac spine	Superior medial surface of tibia (pes anserinus conjoined tendon of sartorius, gracilis and semitendinosus)	Flexion, abduction and laterally (externally) rotates the thigh	Femoral nerve (L2–L3)
Rectus femoris	Anterior head: anterior inferior iliac spine Posterior head: ilium superior to acetabulum	Quadriceps tendon to patella, via ligamentum patellae onto tubercle of tibia	Extension of the knee and flexion of the hip	Femoral nerve (L2–L4)
Vastus lateralis	Lateral lip of linea aspera, intertrochanteric line, and inferior portion of greater trochanter	Quadriceps tendon to patella, via ligamentum patellae onto tubercle of tibia	Extension of the knee	Femoral nerve (L2–L4)
Vastus intermedius	Upper two-thirds of anterior and lateral surface of femur, linea aspera and lateral supracondylar line	Quadriceps tendon to patella, via ligamentum patellae onto tubercle of tibia	Extension of the knee	Femoral nerve (L2–L4)
Vastus medialis	Medial lip of linea aspera, intertrochanteric line and medial supracondylar line	Quadriceps tendon to patella, via ligamentum patellae onto tubercle of tibia	Extension of the knee	Femoral nerve (L2–L4)
Articularis genus	Distal anterior surface of femur	Superior surface of knee capsule	Lifting the suprapatellar bursa during extension of the knee	Femoral nerve (L2–L4)
Gracilis	Ischiopubic ramus	Superior medial surface of tibia (pes anserinus conjoined tendon of sartorius, gracilis and semitendinosus)	Flexion, medially (internally) rotates, and adduction of the thigh	Obturator nerve (L3–L4)
Semimembranosus	Tuberosity of ischium	Medial condyle of tibia	Flexion of the knee and extension of the hip	Tibial portion of sciatic nerve (L5–S2)

(Continued)

Name	Origin	Insertion	Action	Nerve supply
Semitendinosus	Tuberosity of ischium	Superior medial surface of tibia (pes anserinus conjoined tendon of sartorius, gracilis and semitendinosus)	Flexion of the knee and extension of the hip	Tibial portion of sciatic nerve (L5–S2)
Biceps femoris	Long head: ischial tuberosity and sacrotuberous ligament Short head: linea aspera and lateral supracondylar ridge	Lateral (external) portion of fibular head and lateral condyle of tibia	Flexion of the knee and long head assists in extension of the thigh	Long head: tibial portion of sciatic nerve (S1–S3) Short head: common peroneal (fibular) portion of sciatic nerve (L5–S2)
Gastrocnemius	Medial head: popliteal portion of femur and superior angle of medial condyle Lateral head: lateral condyle	Posterior surface of calcaneus via the tendocalcaneus (Achilles) tendon	Plantar flexion of the foot and flexion of the knee	Tibial nerve (S1–S2)
Soleus	Posterior surface of fibula, fibular head and tibia (soleal line)	Posterior surface of calcaneus via the tendocalcaneus (Achilles) tendon	Plantar flexion of the foot	Tibial nerve (S1–S2)
Plantaris	Oblique (popliteal) ligament, lower portion of lateral supracondylar ridge	Posterior surface of calcaneus via the tendocalcaneus (Achilles) tendon	Plantar flexion of the foot and flexion of the knee	Tibial nerve (S1–S2)
Popliteus	Lateral meniscus and lateral surface of lateral condyle of femur	Upper posterior surface of tibia and superior to soleal line	Unlocks the fully extended knee (by medially rotating the lower leg) and weak flexor	Tibial nerve (S1–S2)

Table 13.7
Knee muscles

Techniques: knee

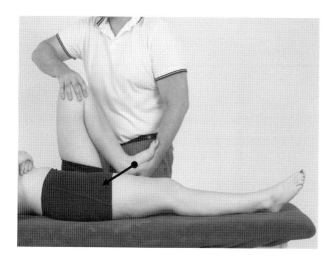

T13.1 Supine flexion of the knee joint

- The patient is positioned on their back, slightly to one side of the plinth.
- Your body is positioned on the side to be examined and your feet are facing the direction of the patient's head.
- Flex their hip and knee to 90°.
- Place your body alongside the patient's outer thigh to support the area.
- Place the hand furthest away from the plinth on the top of the patient's knee and palpate the joint line.
- Your opposite hand is cupping the patient's heel and your forearm is supporting their foot.
- Gently push the patient's foot towards their buttock while keeping the hip at a 90° angle.
- Knee flexion is approximately 130–150°.

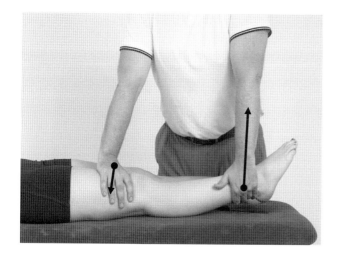

T13.2 Supine extension of the knee joint

- The patient is positioned on their back, slightly to one side of the plinth, with their leg lying flat.
- Your body is positioned on the side to be examined and your feet are facing the direction of the patient's head.
- Place the hand furthest away from the plinth just above the patient's kneecap region to stabilize the knee.
- Your opposite hand is placed behind the patient's ankle region.
- Keeping both arms straight, gently rock your body towards the patient's head. This will cause the patient's foot to be raised off the plinth while your other hand is stabilizing the thigh against the plinth, resulting in extension of the knee.
- Knee extension is approximately 0–5°.

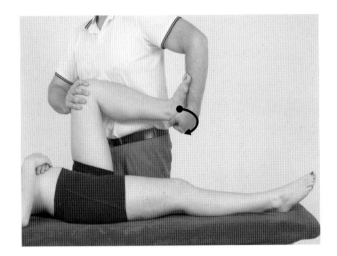

T13.3 Supine medial (internal) rotation of the knee joint

- The patient is positioned on their back, slightly to one side of the plinth.
- Your body is positioned on the side to be examined and your feet are facing the direction of the patient's head.
- Flex their hip and knee to 90° angles. Place your body alongside the patient's outer thigh to support the area.
- Place the hand furthest away from the plinth on the top of the patient's knee and palpate the joint line, feeling for the tibial rotation.
- The hand closest to the plinth is cupping the patient's ankle, while your forearm is supporting the foot and maintaining dorsiflexion.
- By rotating your shoulder forward, the hand closest to the plinth then rotates the ankle towards the patient's opposite leg.
- Medial rotation of the knee is approximately 5°.

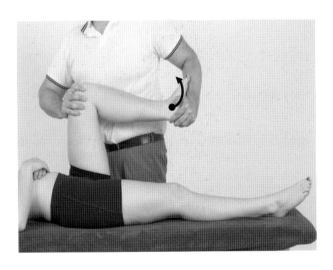

T13.4 Supine lateral (external) rotation of the knee joint

- The patient is positioned on their back, slightly to one side of the plinth.
- Your body is positioned on the side to be examined and your feet are facing the direction of the patient's head.
- Flex their hip and knee to 90° angles.
- Place your body alongside the patient's outer thigh to support the area.
- Place the hand furthest away from the plinth on the top of the patient's knee and palpate the joint line, feeling for the tibial rotation.
- The hand closest to the plinth is cupping the patient's ankle, while your forearm is supporting the foot and maintaining dorsiflexion.
- By rotating your shoulder backward, the hand closest to the plinth then rotates the ankle away from the patient's body.
- Lateral rotation of the knee is approximately 5°.

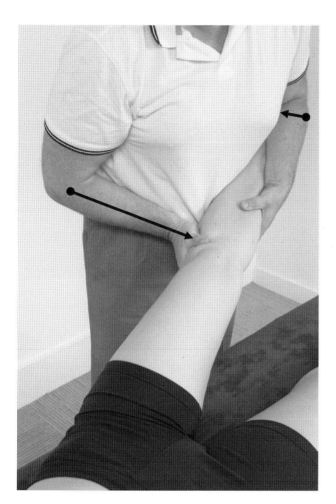

T13.5 Supine medial (internal) gapping of the knee joint

- The patient is positioned on their back, slightly to one side of the plinth, with their leg lying flat.

- Your body is positioned on the side to be examined. Your feet are in a split stance and are facing the patient's opposite shoulder and your upper body is facing the patient's leg.

- Pick up the patient's leg and place it into the side of your body.

- Your hand and forearm closest to the plinth are placed alongside the medial part of the patient's lower leg for support.

- Place the thumb of your other hand below the patient's patella and lightly over the joint line, with your index finger firmly placed along the joint line.

- Compress the leg between your hands and introduce a small degree of flexion into the knee – approximately 5–20° as extension will lock the knee.

- Now rotate your body from your feet towards the patient. This will cause medial gapping of the knee joint.

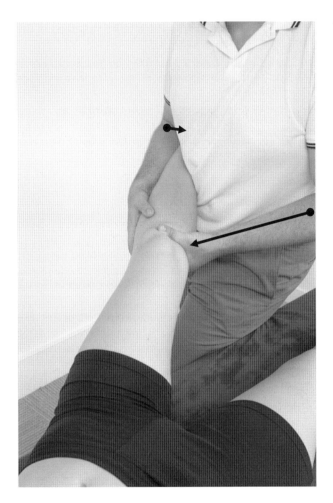

T13.6 Supine lateral (external) gapping of the knee joint

- Work from the medial gapping position.
- Flex the patient's knee and position your body between the plinth and the medial aspect of the knee. (For modesty purposes, bring patient's other leg slightly more into the midline of the plinth.) Now straighten the patient's leg.
- Keep your feet in a split stance, pointing slightly away from the patient towards their head.
- Place your hand and forearm furthest from the plinth alongside the lateral part of the patient's lower leg for support.
- With your other hand, place your thumb below the patella and lightly over the joint line, and your index finger firmly along the joint line.
- Introduce a small degree of flexion into the knee – approximately 5–20° as extension will lock the knee.
- Now rotate your body from your feet, away from the patient. This will cause lateral gapping of the knee joint.

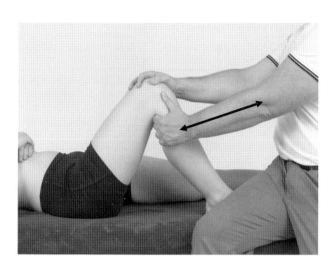

T13.7 Supine examination of the superior tibiofibular joint

- The patient is positioned on their back, slightly to one side of the plinth.
- The patient's knee is raised and flexed, and their foot is placed flat on the plinth, at roughly 90°. Gently sit on the patient's toes.
- The hand closest to the plinth is placed on the top of the patient's knee to stabilize the joint.
- Use your outer hand to palpate the outer part of the top of the patient's calf and gently move the muscles away from the fibula.
- With your outer hand, grip the fibula between your thumb, index and other fingers, keeping your arm straight, and lean slightly out from the plinth and away from the patient. This produces anterior lateral movement of the fibular head.
- Using the same grip, push the fibula towards the patient and slightly towards their opposite shoulder, causing posterior medial movement of the fibular head.

T13.8 Anterior draw test

- The patient is positioned on their back, slightly to one side of the plinth.
- The patient's knee is flexed to approximately 90° and their foot is placed flat on the plinth.
- Gently sit on the patient's toes.
- Place your hands either side of the patient's knee with your fingers cupping the posterior leg below the knee.
- Place your thumbs and thenar eminences on the front of the knee, either side of the tibial tuberosity.
- Gently pull away from the patient, causing anterior movement of the tibia to assess the anterior cruciate ligament.
- The test is positive if there is excessive anterior movement of the tibia or a soft end feel.

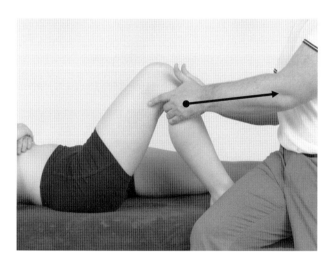

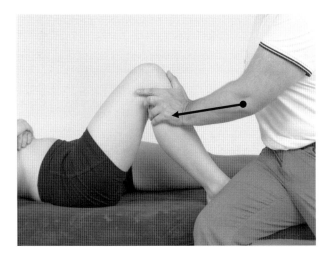

T13.9 Posterior draw test

- The patient is positioned on their back, slightly to one side of the plinth.
- The patient's knee is flexed to approximately 90° and their foot is placed flat on the plinth.
- Gently sit on the patient's toes.
- Place your hands either side of the patient's knee with your fingers cupping the posterior leg below the knee.
- Place your thumbs and thenar eminences on the front of the knee, either side of the tibial tuberosity.
- Gently push forwards towards the patient and table, causing posterior movement of the tibia assessing the posterior cruciate ligament.
- The test is positive if there is excessive posterior movement of the tibia or a soft end feel.

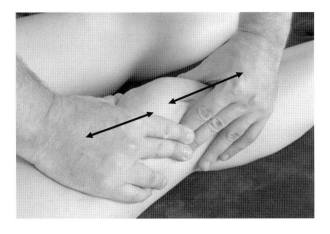

T13.10 Superior and inferior patella tracking

- The patient is positioned on their back in the middle of the plinth with their leg lying flat.
- Your body is positioned opposite the side to be examined and is facing across the plinth.
- Place the thumb and index finger of your hand closest to the patient's feet on the inferior borders of the patella.
- Place the thumb and index finger of your other hand on the superior borders of the patella.
- With both hands simultaneously, push the patellar superiorly towards the patient's head and then inferiorly towards their feet.
- The movements felt should be smooth and even.

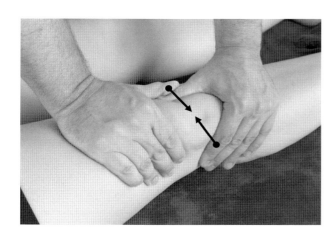

T13.11 Medial (internal) and lateral (external) patellar tracking

- The patient is positioned on their back in the middle of the plinth with their leg lying flat.
- Your body is positioned opposite the side to be examined and is facing across the plinth.
- Place the thumb and index finger of your hand closest to the patient's feet on the inferior borders of the patella.
- Place the thumb and index finger of your other hand on the superior borders of the patella.
- With both hands simultaneously, push the patella laterally away from the patient's knee and medially towards the opposite knee.
- The movements felt should be smooth and even.

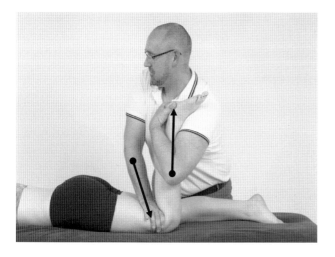

T13.12 Prone traction of the knee joint

- The patient is in the prone position, with the plinth set to a low height.
- Stand on the opposite side from the knee you are treating with your knees slightly flexed.
- Flex the patient's knee to 90°.
- Fix your hand furthest away from the plinth on the distal part of the patient's thigh, towards the crease of the knee.
- Cradle and compress the lower leg between your bicep and shoulder while cupping the heel of the patient's foot with your palm.
- Straighten your legs to standing up while keeping your hand fixed behind the knee crease.

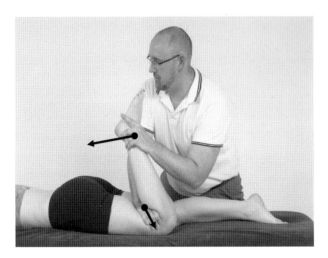

T13.13 Articulation of the superior tibiofibular joint 1

- The patient is in the prone position.
- Stand on the opposite side from the knee you are treating.
- Flex the knee to 90°.
- Fix your hand furthest away from the plinth on the distal part of the patient's thigh, towards the crease of the knee.
- Your other hand grips the front of their ankle.
- Maintain the fixing of your hand on the patient's thigh and knee crease, using this as a fulcrum to the knee.
- Use your other hand to flex the lower leg towards the patient's buttocks in an arching motion.

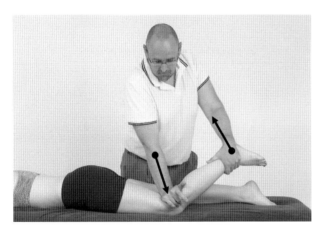

T13.14 Articulation of the superior tibiofibular joint 2

- With one hand gripping around the patient's ankle, use your other hand to compress behind the fibular head on the posterior surface.
- Note: be careful not to compress on the common fibular (peroneal) nerve as it passes the fibular head. If you do, simply adjust where you are compressing to release the nerve.
- As you lift the patient's ankle, thus flexing the knee, compress through your other hand in an oblique direction to articulate the superior tibiofibular joint.
- In addition, to target the joint line more effectively, slightly medially rotate the lower leg while flexing the knee.

REFERENCES

Ackerman IN, Bennell KL (2004). Does pre-operative physiotherapy improve outcomes from lower limb joint replacement surgery? A systematic review. Australian Journal of Physiotherapy 50(1):25-30.

Arden N, Nevitt MC (2006). Osteoarthritis: epidemiology. Best Practice and Research. Clinical Rheumatology 20(1):3-25.

Baxter RE (2003). Pocket Guide to Musculoskeletal Assessment. Philadelphia: WB Saunders; 110-114.

Bohensky MA, Sundararajan V, Andrianopoulos N et al (2012). Trends in elective knee arthroscopies in a population-based cohort, 2000–2009. The Medical Journal of Australia 197:399-403.

Boles CA, Martin DF (2001). Synovial plicae in the knee. American Journal of Roentgenology 177(1):221-227.

Boling M, Padua D, Marshall S et al (2010). Gender differences in the incidence and prevalence of patellofemoral pain syndrome. Scandinavian Journal of Medicine and Science in Sports 20(5):725-730.

Boonen B, Kort N, Kerens B (2015). Knee examination: overview, periprocedural care, technique. Available from: http://emedicine.medscape.com [Accessed 10 August 2015].

Calmbach WL, Hutchens M (2003a). Evaluation of patients presenting with knee pain: Part I. History, physical examination, radiographs, and laboratory tests. American Family Physician 68(5):907-912.

Calmbach WL, Hutchens M (2003b). Evaluation of patients presenting with knee pain: Part II. Differential diagnosis. American Family Physician 68(5):917-922.

Christensen R, Astrup A, Bliddal H (2005). Weight loss: the treatment of choice for knee osteoarthritis? A randomized trial. Osteoarthritis Cartilage 13:20-27.

Christoforakis JJ, Sanchez-Ballester J, Hunt N et al (2006). Synovial shelves of the knee: association with chondral lesions. Knee Surgery, Sports Traumatology, Arthroscopy 14(12):1292-1298.

Collins NJ, Bisset LM, Crossley KM et al (2012). Efficacy of nonsurgical interventions for anterior knee pain. Sports Medicine 42(1):31-49.

Corti MC, Rigon C (2003). Epidemiology of osteoarthritis: prevalence, risk factors and functional impact. Aging Clinical and Experimental Research 15(5):359-363.

Cothran RL, McGuire PM, Helms CA et al (2003). MR imaging of infra-patellar plica injury. American Journal of Roentgenology 180(5)1443-1447.

Crossley K, Bennell K, Green S et al (2002). Physical therapy for patellofemoral pain: a randomized, double-blinded, placebo-controlled trial. The American Journal of Sports Medicine 30(6):857-865.

Dawson J, Fitzpatrick R, Fletcher J et al (2004). Osteoarthritis Affecting the Hip and Knee. Health Needs Assessment.

De Filippis L, Gulli S, Caliri A et al (2004). Epidemiology and risk factors in osteoarthritis: literature review data from 'OASIS' study. Reumatismo 56(3):169-184.

Demirag B, Ozturk C, Karakayali M (2006). Symptomatic infrapatellar plica. Knee Surgery, Sports Traumatology, Arthroscopy 14(2):156-160.

Deyle GD, Henderson NE, Matekel RL et al (2000). Effectiveness of manual physical therapy and exercise in osteoarthritis of the knee: a randomized, controlled trial. Annals of Internal Medicine 132(3):173-181.

Du H, Chen SL, Bao CD et al (2005). Prevalence and risk factors of knee osteoarthritis in Huang-Pu District, Shanghai, China. Rheumatology International 25(8):585-590.

Dupont JY (1997). Synovial plicae of the knee: controversies and review. Clinics in Sports Medicine 16(1):87-122.

Duri ZA, Patel DV, Aichroth PM (2002). The immature athlete. Clinics in Sports Medicine 21(3):461-482.

El-Metwally A, Salminen JJ, Auvinen A et al (2006). Risk factors for traumatic and non-traumatic lower limb pain among preadolescents: a population-based study of Finnish schoolchildren. BMC Musculoskeletal Disorders 7(1):3.

Englund M, Guermazi A, Gale D et al (2008). Incidental meniscal findings on knee MRI in middle-aged and elderly persons. New England Journal of Medicine 359:1108-1115.

Feldesman MR, Kleckner JG, Lundy JK (1990). Femur/stature ratio and estimates of stature in mid-and late-Pleistocene fossil hominids. American Journal of Physical Anthropology 83(3):359-372.

Flynn JM, Kocher MS, Ganley TJ (2004). Osteochondritis dissecans of the knee. Journal of Pediatric Orthopaedics 24(4):434-443.

Fransen M, Crosbie J, Edmonds J (2001). Physical therapy is effective for patients with osteoarthritis of the knee: a randomized controlled clinical trial. The Journal of Rheumatology 28(1):156-164.

Fulkerson JP, Buuck DA, Post WR (2004). Disorders of the Patellofemoral Joint. Philadelphia: Lippincott Williams & Wilkins; 129-142.

Gage BE, McIlvain NM, Collins CL et al (2012). Epidemiology of 6.6 million knee injuries presenting to United States emergency departments from 1999 through 2008. Academic Emergency Medicine 19(4):378-385.

Grella RJ (2013). Continuous passive motion following total knee arthroplasty: a useful adjunct to early mobilisation? Physical Therapy Reviews.

Gupta MN, Sturrock RD, Field M (2001). A prospective 2-year study of 75 patients with adult-onset septic arthritis. Rheumatology 40(1):24-30.

Hartley A (1995). Practical Joint Assessment: Lower Quadrant: A Sports Medicine Manual, 2nd ed. Mosby Year Book; 160-184.

Harris IA, Madan NS, Naylor JM et al (2013). Trends in knee arthroscopy and subsequent arthroplasty in an Australian population: a retrospective cohort study. BMC Musculoskeletal Disorders 14(1):143.

Helmick CG, Felson DT, Lawrence RC et al (2008). Estimates of the prevalence of arthritis and other rheumatic conditions in the United States: Part I. Arthritis and Rheumatism 58(1):15-25.

Hoogeboom TJ, Oosting E, Vriezekolk JE et al (2012). Therapeutic validity and effectiveness of preoperative exercise on functional recovery after joint replacement: a systematic review and meta-analysis. Public Library of Science One 7(5):e38031.

Jacobs B (1992). Knee osteochondritis dissecans. Journal of Bone and Joint Surgery 66:1242-1245.

Jinks C, Jordan K, Ong BN et al (2004). A brief screening tool for knee pain in primary care (KNEST). 2. Results from a survey in the general population aged 50 and over. Rheumatology 43(1):55-61.

Katz JN, Brophy RH, Chaisson CE et al (2013). Surgery versus physical therapy for a meniscal tear and osteoarthritis. New England Journal of Medicine 368(18):1675-1684.

Kent M, Khanduja V (2010). Synovial plicae around the knee. The Knee 17(2):97-102.

Kim K-I, Egol KA, Hozack WJ, et al (2006). Periprosthetic fractures after total knee arthroplasties. Clinical Orthopaedics & Related Research 446(3):167-175.

Kim S, Bosque J, Meehan JP et al (2011). Increase in outpatient knee arthroscopy in the United States: a comparison of National Surveys of Ambulatory Surgery, 1996 and 2006. Journal of Bone and Joint Surgery, American Volume 93(11):994-1000.

Kishner S, Courseault J, Authement A (2015). Knee joint anatomy: overview, gross anatomy, natural variants. Available from: http://emedicine.medscape.com [Accessed 31 July 2015].

Lachance L, Sowers MF, Jamadar D et al (2002). The natural history of emergent osteoarthritis of the knee in women. Osteoarthritis Cartilage 10:849–854.

Lankhorst NE, Bierma-Zeinstra SM, van Middelkoop M (2012). Risk factors for patellofemoral pain syndrome: a systematic review. Journal of Orthopaedic and Sports Physical Therapy 42(2):81-94.

Lavine R (2010). Iliotibial band friction syndrome. Current Reviews in Musculoskeletal Medicine 3(1-4):18-22.

Lawrence RC, Felson DT, Helmick CG et al (2008). Estimates of the prevalence of arthritis and other rheumatic conditions in the United States: Part II. Arthritis and Rheumatism 58(1):26-35.

Leeds Community Healthcare (2012). Differential diagnosis for internal derangement injuries in the knee. NHS Trust. Available from: http://www.leedscommunityhealthcare.nhs.uk/document.php?o=1869 [Accessed 11 March 2016].

McGee SR, Boyko EJ (1998). Physical examination and chronic lower-extremity ischemia: a critical review. Archives of Internal Medicine 158(12):1357-1364.

McRae R (2010). Clinical Orthopaedic Examination, 6th ed. Edinburgh: Elsevier Health Sciences; 201-230.

Mader SS (2004). Understanding Human Anatomy and Physiology. New York: McGraw-Hill Science.

Messier S, Loeser R, Mitchell M et al (2000). Exercise and weight loss in obese older adults with knee osteoarthritis: a preliminary study. Journal of the American Geriatrics Society 48:1062-1072.

Miyasaka KC, Daniel DM, Stone ML et al (1991). The incidence of knee ligament injuries in the general population. American Journal of Knee Surgery 4(1):3-8.

Moss P, Sluka K, Wright A (2007). The initial effects of knee joint mobilisations on osteoarthritic hyperalgesia. Manual Therapy 12:109-18.

National Institute for Health and Clinical Excellence (NICE) (2008). Osteoarthritis: National Clinical Guideline for Care and Management in Adults. Clinical guideline 59.

Nakayama A, Sugita T, Aizawa T et al (2011). Incidence of medial plica in 3,889 knee joints in the Japanese population. Arthroscopy 11:1523-1527.

Nicholl JP, Coleman P, Williams BT (1991). Pilot study of the epidemiology of sports injuries and exercise-related morbidity. British Journal of Sports Medicine 25(1):61-66.

OpenStax College (2013). Anatomy and physiology. Available from: http://cnx.org/content/col11496/latest [Accessed 8 February 2016].

Peat G, McCarney R, Croft P (2001). Knee pain and osteoarthritis in older adults: a review of community burden and current use of primary health care. Annals of the Rheumatic Diseases 60(2):91-97.

Pollard H, Ward G, Hoskins W et al (2008). The effect of a manual therapy knee protocol on osteoarthritic knee pain: a randomised controlled trial. The Journal of the Canadian Chiropractic Association 52(4):229.

Schindler OS (2004). Synovial plicae of the knee. Current Orthopaedics 18(3):210-219.

Schindler OS (2014). 'The Sneaky Plica' revisited: morphology, pathophysiology and treatment of synovial plicae of the knee. Knee Surgery, Sports Traumatology, Arthroscopy 22(2):247-262.

Schünke M, Ross LM, Schulte E et al (2006). Thieme Atlas of Anatomy: General Anatomy and Musculoskeletal System. Stuttgart: Thieme.

Sluka KA, Skyba DA, Radhakrishnan R et al (2006). Joint mobilization reduces hyperalgesia associated with chronic muscle and joint inflammation in rats. The Journal of Pain 7(8):602-607.

Soucie JM, Wang C, Forsyth A et al (2011). Range of motion measurements: reference values and a database for comparison studies. Haemophilia 17(3):500-507.

Stakes NO, Myburgh C, Brantingham JW et al (2006). A prospective randomized clinical trial to determine efficacy of combined spinal manipulation and patella mobilization compared to patella mobilization alone in the conservative management of patellofemoral pain syndrome. Journal of the American Chiropractic Association 43(7):11-18.

Standring S (2008). Gray's Anatomy: The Anatomical Basis of Clinical Practice, 40th ed. Edinburgh: Churchill Livingstone.

Tate P (2009). Anatomy of Bones and Joints. Seeley's Principles of Anatomy and Physiology. New York: McGraw-Hill; 149-196.

Taylor KE, Brantingham JW (2003). An investigation into the effect of exercise combined with patella mobilization/manipulation in the treatment of patellofemoral pain syndrome: a randomized, accessor-blinded, controlled clinical pilot trial. European Journal of Chiropractic 51(1):5-18.

Thorlund JB, Hare KB, Lohmander LS (2014). Large increase in arthroscopic meniscus surgery in the middle-aged and older population in Denmark from 2000 to 2011. Acta Orthopaedica 85(3):287-292.

Ulmer T (2002). The clinical diagnosis of compartment syndrome of the lower leg: are clinical findings predictive of the disorder? Journal of Orthopaedic Trauma 16(8):572-577.

Vassiou K, Vlychou M, Zibis A et al (2015). Synovial plicae of the knee joint: the role of advanced MRI. Postgraduate Medical Journal 91(1071):35-40.

Wallis JA, Taylor NF (2011). Pre-operative interventions (non-surgical and non-pharmacological) for patients with hip or knee osteoarthritis awaiting joint replacement surgery – a systematic review and meta-analysis. Osteoarthritis and Cartilage 19(12):1381-1395.

Webb R, Brammah T, Lunt M et al (2004). Opportunities for prevention of 'clinically significant' knee pain: results from a population-based cross sectional survey. Journal of Public Health 26(3):277-284.

Williams AM, Lloyd JM, Watts MC et al (2012). The arthroscopic features of the pathological medial plica of the knee: a classification based on an analysis of 3,017 arthroscopies. European Orthopaedics and Traumatology 3(1):43-47.

UW Health (2011). Rehabilitation guidelines for knee arthroscopy. University of Wisconsin Sports Medicine. Available from: http://www.uwhealth.org/files/uwhealth/docs/sportsmed/SM_knee_arthroscopy.pdf (Accessed 8 February 2016).

Yim JH, Seon JK, Song EK et al (2013). A comparative study of meniscectomy and non-operative treatment for degenerative horizontal tears of the medial meniscus. The American Journal of Sports Medicine 41(7):1565-1570.

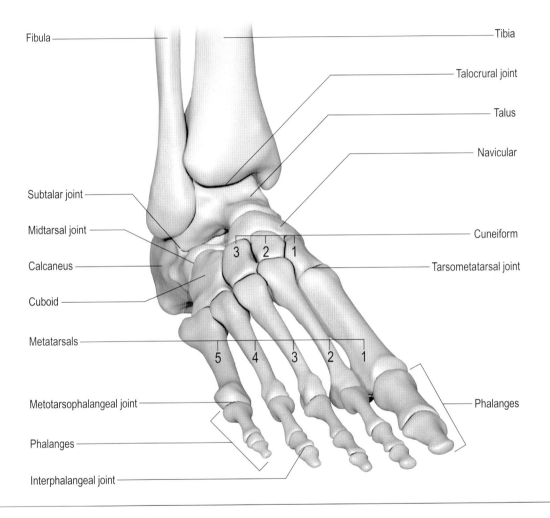

Fibula

Tibia

Talocrural joint

Talus

Navicular

Subtalar joint

Midtarsal joint

Calcaneus

Cuboid

Cuneiform

Tarsometatarsal joint

3 2 1

Metatarsals

5 4 3 2 1

Metotarsophalangeal joint

Phalanges

Phalanges

Interphalangeal joint

Figure 14.1
The ankle and foot

Introduction

The ankle is the second most common area to be affected by sport injuries after the knee (Fong et al 2007). Lateral ankle sprains are so common that in the United States they alone have an annual health-care cost of $4 billion (Curtis et al 2008, Waterman et al 2010). Ankle sprains have been recorded to require more than 23,000 Americans to seek medical attention daily (Court-Brown & Caesar 2006). In addition, a recent study by You et al (2016) using MRI investigations found that between 15.8% and 20.5% of individuals who experienced ankle tendon and ligament injuries also had corresponding osteochondral lesions of the distal tibia and fibula and talus, thus leading to the possibility of recurrent issues.

As well as sports-related foot injuries, the increase in levels of obesity has been associated with an increase in foot and ankle complications including tendonitis, plantar fasciitis and osteoarthritic changes (Gross et al 2015, Mickle & Steele 2015). Nkhata et al (2015) postulated that obesity was one of the contributing factors in their investigation of work-related disorders among nurses when they discovered that the most commonly affected body parts were ankles and feet (54.8%). Biomechanical compensations from other joints can also lead to foot pain, as reported by Paterson et al (2015) who found that foot pain, both bilateral and ipsilateral, is commonly observed with osteoarthritic changes of the knee. For these reasons, it is important to investigate other joints rather than focus solely on the primary presentation when treating foot symptoms.

Martins et al (2012, 2013) found that 9 minutes of articulation based on a grade 3 articulation (Maitland scale) of the ankle joint over a period of 5 days decreased postoperative pain in the ankle. The effect is thought to be via both peripheral and central neurological receptors. Martins et al (2011) also found that ankle articulation helped produce 'pronounced

and long-lasting analgesic effects' in rats with sciatic nerve crush causing neuropathic pain. Green et al (2001) performed passive articulation to ankle joints following an acute ankle sprain and found that it greatly improved the pain-free movement of the ankle when compared to a control group. Collins et al (2004) also found that articulation of the ankle joint with a sub-acute sprain helped improve the range of movement of the joint. Hoch et al (2012) performed anterior–posterior articulation of the talocrural joint over a period of 2 weeks on participants with a history of ankle sprains and found that it improved self-reported function of the ankle and foot, increased dorsiflexion and improved balance. This is also reported in Mulligan articulation of the ankle joint, where the talus is believed to be anteriorized and inverted following ankle sprains, therefore restricting dorsiflexion and making the ankle prone to respraining (Collins et al 2004).

Hallux limitus, or turf toe, causes loss of motion in the big toe joint and is the third most common injury reported to prevent participation in athletics (Adelaar & Anderson 1997), but it is a condition that can easily be overlooked. Being unable to push off properly with the foot can lead to further issues within not only the hallux (big toe) itself but also the ankle and knee, particularly in sportspeople (McCormick & Anderson 2009, Anderson et al 2010, Frimenko et al 2012). As with most sprains, the initial treatment suggestions are rest, ice, compression and elevation (RICE), with appropriate non-steroidal anti-inflammatory drugs (NSAIDs) and strapping of the joint when needed. In the sub-acute phase of turf toe, articulation of the hallux is recommended (Fritz 1999, Shamus et al 2004, McCormick & Anderson 2009). Shamus et al (2004) also looked at articulation of the sesamoid bones of the hallux with flexor hallucis strengthening and found a great improvement in symptoms with patients suffering with hallux limitus. In some circumstances surgery is needed for turf toe (VanPelt et al 2012), but not all evidence supports the overall effectiveness of surgery (Maffulli et al 2011). Evidence shows that post-surgical articulation of the hallux can be more beneficial than surgery alone (Grady et al 2013).

Plantar fasciitis (also known as plantar fasciosis or jogger's heel) is one of the most common causes of heel and foot pain, affecting 10% of the general population in their lifetime (Li et al 2013, Beeson 2014), and classically originating from repetitive trauma to the calcaneus. Prakash and Misra (2014) found that manual therapy 'is a superior approach in improving pain and disability in individuals with plantar fasciitis', a finding supported by Cleland et al (2009). Patla et al (2015) suggested that articulation of the cuboid and exercise management can help with tibialis posterior tendinopathy, but the findings from this case report require further research.

Anatomy

The ankle and foot are the most distal part of the lower limb of the appendicular skeleton. The bones, ligaments, tendons and muscles of the ankle and foot are highly developed, complex structures. The joints here are unlike many other joints in the body, because they are at times mobile and at other times quite stable. These structures articulate together to provide functional mobility and stability and enable us to perform diverse activities, including walking, running, standing and jumping (Riegger 1988).

Ankle

In medical usage, the term 'ankle' usually refers specifically to the talocrural joint. However, in common usage, it often refers to the region or angle between the foot and leg. The ankle is made up of the articulation of three bones (the tibia, fibula and talus) and includes three joints (the talocrural, subtalar and inferior tibiofibular joints). The ankle allows dorsiflexion and plantar flexion movements of the foot (Moore et al 2013).

Foot

The foot, in contrast, is an intricate, biomechanically complex structure that supports the body weight, allows locomotion and withstands forces during propulsion. In addition to the tibia and fibula, there are 26 bones in each foot. These bones form a series of arches in the foot. They can be divided into three groups: the tarsal

bones (7), the metatarsal bones (5), and the phalanges (14). The seven tarsal bones – the calcaneus, talus, navicular, cuboid bones and the medial, intermediate and lateral cuneiforms – are located at the proximal portion of the foot. The long metatarsals and the phalanges are located just anterior to the tarsals (OpenStax 2013).

The foot has a number of joints, which afford it stability and mobility. Although the total number of joints is not universally agreed, it is estimated that there are more than 30 in the foot. Some of the most important include the talocrural (ankle), subtalar, transverse tarsal, tarsometatarsal, metatarsophalangeal and interphalangeal joints (Tate 2009).

Structurally, the foot is subdivided into three main parts: the hindfoot, the midfoot and the forefoot. The hindfoot is the region closest to the center of the body. It is composed of three joints and contains two of the seven tarsal bones (the talus and the calcaneus). The midfoot constitutes the arches of the foot and works as a shock-absorber. This is made up of the remaining five tarsal bones (three cuneiform and the cuboid and navicular bones). The forefoot comprises five toes (phalanges), the corresponding five metatarsals and associated soft-tissue structures (Standring 2008).

Bony and joint anatomy

Tarsals

The tarsal bones, also known as the tarsus, are a cluster of seven articulating bones that form the posterior half of the foot. In a similar arrangement to the carpal bones of the wrist, tarsal bones are in proximal and distal rows; however, there is an extra element present medially in the tarsus – the navicular. The proximal row is composed of the talus and the calcaneus, and the distal row contains the three cuneiform and the cuboid (Moore et al 2013).

The talus is the most superior of the tarsal bones. It is an unusual bone, in that no muscle or tendon attaches with it. It forms the ankle joint, articulating with the tibia and fibula. The calcaneus is the largest bone of the foot. It forms the heel and serves as the attachment site for the large calf muscles. The cuboid is a relatively square-shaped bone located at the anterior end of the calcaneus. It articulates posteriorly with the calcaneus bone and medially with the navicular and lateral cuneiform bones. The navicular is a small bone that is located in front of the talus. It articulates posteriorly with the talus and anteriorly with the three cuneiforms. The cuneiforms are wedge-shaped bones that have an extensive superior surface but a narrow inferior surface (OpenStax 2013).

Metatarsals

The metatarsal bones, also known as the metatarsus, are dorsally convex, elongated bones (numbered 1–5) that form the anterior half of the foot. The second of these bones is the longest of all; the first is thicker and shortest. They are located between the tarsus and the phalanges. Like the metacarpal bones of the hand, they have a shaft or body, proximal base and distal head. The shaft is prismatic in form, which tapers distally from the tarsal to the phalangeal extremity. The base is wedge-shaped and articulates with the cuboid or cuneiform bones. The head is the extended distal end of each metatarsal bone. It forms the ball of the foot and articulates with the proximal phalanx of a toe (Panchbhavi 2013).

Phalanges

The phalanges of the foot resemble those of the hand in number and structural arrangement. However, they are shorter than the finger phalanges and, those of the first row especially, are compressed laterally. The foot contains a total of 14 phalanx bones, which are distributed in five toes (numbered 1–5). The big toe (hallux) is analogous to the thumb, with two phalanx bones: the proximal and distal phalanges. The other toes contain three phalanx bones: proximal, middle and distal phalanges (Standring 2008).

Joints

Table 14.1 lists the major joints that provide the functional mobility and stability of the ankle and foot.

Ligaments

The ligaments of the ankle and foot complex can be divided into a number of groups, depending on their anatomical position. They include the lateral and medial collateral ligaments, the tibiofibular syndesmotic ligaments, the ligaments of the subtalar and talocalcaneal joints, the talonavicular and plantar calcaneonavicular ligaments, the ligaments of the calaneocuboid joint, the intermetatarsal ligaments, and many more (Standring 2008, Golanó et al 2010). The most important are summarized in Table 14.2.

Joint	Characteristics
Talocrural joint	A synovial hinge joint that joins the upper surface (trochlea) of the talus with the tibia and fibula
	Permits dorsiflexion and plantar flexion movements via axis in the talus
Subtalar joint	A modified multiaxial joint, allowing anterior and posterior articulations between the talus and the calcaneus
	Permits inversion and eversion motions of the foot
Talocalcaneonavicular joint	A compound multiaxial joint, which forms when the rounded head of the talus connects with the navicular and the calcaneus
	Allows plantar flexion of talus on the navicular
Calcaneocuboid joint	A biaxial joint formed by the articulation between the heel bone (calcaneus) and the cuboid bone
	Allows a movement that is best referred to as obvolution–involution
Interphalangeal joints	Ginglymoid (hinge) joints formed by the articulations between the superior surfaces on the phalangeal heads and the adjacent phalangeal bases
	Permit flexion and extension movements

Table 14.1

Important joints of the ankle and foot complex

Data from Riegger (1988), Standring (2008), Norkin & White (2009)

Name	Description
Lateral collateral ligament (complex)	Consists of the anterior and posterior talofibular ligaments and the calcaneofibular ligament
	Originates from the lateral malleolus of the fibula to the talus and calcaneus
	Serves to stabilize the ankle joint
Medial collateral ligament	A fan-shaped, multifascicular ligament that is composed of a superficial and deep layer
	Commonly known as the deltoid ligament
	Originates from the medial malleolus (the bottom portion of the tibia) to the talus, calcaneus and navicular bone
	Stabilizes the inside of the ankle
Tibiofibular syndesmotic ligament (complex)	Consists of four ligaments: the anterior tibiofibular, posterior tibiofibular, inferior transverse and interosseous
	Serves to stabilize the tibiofibular syndesmosis
	Provides stability between the distal tibia and the fibula
	Fights forces (e.g. axial, translational or rotational) that attempt to separate the distal (inferior) tibiofibular joint
Cervical ligament	Also known as the subtalar ligament
	Originates from the superior calcaneal surface to the inferolateral tubercle of the talus
	Serves to hold the calcaneous in order to stabilize the subtalar joint
Bifurcate ligament	Originates from the anterior aspect of the calcaneus to the dorsomedial surface of the cuboid and navicular bones
	Serves to stabilize the calcaneocuboid joint
Intermetatarsal interosseus ligaments	Run between the lateral four metatarsal bones
	Serve to stabilize the intermetatarsal joints
	Hold together the metatarsals so that they can move in sync

Table 14.2

Important ligaments of the ankle and foot complex

Data from Milner & Soames (1998), Standring (2008), Boonthathip et al (2010), Golanó et al (2010), Moore et al (2013)

These ligaments primarily serve to hold the tendons in place and stabilize the joints of the foot and ankle (Standring 2008).

Range of motion

Ankle

The axis of rotation of the ankle is dynamic because of the complex morphology of the talocrural joint. The ankle shifts during dorsi- and plantar flexion, but there is a wide range of variability in reported values of normal dorsiflexion and plantar flexion (see Tables 14.3 and 14.4).

Foot

The range of motion of the foot joints is complex. The motion of the subtalar joint is triplanar, providing pronation and supination. The joint allows 1° of freedom. The transverse tarsal joint is reported to permit some degrees of inversion and eversion, but it mainly serves to amplify

Movement type	Range of motion (°)	Reference
Normal dorsiflexion	0–50	Clarkson (2000)
Normal plantar flexion	0–20	
Dorsiflexion, knee extended	14–48	Spink et al (2011)
Dorsiflexion, knee flexed	16–60	

Table 14.3

Approximate range of motion of the ankle

Movement type	Reported variation in range of motion (°)	Reference
Dorsiflexion	10–30	Oatis (1988)
Plantar flexion	45–65	
Dorsiflexion	13–33	Roaas & Andersson (1982), Lindsjo et al (1985), Lundberg et al (1989), Valderrabano et al (2003)
Plantar flexion	40–56	

Table 14.4

Variation in reference values reported for range of motion of the ankle

Joint	Movement type	Range of motion (°)
Subtalar joint	Inversion	0–50
	Eversion	0–26
Metatarsophalangeal joints	Flexion (big/great toe)	0–45
	Flexion (lesser toes)	0–40
	Extension (big/great toe)	0–80
	Extension (lesser toes)	0–70
Interphalangeal joints	Flexion (big/great toe)	0–90
	Flexion (lesser toes)	0–30
	Extension (big/great toe and other toes)	0–80

Table 14.5

Range of motion of the foot joints

Data from Oatis (1988), Norkin & White (2009)

the motions of the talocrural joint and the subtalar joint (Oatis 1988). The motion of the tarsometatarsal joints is translatory or planar. They are presumed to continue the compensating movement produced at the transverse tarsal joint when it reaches its maximum range of motion. The metatarsophalangeal joints allow 2° of freedom, providing motion in the sagittal and transverse planes. The interphalangeal (IP) joints permit motion in the sagittal plane, allowing pure flexion and extension (Norkin & White 2009). The range of motion of the joints of the foot is summarized in Table 14.5.

Epidemiology

Ankle injuries

Ankle injury is a very common musculoskeletal injury, accounting for 25% of all sports-related injuries, and it can affect anyone, regardless of age and sex (Fong et al 2007). The most common type of ankle injury is the sprain of the lateral ligament complex, involved in up to 80% of all ankle sprains (O'Loughlin et al 2009). These injuries can occur when participating in athletic activities such as running or jumping sports, or when simply stepping down at an angle or onto an uneven surface. In the UK, the incidence of ankle sprain is roughly 61 per 10,000 individuals. This equates to a total of about 302,000 people and 42,000 (severe) new ankle sprain patients visiting accident and emergency departments every year (Bridgman et al 2003). The main precursor for ankle sprains is a history of sprains (Noronha et al 2013), but a restriction in dorsiflexion of the talocrural joint can also predispose a person to ankle sprains and fractures of the ankle (Tabrizi et al 2000, Willems et al 2005).

Ankle sprain can happen to both non-athletes and athletes. People of all ages, including children, adolescents and older adults, are all at risk of ankle sprains. Overall, males of 15–24 years of age and females over 30 years of age come in the highest-risk category. However, females have a greater risk of spraining their ankle than males (13.6 versus 6.94 per 1000 exposures), and children are more likely than teenagers and older adults (2.85, 1.94 and 0.72 per 1000 exposures, respectively) (Waterman et al 2010, Doherty et al 2014).

Condition	Description	Reference
Tibial posterior tendonitis	The most common cause of ankle pain of the medial portion Causes acquired flatfoot deformity in adults Seriously affects gait and balance Occurs because of prolonged stretching into eversion Often linked to extreme subtalar pronation Most commonly affects women over 40 years of age Symptoms include flattening of the foot, change in foot shape, pain and swelling at the medial hindfoot, an abducted forefoot and a valgus heel	Kohls-Gatzoulis et al (2004), Trnka (2004)
Peroneal tendonitis	The most common overuse injury that causes ankle pain of the lateral portion Causes inflammation of the peroneal tendons Often occurs as a result of excessive eversion and pronation Commonly affects sport athletes, particularly those whose sport involves repetitive ankle motion	Wang et al (2005)
Hallux valgus (bunion)	Progressive and commonest forefoot deformity, also called a bunion Causes a valgus angulation of the proximal phalanx of the big toe Often leads to painful motion of the joint (pronation problems), trouble with footwear, and painful swelling on the big toe during weight-bearing Occurs most commonly in adolescents, particularly in girls Estimated prevalence: 23–35%	Hartley (1995), Nix et al (2010)
Plantar fasciitis	A degenerative disease of the plantar fascia The most common cause of stabbing pain in the heel and bottom of the foot Commonly affects middle-aged people About 10% of individuals develop it at some time during their lives Risk factors include leg length inconsistency, nerve entrapment, muscle tightness, excessive pronation, over-training and using ill-fitting footwear	Li et al (2013), Beeson (2014)

(Continued)

Condition	Description	Reference
Tarsal tunnel syndrome	Occurs due to compression of the posterior tibial nerve in the tarsal tunnel (canal formed between the flexor retinaculum and the medial malleolus) Often occurs because of having flat feet or fallen arches, trauma, an underlying disease (such as diabetes or arthritis) or excessive pronation Symptoms include shooting pain radiating into the heel, toes and arch of the foot, tingling or burning sensation and numbness on the plantar aspect	Reade et al (2001), Franson & Baravarian (2006)
Morton's neuroma (Morton's metatarsalgia or interdigital neuroma)	Commonly affects one foot, but can occasionally be both feet Normally affects the nerve between the third and fourth metatarsals, but occasionally the second and third toes Can occur at any age, but most often affects middle-aged women (perhaps because of footwear) Higher incidence in runners Symptoms initially start with tingling that gradually gets worse, developing to a sharp, shooting pain	Owens et al (2011), Pastides et al (2012)
Turf toe (hallux limitus)	Involves the metatarsophalangeal joint of the hallux (big toe) Chronic pain and loss of strength when pushing off Can lead to joint degeneration Loss of range of movement can lead to lack of ability to push off in gait cycle and eventually lead to ankle and knee issues Common in sports such as, soccer, American football and athletics Can be divided into three categories: hyperextension, hyperflexion and dislocation	McCormick & Anderson (2009), Anderson et al (2010), Frimenko et al (2012)

Table 14.6
Common disorders of the ankle and foot

As discussed in Chapter 1, meniscoids can develop in the embryo or after trauma to the ankle joint (Lahm et al 1998, Baums et al 2006, Glazebrook et al 2009). This can lead to long-term symptoms such as locking, decreased range of movement and pain in the ankle. In a similar way to plica in the knee (see Chapter 13, The knee), meniscoids can only be fully diagnosed after imaging or arthroscopy (Valkering et al 2013). Also like plica, although manual therapy can be effective in treating the area, surgery may also be a viable treatment mode (Brennan et al 2012).

Foot pain

Foot pain is an extremely common problem. It is associated with balance and gait problems, high risk of falls, and reduced ability to execute activities of daily living. Risk factors for foot pain include age, sex, heredity, obesity, generalized osteoarthritis, intrinsic foot conditions (such as toe deformity, hallux valgus, calluses and corns), extreme exercise and ill-fitting footwear (Menz et al 2006). Foot pain is highly prevalent in elderly people and is estimated to affect around 20–30% of adults aged 65 and over (Benvenuti et al 1995, Dunn et al 2004, Thomas et al 2004). The prevalence of foot pain in other age groups, however, has not been so widely studied to date. Nevertheless, women are known to be 40% more likely than men to have foot pain (Hill et al 2008). The prevalence of disabling foot pain in subjects reporting foot pain in the past month is about 9.5% (Garrow et al 2004). Common disorders of the ankle and foot are described in Table 14.6.

Ankle and foot examination

Medical history

During the ankle and foot examination, a detailed medical history of the patient should be taken to characterize the severity of the pain, narrow down the differential diagnosis, and facilitate the physical examination. While interviewing the patient, the ankle and foot must be exposed as much as possible, so that visual observation can be made. The examiner should review prior injuries and/or surgeries, past medical history, previous diagnostic reports, recreational and occupational activities, medications, allergies and social history. The patient should also be asked about the severity and location of pain, presence of swelling, duration of symptoms, exacerbating and relieving factors, and functional difficulty, such as inability to walk, run and jump.

Red flags

Table 14.7 details the red flag conditions that the examiner should note in particular from the patient's narrative and examination.

Condition	Signs and symptoms
Fractures	History of recent trauma such as a crush injury, an ankle injury or a fall from height
	Pain, bruising or swelling on affected leg
	Persistent synovitis
	Point tenderness over involved tissues
	Inability to walk or bear weight on involved leg
Deep vein thrombosis (DVT)	History of recent surgery
	Calf pain
	Redness of the skin
	Swelling and tenderness on affected leg
	Pain intensified with walking or standing and reduced by elevation and rest
Septic arthritis	Fever, chills
	History of recent bacterial infection
	Constant aching and/or throbbing pain
	Coexisting immunosuppressive disorder
	Red, swollen joint with no history of trauma
Compartment syndrome	History of trauma or crush injury
	Pain with dorsiflexion of toes
	Pain intensified with stretch applied to affected muscles
	Swelling, tightness and bruising of involved compartment
Cancer	Previous history of cancer (e.g. prostate, breast or any reproductive cancer)
	Systemic symptoms such as fever, chills, malaise and weakness
	Sudden loss of weight with no valid reason
	Suspected malignancy
	Unexplained deformity, mass, or swelling

Table 14.7

Red flags for serious pathology in the ankle and foot complex

Data from McGee & Boyko (1998), Gupta et al (2001), Judd & Kim (2002), Ulmer (2002), Hatch & Hacking (2003)

Physical examination

Physical examinations of the ankle and foot should be carried out in a systematic manner to help confirm initial findings, fully explore the nature and extent of the problem, and make judgments. A general evaluation of the ankle and foot should include inspection, palpation, range of motion, neurovascular assessment and special tests.

Inspection

The physical examination of the ankle and foot should start with a careful visual inspection of the patient's stance and gait, with and without shoes. Next, the examiner should check the alignment and foot and toe shape, and note whether the foot is normally proportioned or has any prominence. If any abnormality, such as valgus, varus, flatfoot, cavus foot, clawed toes, hammertoe and mallet toe is observed, it should be noted immediately. The examiner should also inspect the ankle and foot carefully to identify any sign of infection, scars, abrasions, plantar callosities, swelling, bruising, deformity and discoloration.

Palpation

While examining the ankle and foot, several bony anatomical landmarks and all ligamentous structures

Test	Procedure	Positive sign	Interpretation
Single leg heel rise	The patient stands on the test limb only, with the knee extended. The patient then plantar flexes the ankle and raises the heel from the floor, standing on their toes.	Absence of heel inversion during plantar flexion	Posterior tibial tendon dysfunction
Talar tilt test	The patient is seated, with the ankle unsupported and the foot in 10–20° of plantar flexed position. The examiner stabilizes the distal lower leg, just proximal to the medial malleolus, with one hand and applies an inversion force to the hindfoot with the other hand. The examiner tilts the talus side to side during inversion of the foot.	Increased joint laxity or increased talar tilt compared with the contralateral side	Compromised calcaneofibular ligament
Thompson test	The patient lies prone, with the knee bent to 90°. The examiner squeezes the calf muscle and looks for the presence of ankle plantar flexion.	Absence of ankle plantar flexion	Ruptured Achilles tendon
Anterior drawer test	The patient lies prone on the table, with the ankle in a neutral position and foot in 20° of plantar flexed position. The examiner stabilizes the distal tibia with one hand and applies an anterior force to the calcaneus (heel) with the other hand.	Increased anterior translation compared to the contralateral side	Compromised anterior talofibular ligament
Kleiger's test	The patient is seated, with the knee flexed over the edge of the table by 90°. The examiner stabilizes the distal tibia with one hand and applies a rotational force externally to the affected foot.	Medial and lateral joint pain or tibiofibular joint pain	Damage to distal tibiofibular syndesmosis (tib–fib joint pain) Compromised deltoid ligament (medial/lateral joint pain)

Table 14.8

Special tests for the ankle and foot examination

Data from Baxter (2003), Young et al (2005), Simpson & Howard (2009)

should be palpated to identify the areas of pathology. The examiner should be able to recognize the following important structures: calcaneum, lateral and medial malleoli, tibiofibular syndesmosis, talofibular ligaments, deltoid ligament complex, navicular bone, sustentaculum tail and metatarsal heads. The process should start with palpation of the metatarsophalangeal joints. Point tenderness of structures should also be assessed, especially at the ankle, subtalar joint, calcaneus (heel bone), Achilles tendon and midfoot.

Range of motion

The examiner should carefully assess all the movements of the ankle and foot. These include dorsiflexion (both knee flexed and knee extended), plantar flexion of the ankle, inversion and eversion of the subtalar joint, flexion, and extension of the metatarsophalangeal and interphalangeal joints. The strength of the big toe and other toes should also be assessed. The examiner may use a hand goniometer or radiographic goniometry to assess the range of motion. After measuring the range of motion, the examiner should compare the collected data with reliable standards (see Tables 14.3, 14.4 and 14.5).

Special tests

See Table 14.8.

Ankle and foot muscles

Name	Origin	Insertion	Action	Nerve supply
Gastrocnemius	Medial head: popliteal portion of femur and superior angle of medial condyle Lateral head: lateral condyle	Posterior surface of calcaneus via the tendocalcaneus (Achilles) tendon	Plantar flexion of the foot and flexion of the knee	Tibial nerve (S1–S2)
Soleus	Posterior surface of fibula, fibula head and tibia (soleal line)	Posterior surface of calcaneus via the tendocalcaneus (Achilles) tendon	Plantar flexion of the foot	Tibial nerve (S1–S2)
Plantaris	Oblique (popliteal) ligament, lower portion of lateral supracondylar ridge	Posterior surface of calcaneus via the tendocalcaneus (Achilles) tendon	Plantar flexion of the foot and flexion of the knee	Tibial nerve (S1–S2)
Fibularis (peroneus) longus	Fibula head and superior two-thirds of lateral surface of fibula	Base of fifth metatarsal and medial cuneiform	Everts the foot and plantar flexes the ankle	Superficial fibular (peroneal) nerve (L5–S2)
Fibularis (peroneus) brevis	Inferior two-thirds of fibula	Base of fifth metatarsal	Everts the foot and plantar flexes the ankle	Superficial fibular (peroneal) nerve (L5–S2)
Tibialis anterior	Superior lateral half of tibia, lateral condyle of tibia and interosseous membrane	Medial and inferior (plantar) surfaces of medial cuneiform and base of first metatarsal	Dorsiflexes and inverts the foot	Deep fibular (peroneal) nerve (L4–S1)
Extensor hallucis longus	Middle anterior surface of fibular and interosseous membrane	Dorsal surface of distal phalanx of hallux (big toe)	Extends the hallux and dorsiflexes the ankle	Deep fibular (peroneal) nerve (L5–S1)
Extensor digitorum longus	Superior three-quarters of anterior surface of fibular, interosseous membrane and lateral condyle of tibia	Dorsal surface of second and fifth middle and distal phalanges	Extends (dorsiflexes) the toes, dorsiflexes the ankle and everts the foot	Deep fibular (peroneal) nerve (L4–S1)
Fibularis (peroneus) tertius	Inferior third of anterior surface of fibula and interosseous membrane	Base of fifth metatarsal	Everts the foot and plantar flexes the ankle	Superficial fibular (peroneal) nerve (L5–S2)

(Continued)

Name	Origin	Insertion	Action	Nerve supply
Flexor hallucis longus	Inferior two-thirds of posterior surface of fibula and interosseous membrane	Base of distal phalanx of hallux (big toe)	Flexes (plantar flexes) the hallux, plantar flexes the ankle and inverts the foot	Tibial nerve (L5–S2)
Flexor digitorum longus	Medial portion of posterior surface of tibia	Base of distal phalanges of second to fifth digits	Flexes (plantar flexes) the second to fifth toes, inverts the foot	Tibial nerve (L5–S1)
Tibialis posterior	Posterior lateral part of tibia, interosseous membrane and posterior superior half of fibula	Navicular tuberosity, plantar surfaces of cuboid, cuneiforms, and second to fourth metatarsals and sustentaculum tali	Plantar flexes and inverts the foot	Tibial nerve (L5–S1)
Extensor digitorum brevis	Anterior and lateral surface of calcaneus, lateral talocalcaneal ligament and inferior extensor retinaculum	Base of proximal phalanx of hallux (big toe), tendons of extensor digitorum longus	Extends the first to fourth toes	Deep fibular (peroneal) nerve (L5–S1)
Abductor hallucis	Tuberosity of calcaneus, plantar aponeurosis and flexor retinaculum	Medial side of base of proximal phalanx of hallux (big toe)	Abducts the hallux (big toe)	Medial plantar nerve (L4–L5)
Flexor digitorum brevis	Calcaneus tuberosity and plantar aponeurosis	Medial and lateral surface of second and fifth phalanges	Flexes the proximal phalanges and extends the distal phalanges of the second to fifth toes	Medial plantar nerve (L4–L5)
Abductor digiti minimi	Calcaneus tuberosity and plantar aponeurosis	Lateral surface of proximal phalanx of fifth toe	Abducts the fifth toe	Lateral plantar nerve (S1–S2)
Quadratus plantae	Medial head: medial surface of calcaneus Lateral head: inferior lateral surface of calcaneus	Lateral part of flexor digitorum longus tendon	Flexes the distal phalanges of the second to fifth digits	Lateral plantar nerve (S1–S2)
Lumbricales	Flexor digitorum longus tendon	Proximal phalanges	Flexes the proximal phalanges of the second to fifth digits	First lumbricalis: medial plantar nerve (L4–L5) Second to fifth lumbricales: lateral plantar nerve (S1–S2)

(Continued)

Name	Origin	Insertion	Action	Nerve supply
Flexor hallucis brevis	Cuboid and lateral cuneiform	Medial section: medial portion of proximal phalanx of hallux (big toe) Lateral section: lateral portion of proximal phalanx of hallux (big toe)	Flexes the hallux (big toe)	Medial plantar nerve (L4–S1)
Adductor hallucis	Oblique portion: second to fourth metatarsal and sheath of peroneus longus tendon Transverse portion: metatarsophalangeal ligaments of third to fifth digits and transverse metatarsal ligaments	Lateral portion of base of proximal phalanx of hallux (big toe)	Adducts the hallux (big toe)	Lateral plantar nerve (S1–S2)
Flexor digiti minimi brevis	Base of fifth metatarsal and tendon of peroneus longus	Lateral portion of base of proximal phalanx of fifth toe	Flexes the fifth digit	Lateral plantar nerve (S1–S2)
Dorsal interossei	Adjacent portion of metatarsal	Base of proximal phalanx First: medial surface of proximal phalanx of second digit Second to fourth: lateral sides of proximal phalanges of second to fourth digits	Abduct the digits, flex the proximal phalanges	Lateral plantar nerve (S1–S2)
Plantar interossei	Medial base of third to fifth metatarsals	Medial base of proximal phalanges	Abduct the digits, flex the proximal phalanges	Lateral plantar nerve (S1–S2)

Table 14.9
Ankle and foot muscles

Techniques: ankle and foot

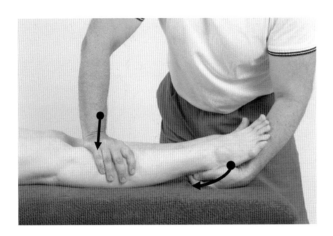

T14.1 Plantar flexion of the talocrural joint

- Stabilize the patient's leg on the plinth.
- Cup the patient's calcaneum with the sole of the foot resting on your forearm.
- Scoop the calcaneum posteriorly to articulate the talocrural joint into plantar flexion.

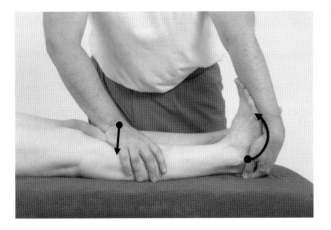

T14.2 Dorsiflexion of the talocrural joint

- Stabilize the patient's leg on the plinth.
- Cup the patient's calcaneum with the sole of the foot resting on your forearm.
- Place pressure through the foot and pull the calcaneum, inducing dorsiflexion.

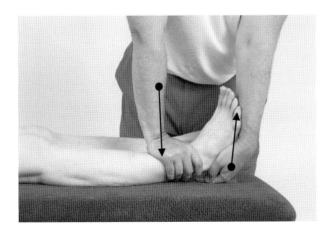

T14.3 Anterior glide of the talocrural joint

- Stand at the lower side of the plinth in a split stance.
- Cup under the patient's calcaneum with one hand and fix across the distal tibia and fibula with the other.
- With straight arms, rock onto your back foot to initiate an anterior glide of the talus against the tibia and fibula.

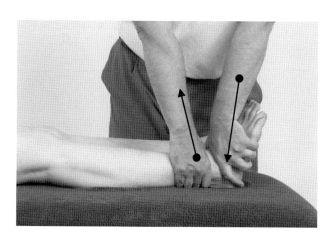

T14.4 Posterior glide of the talocrural joint

- Stand at the lower side of the plinth in a split stance.
- Stabilize the patient's foot into the plinth in a neutral position with your lower hand.
- Grasp around the tibia and fibula with the other hand.
- Drop your weight through the lower hand to glide the talus posterior to the tibia and fibula.

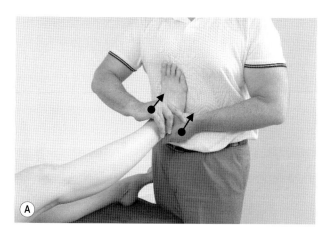

T14.5 Traction to the talocrural joint supine

- Standing at the end of the plinth, cup under the patient's calcaneum with one hand and around the talus with the other.
- With a split stance and keeping your arms close to your body, shift your weight onto your back leg to create traction at the talocrural joint.

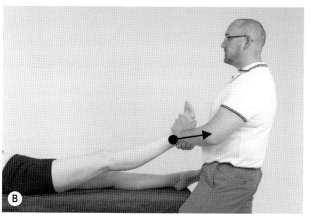

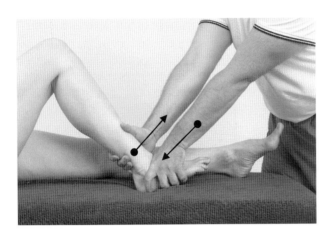

T14.6 Anterior articulation of the talocrural joint

- Stand at the foot of the plinth in a split stance.
- Flex the patient's knee and foot to 90° angles.
- Stabilize the foot around the talus with one hand.
- With your other hand, grip the patient's lower leg around the tibia.
- With straight arms, shift your weight onto the back leg to drive the tibia and fibula anterior to the talus.

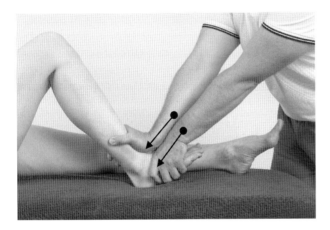

T14.7 Posterior articulation of the talocrural joint

- Stand at the foot of the plinth in a split stance.
- Flex the patient's knee and foot to 90° angles.
- Stabilize the foot around the talus with one hand.
- With your other hand, grip anteriorly around the patient's tibia.
- With straight arms, shift your weight onto the front leg to drive the tibia and fibula posterior to the talus.

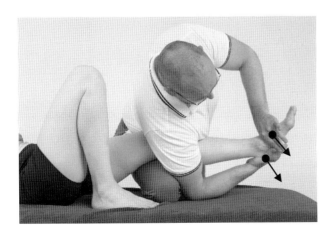

T14.8 Traction to the talocrural joint, supine

- Place the patient's knee over your flexed knee on the plinth.
- With your elbow supported against your knee, fix your lower hand behind the patient's calcaneum.
- Use your upper hand to dorsiflex the foot and drive it downward towards the plinth.

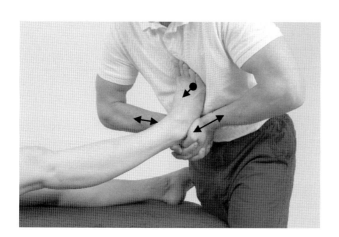

T14.9 Subtalar inversion/eversion

- Standing at the end of the plinth, brace the patient's foot against your lower sternum. Lean forward to dorsiflex the foot.
- Interlock your fingers and cup them around the calcaneum.
- In this fixed position, rotate your torso to create inversion and eversion of the subtalar joint.

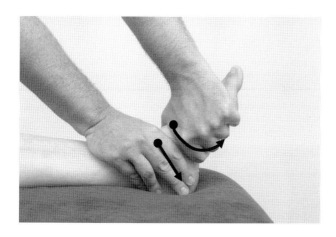

T14.10 Talonavicular joint

- Facing away from the patient, fix the patient's foot in a neutral position with your index finger posterior to the navicular.
- Grasp the foot with your other hand, aligning your index fingers.
- With straight arms, use your body weight to articulate through the talonavicular joint.

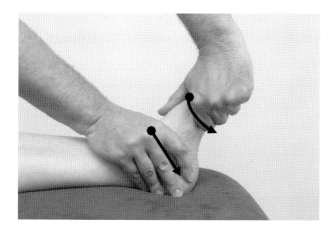

T14.11 Naviculocuneiform joint

- Facing away from the patient, fix the patient's foot in a neutral position with your index finger on the navicular.
- Grasp the foot with your other hand, covering the cuneiform and metatarsals.
- With straight arms, use your body weight to articulate through the naviculocuneiform joint.

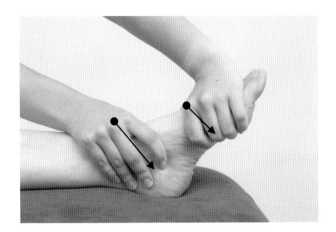

T14.12 Tarsometatarsal joint

- Facing away from the patient, fix the patient's foot in a neutral position, covering the navicular and medial cuneiform.
- Grasp the foot with your other hand, covering the first metatarsal.
- With straight arms, use your body weight to articulate through the tarsometatarsal joint.

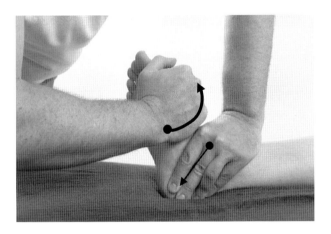

T14.13 Medial border

- Standing at the end of the plinth, fix with one hand around the patient's talus and navicular.
- With the other hand, grasp around the medial aspect of the foot to articulate the medial cuneiform on the navicular.

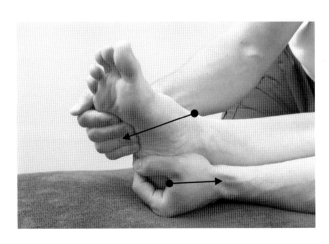

T14.14 Calcaneum–cuboid articulation

- Stand at the side of the plinth, facing away from the patient's head.
- Cup under the patient's calcaneum on the medial side of their leg with your forearm resting on the plinth.
- With the thenar eminence and fingers of your corresponding hand, grip around the cuboid and fourth and fifth metatarsals.
- With straight arms, transfer your weight from your front foot to your back foot to articulate the cuboid on the calcaneum.

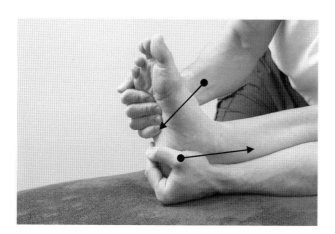

T14.15 Cuboid–metatarsal articulation

- Stand at the side of the plinth, facing away from the patient's head.
- Cup under the patient's calcaneum and cuboid on the medial side of their leg with your forearm resting on the plinth.
- With the thenar eminence and fingers of your corresponding hand, grip around the fourth and fifth metatarsals.
- With straight arms, transfer your weight from your front foot to your back foot to articulate the metatarsals on the cuboid.

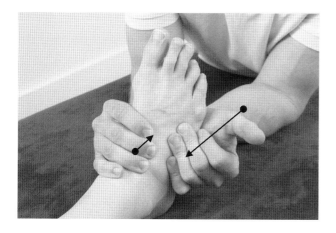

T14.16 Lateral border articulation

- Stand at the foot of the plinth.
- Grasp the medial aspect of the patient's foot, keeping it in a neutral position with your thumb fixed on the cuboid.
- Hold the fourth and fifth metatarsals between your thenar eminence and fingers.
- Articulate the metatarsals against the fixed cuboid.

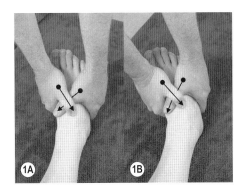

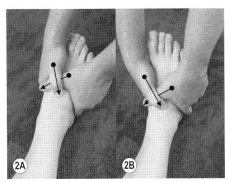

T14.17 Cuneiform articulation

1 Intermediate cuneiform

- Stand at the foot of the plinth.
- Grasp around the foot with both hands, crossing your thumbs on the dorsum of the foot over the targeted cuneiform.
- Articulate the targeted joint (intermediate, medial or lateral cuneiform) in an imaginary 'figure of eight' motion, as demonstrated in the photographs.

2 Medial cuneiform

3 Lateral cuneiform

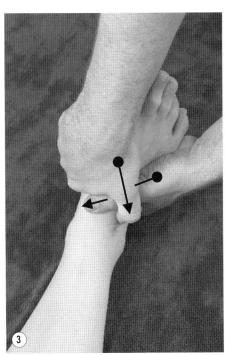

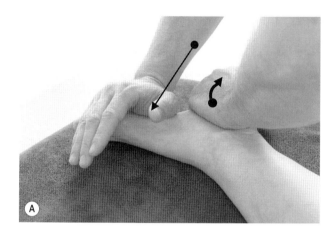

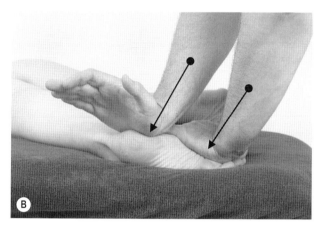

T14.18 Medial border articulation side-lying

- Stand at the end of the plinth with the patient lying on the affected side with the knee bent.
- Use a cross-hand technique on the calcaneum to fix the patient's foot into dorsiflexion.
- With your other hand, invert the foot by applying pressure over the navicular.
- Adjust the pressure between your hands to articulate the subtalar joint.

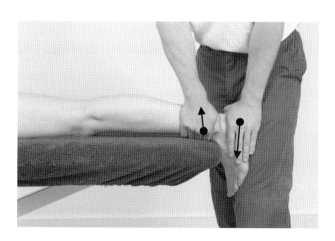

T14.19 Talocrural prone shift

- Stand at the end of the plinth, medial to the patient's leg, with the patient's foot off the end of the plinth.
- Hook under the tibia with one hand and place your corresponding hand webbed around the posterior aspect of the patient's calcaneum.
- With a split stance, drop your weight through the calcaneum towards the floor to glide the talus forward on the tibia.

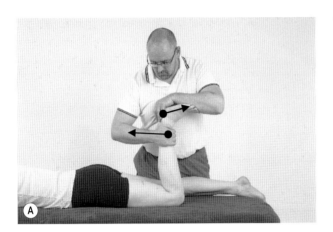

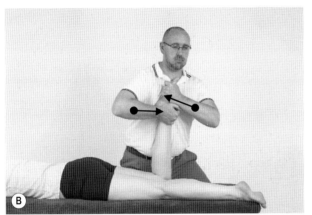

T14.20 Talocrural shearing

- Stand at the side of the plinth with the patient prone.
- Flex the patient's knee and foot to 90°.
- Grasp around the anterior aspect of the patient's ankle with your other hand on the posterior aspect of the calcaneum.
- Apply opposing forces with your arms to create shearing at the talocrural joint.

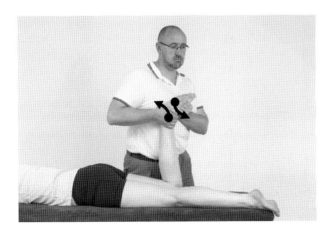

T14.21 Prone medial border articulation

- Stand at the side of the plinth with the patient's nearest leg flexed to 90° at the knee.
- Fix around the medial ankle.
- Grasp around the navicular and medial cuneiform and use a scooping motion to articulate the talonavicular joint.
- Slide your hands along to articulate the naviculocuneiform and cuneiform–metatarsal joints.

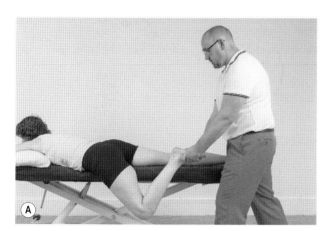

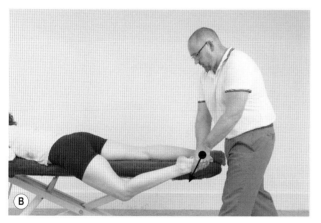

T14.22 Cuboid prone articulation

- Stand at the lower corner of the plinth.
- With the patient's knee off the table, grasp their foot with both hands, crossing your thumbs over the plantar aspect of the cuboid.
- Articulate from a dorsiflexed to a plantarflexed position by extending the hip and the knee, driving through the tibia.
- Maintain abduction, inversion and compression with your fingers.

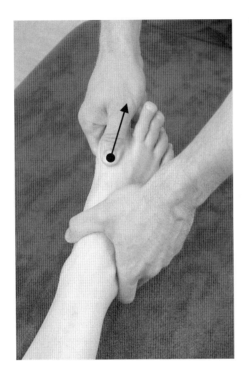

T14.23 Hallux traction

- Stand at the foot of the plinth. Support the patient's foot with one hand around the metatarsals.
- Grasp the metatarsophalangeal joint of the hallux with your thumb over the joint.
- Articulate the joint by applying traction and circumduction forces.

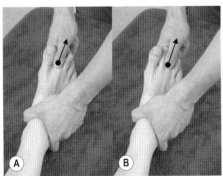

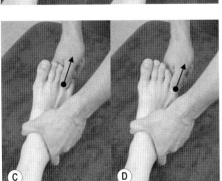

T14.24 Toe traction

- Stand at the end of the plinth. Support the patient's foot with one hand around the metatarsals.
- Grasp the metatarsophalangeal joint with your thumb over the joint.
- Articulate the joint by applying traction and circumduction forces.

REFERENCES

Adelaar RS, Anderson RB eds (1997). Disorders of the Great Toe. American Academy of Orthopaedic Surgeons.

Anderson RB, Hunt KJ, McCormick JJ (2010). Management of common sports-related injuries about the foot and ankle. Journal of the American Academy of Orthopaedic Surgeons 18(9):546-556.

Baums MH, Kahl E, Schultz W et al (2006). Clinical outcome of the arthroscopic management of sports-related 'anterior ankle pain': a prospective study. Knee Surgery, Sports Traumatology, Arthroscopy 14(5):482-486.

Baxter RE (2003). Pocket Guide to Musculoskeletal Assessment. Philadelphia: WB Saunders; 123-130.

Beeson P (2014). Plantar fasciopathy: revisiting the risk factors. Foot and Ankle Surgery 20(3):160-165.

Benvenuti F, Ferrucci L, Guralnik JM et al (1995). Foot pain and disability in older persons: an epidemiologic survey. Journal of the American Geriatrics Society 43(5):479-484.

Boonthathip M, Chen L, Trudell DJ et al (2010). Tibiofibular syndesmotic ligaments: MR arthrography in cadavers with anatomic correlation 1. Radiology 254(3):827-836.

Brennan SA, Rahim F, Dowling J et al (2012). Arthroscopic debridement for soft tissue ankle impingement. Irish Journal of Medical Science 181(2):253-256.

Bridgman SA, Clement D, Downing A et al (2003). Population-based epidemiology of ankle sprains attending accident and emergency units in the West Midlands of England, and a survey of UK practice for severe ankle sprains. Emergency Medicine Journal 20(6):508-510.

Clarkson HM (2000). Musculoskeletal Assessment: Joint Range of Motion and Manual Muscle Strength. Philadelphia: Lippincott Williams & Wilkins.

Cleland JA, Abbott JH, Kidd MO et al (2009). Manual physical therapy and exercise versus electrophysical agents and exercise in the management of plantar heel pain: a multicenter randomized clinical trial. Journal of Orthopaedic and Sports Physical Therapy 39:573-585.

Collins N, Teys P, Vicenzino B (2004). The initial effects of a Mulligan's mobilization with movement technique on dorsiflexion and pain in subacute ankle sprains. Manual Therapy 9(2):77-82.

Court-Brown CM, Caesar B (2006). Epidemiology of adult fractures: a review. Injury 37(8):691-697.

Curtis CK, Laudner KG, McLoda TA et al (2008). The role of shoe design in ankle sprain rates among collegiate basketball players. Journal of Athletic Training 43(3):230.

Doherty C, Delahunt E, Caulfield B et al (2014). The incidence and prevalence of ankle sprain injury: a systematic review and meta-analysis of prospective epidemiological studies. Sports Medicine 44(1):123-140.

Dunn JE, Link CL, Felson DT et al (2004). Prevalence of foot and ankle conditions in a multiethnic community sample of older adults. American Journal of Epidemiology 159(5):491-498.

Fong DTP, Hong Y, Chan LK et al (2007). A systematic review on ankle injury and ankle sprain in sports. Sports Medicine 37(1):73-94.

Franson J, Baravarian B (2006). Tarsal tunnel syndrome: a compression neuropathy involving four distinct tunnels. Clinics in Podiatric Medicine and Surgery 23(3):597-609.

Frimenko RE, Lievers WB, Coughlin MJ et al (2012). Etiology and biomechanics of first metatarsophalangeal joint sprains (turf toe) in athletes. Critical Reviews™ in Biomedical Engineering 40(1):43-61.

Fritz JM (1999). Rehabilitation in sports medicine: a comprehensive guide. Journal of Athletic Training 34(1):68.

Garrow AP, Silman AJ, Macfarlane GJ (2004). The Cheshire Foot Pain and Disability Survey: a population survey assessing prevalence and associations. Pain 110(1):378-384.

Glazebrook MA, Ganapathy V, Bridge MA et al (2009). Evidence-based indications for ankle arthroscopy. Arthroscopy 25(12):1478-1490.

Golanó P, Vega J, De Leeuw PA et al (2010). Anatomy of the ankle ligaments: a pictorial essay. Knee Surgery, Sports Traumatology, Arthroscopy 18(5):557-569.

Grady JF, Smith AM, Boumendjel Y et al (2013). Hallux rigidus: the valenti arthroplasty. In: Sports Medicine and Arthroscopic Surgery of the Foot and Ankle. London: Springer; 29-39.

Green T, Refshauge K, Crosbie J et al (2001). A randomised controlled trial of a passive accessory joint mobilisation on acute ankle inversion sprains. Physical Therapy 81(4):984-994.

Gross CE, Lampley A, Green CL et al (2015). The effect of obesity on functional outcomes and complications in total ankle arthroplasty. Foot and Ankle International, 1071100715606477.

Gupta MN, Sturrock RD, Field M (2001). A prospective 2-year study of 75 patients with adult-onset septic arthritis. Rheumatology 40(1):24-30.

Hartley A (1995). Practical Joint Assessment: Lower Quadrant: A Sports Medicine, 2nd ed. Mosby Year Book; 260-284.

Hatch RL, Hacking S (2003). Evaluation and management of toe fractures. American Family Physician 68(12).

Hill CL, Gill TK, Menz HB et al (2008). Prevalence and correlates of foot pain in a population-based study: the North West Adelaide health study. Journal of Foot and Ankle Research 1(2):1-7.

Hoch MC, Andreatta RD, Mullineaux DR et al (2012). Two-week joint mobilization intervention improves self-reported function, range of motion, and dynamic balance in those with chronic ankle instability. Journal of Orthopaedic Research 30(11):1798-1804.

Judd DB, Kim DH (2002). Foot fractures frequently misdiagnosed as ankle sprains. American Family Physician 66(5):785-794.

Kohls-Gatzoulis J, Angel JC, Singh D et al (2004). Tibialis posterior dysfunction: a common and treatable cause of adult acquired flatfoot. British Medical Journal 329(7478):1328-1333.

Lahm A, Erggelet C, Reichelt A (1998). Ankle joint arthroscopy for meniscoid lesions in athletes. Arthroscopy 14(6):572-575.

Li Z, Jin T, Shao Z (2013). Meta-analysis of high-energy extracorporeal shock wave therapy in recalcitrant plantar fasciitis. Swiss Medical Weekly 143:w13825.

Lindsjo U, Danckwardt-Lilliestrom G, Sahlstedt B (1985). Measurement of the motion range in the loaded ankle. Clinical Orthopaedics and Related Research 199:68-71.

Lundberg A, Goldie I, Kalin B et al (1989). Kinematics of the ankle/foot complex: plantarflexion and dorsiflexion. Foot and Ankle International 9(4):194-200.

McCormick JJ, Anderson RB (2009). The great toe: failed turf toe, chronic turf toe, and complicated sesamoid injuries. Foot and Ankle Clinics 14(2):135-150.

McGee SR, Boyko EJ (1998). Physical examination and chronic lower-extremity ischemia: a critical review. Archives of Internal Medicine 158(12):1357-1364.

Maffulli N, Papalia R, Palumbo A et al (2011). Quantitative review of operative management of hallux rigidus. British Medical Bulletin 98(1):75-98.

Martins DF, Mazzardo-Martins L, Gadotti VM et al (2011). Ankle joint mobilization reduces axonotmesis-induced neuropathic pain and glial activation in the spinal cord and enhances nerve regeneration in rats. Pain 152(11):2653-2661.

Martins DF, Bobinski F, Mazzardo-Martins L et al (2012). Ankle joint mobilization decreases hypersensitivity by activation of peripheral opioid receptors in a mouse model of postoperative pain. Pain Medicine 13(8):1049-1058.

Martins DF, Mazzardo-Martins L, Cidral-Filho FJ et al (2013). Ankle joint mobilization affects postoperative pain through peripheral and central adenosine A1 receptors. Physical Therapy 93(3):401-412.

Menz HB, Tiedemann A, Kwan MMS et al (2006). Foot pain in community-dwelling older people: an evaluation of the Manchester Foot Pain and Disability Index. Rheumatology 45(7):863-867.

Mickle KJ, Steele JR (2015). Obese older adults suffer foot pain and foot-related functional limitation. Gait and Posture 42(4):442-447.

Milner CE, Soames RW (1998). Anatomy of the collateral ligaments of the human ankle joint. Foot and Ankle International 19(11):757-760.

Moore KL, Dalley AF, Agur AM (2013). Lower limb. In: Clinically Oriented Anatomy, 7th ed. Philadelphia: Lippincott Williams & Wilkins, 519-525.

Nix S, Smith M, Vicenzino B (2010). Prevalence of hallux valgus in the general population: a systematic review and meta-analysis. Journal of Foot and Ankle Research 3(1):21.

Nkhata LA, Esterhuizen TM, Siziya S et al (2015). The prevalence and perceived contributing factors for work-related musculoskeletal disorders among nurses at the University Teaching Hospital in Lusaka, Zambia. Science 3(4):508-513.

Norkin CC, White DJ (2009). Measurement of Joint Motion: A Guide to Goniometry. Philadelphia: FA Davis.

Noronha MD, França LC, Haupenthal A et al (2013). Intrinsic predictive factors for ankle sprain in active university students: a prospective study. Scandinavian Journal of Medicine and Science in Sports 23(5):541-547.

Oatis CA (1988). Biomechanics of the foot and ankle under static conditions. Physical Therapy 68(12):1815-1821.

O'Loughlin PF, Murawski CD, Egan C et al (2009). Ankle instability in sports. The Physician and Sportsmedicine 37(2):93-103.

OpenStax College (2013). Anatomy and physiology. Available from: http://cnx.org/content/col11496/latest [Accessed 11 February 2016].

Owens R, Gougoulias N, Guthrie H et al (2011). Morton's neuroma: clinical testing and imaging in 76 feet, compared to a control group. Foot and Ankle Surgery 17(3):197-200.

Panchbhavi V (2013). Foot bone anatomy: overview; Tarsal bones – gross anatomy; Metatarsal bones – Gross anatomy. Available from: http://emedicine.medscape.com/article/1922965-overview#showall [Accessed 11 February 2016].

Pastides P, El-Sallakh S, Charalambides C (2012). Morton's neuroma: a clinical versus radiological diagnosis. Foot and Ankle Surgery 18(1):22-24.

Paterson KL, Hinman RS, Hunter DJ et al (2015). Concurrent foot pain is common in people with knee osteoarthritis and impacts health and functional status: data from the Osteoarthritis Initiative. Arthritis Care and Research 67(7):989.

Patla C, Lwin J, Smith L et al (2015). Cuboid manipulation and exercise in the management of posterior tibialis tendonopathy: A case report. International Journal of Sports Physical Therapy 10(3):363-370.

Prakash S, Misra A (2014). Effect of manual therapy versus conventional therapy in patients with plantar fasciitis – comparative study. International Journal of Physiotherapy Research 2(1):378-382.

Reade BM, Longo DC, Keller MC (2001). Tarsal tunnel syndrome. Clinics in Podiatric Medicine and Surgery 18(3):395-408.

Riegger CL (1988). Anatomy of the ankle and foot. Physical Therapy 68(12):1802-1814.

Roaas A, Andersson GB (1982). Normal range of motion of the hip, knee and ankle joints in male subjects, 30–40 years of age. Acta Orthopaedica 53(2):205-208.

Shamus J, Shamus E, Gugel RN et al (2004). The effect of sesamoid mobilization, flexor hallucis strengthening, and gait training on reducing pain and restoring function in individuals with hallux limitus: a clinical trial. Journal of Orthopaedic and Sports Physical Therapy 34(7):368-376.

Simpson MR, Howard TM (2009). Tendinopathies of the foot and ankle. American Family Physician 80(10):1107-1114.

Spink MJ, Fotoohabadi MR, Wee E et al (2011). Foot and ankle strength, range of motion, posture, and deformity are associated with balance and functional ability in older adults. Archives of Physical Medicine and Rehabilitation 92(1):68-75.

Standring S (2008). Gray's Anatomy: The Anatomical Basis of Clinical Practice, 40th ed. Edinburgh: Churchill Livingstone.

Tabrizi P, McIntyre WMJ, Quesnel MB et al (2000). Limited dorsiflexion predisposes to injuries of the ankle in children. Journal of Bone and Joint Surgery (British Volume) 82(8):1103-1106.

Tate P (2009). Anatomy of Bones and Joints. Seeley's Principles of Anatomy and Physiology. New York: McGraw-Hill; 149-196.

Thomas E, Peat G, Harris L et al (2004). The prevalence of pain and pain interference in a general population of older adults: cross-sectional findings from the North Staffordshire Osteoarthritis Project (NorStOP). Pain 110(1):361-368.

Trnka HJ (2004). Dysfunction of the tendon of tibialis posterior. Journal of Bone and Joint Surgery (British Volume) 86-B(7):939-946.

Ulmer T (2002). The clinical diagnosis of compartment syndrome of the lower leg: are clinical findings predictive of the disorder? Journal of Orthopaedic Trauma 16(8): 572-577.

Valderrabano V, Hintermann B, Nigg BM et al (2003). Kinematic changes after fusion and total replacement of the ankle: part 1: Range of motion. Foot and Ankle International 24:881-887.

Valkering KP, Golanó P, van Dijk CN et al (2013). 'Web impingement' of the ankle: a case report. Knee Surgery, Sports Traumatology, Arthroscopy 21(6):1289-1292.

VanPelt MD, Saxena A, Allen MA (2012). Turf toe injuries. In: International Advances in Foot and Ankle Surgery. London: Springer; 219-228.

Wang XT, Rosenberg ZS, Mechlin MB et al (2005). Normal variants and diseases of the peroneal tendons and superior peroneal retinaculum: MR Imaging features 1. Radiographics 25(3):587-602.

Waterman BR, Owens BD, Davey S et al (2010). The epidemiology of ankle sprains in the United States. Journal of Bone and Joint Surgery 92(13):2279-2284.

Willems TM, Witvrouw E, Delbaere K et al (2005). Intrinsic risk factors for inversion ankle sprains in male subjects: a prospective study. American Journal of Sports Medicine 33(3):415-423.

You JY, Lee GY, Lee JW et al (2016). An osteochondral lesion of the distal tibia and fibula in patients with an osteochondral lesion of the talus on MRI: prevalence, location, and concomitant ligament and tendon injuries. American Journal of Roentgenology 206(2):366-372.

Young CC, Niedfeldt MW, Morris GA et al (2005). Clinical examination of the foot and ankle. Primary Care: Clinics in Office Practice 32(1):105-132.

Note: Page number followed by f and/or t indicates figure and table respectively.